THE

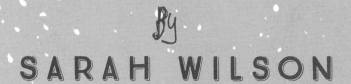
I QUIT SUGAR

COOKBOOK

By

SARAH WILSON

CLARKSON POTTER / PUBLISHERS
NEW YORK

When my seriously lovely publisher Ingrid "invited" me to write this book, I said, "Only if we can make it fun!" I also added that it would have to be really AUTHENTIC.

→ this meant doing meetings over breakfast or martinis (like-minded) favorite cafes.

We'd have to cook with SCRAPS, grow leftovers, enlist community + be TRANSPARENT.

WHich is why the props in the photographs are actually my everyday things, the garnishes are offcuts from other shoots + this messy handwriting + the "naive" illustrations are mine. To keep things real(ish).

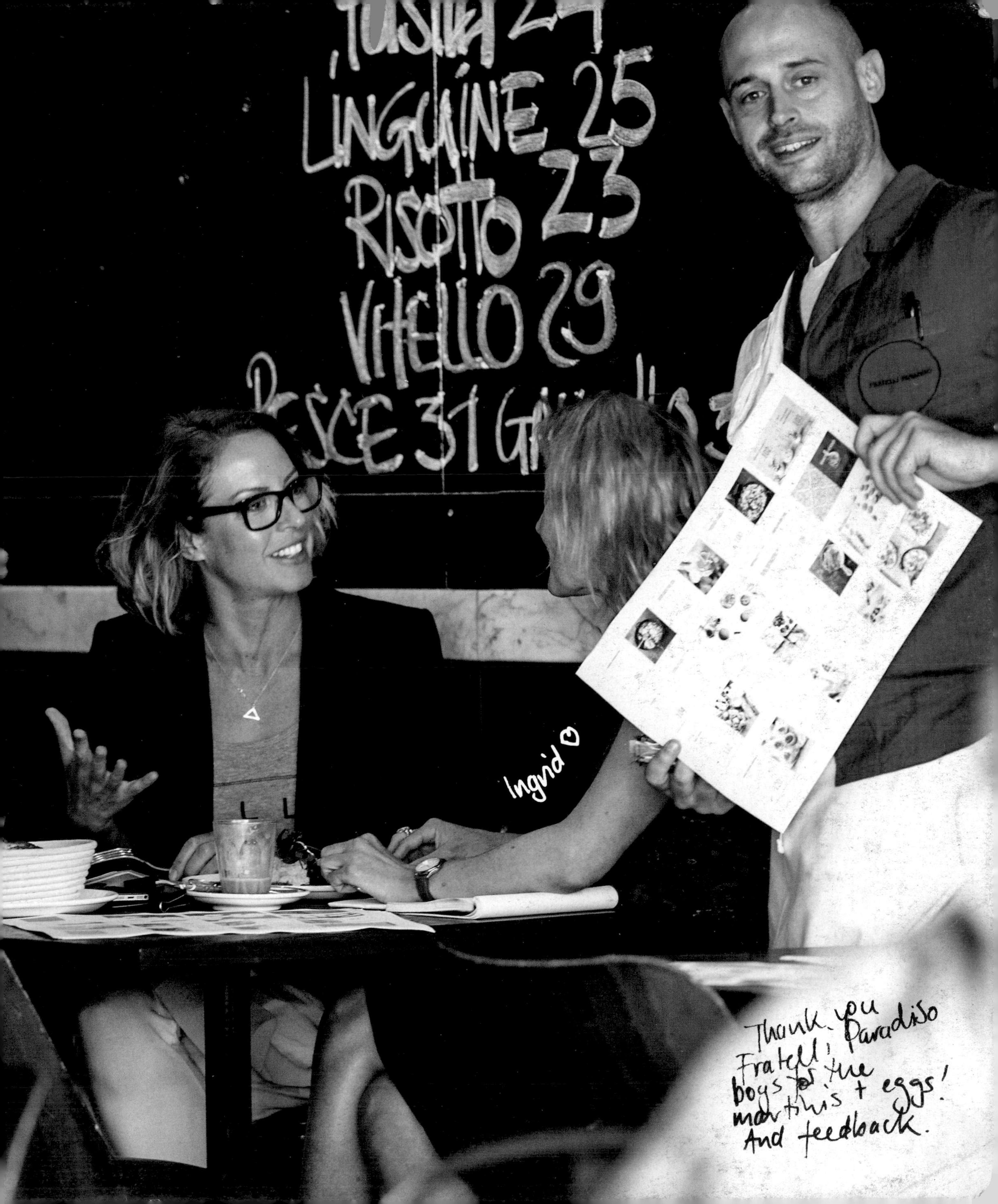

TOSTA 24
LINGUINE 25
RISOTTO 23
VITELLO 29
PESCE 31 G

Ingrid ♡

Thank you
Fratelli Paradiso
boys for the
martinis + eggs!
And feedback.

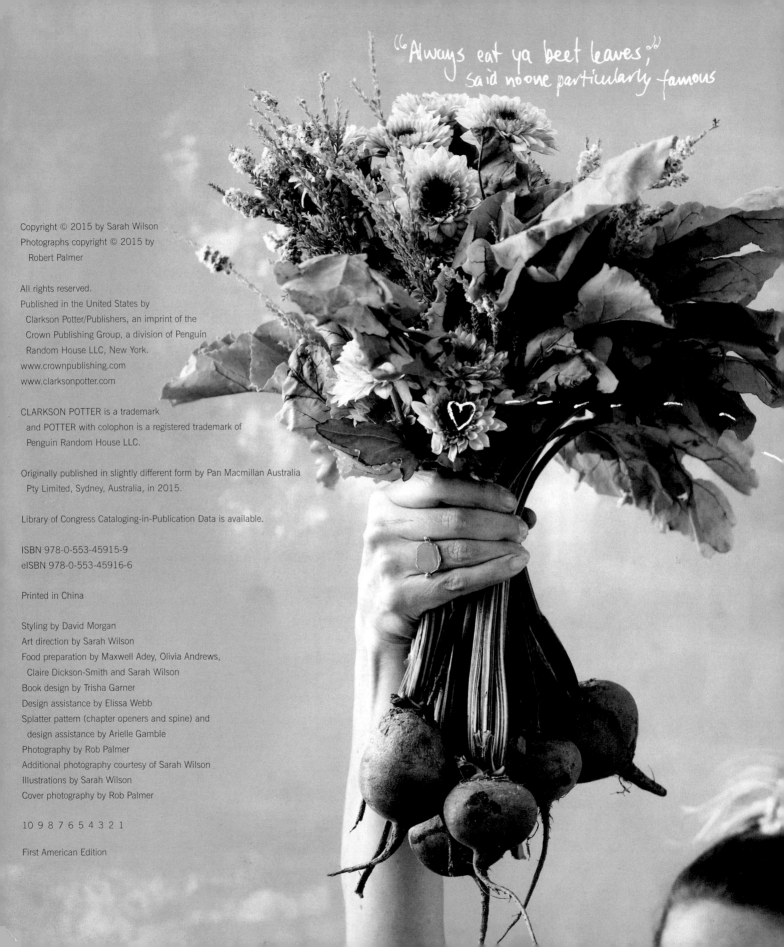

"Always eat ya beet leaves,"
said no one particularly famous

Published in the United States by
Clarkson Potter/Publishers, an imprint of the
Crown Publishing Group, a division of Penguin
Random House LLC, New York.
www.crownpublishing.com
www.clarksonpotter.com

CLARKSON POTTER is a trademark
and POTTER with colophon is a registered trademark of
Penguin Random House LLC.

Originally published in slightly different form by Pan Macmillan Australia
Pty Limited, Sydney, Australia, in 2015.

Library of Congress Cataloging-in-Publication Data is available.

ISBN 978-0-553-45915-9
eISBN 978-0-553-45916-6

Printed in China

Styling by David Morgan
Art direction by Sarah Wilson
Food preparation by Maxwell Adey, Olivia Andrews,
Claire Dickson-Smith and Sarah Wilson
Book design by Trisha Garner
Design assistance by Elissa Webb
Splatter pattern (chapter openers and spine) and
design assistance by Arielle Gamble
Photography by Rob Palmer
Additional photography courtesy of Sarah Wilson
Illustrations by Sarah Wilson
Cover photography by Rob Palmer

10 9 8 7 6 5 4 3 2 1

First American Edition

The bit where I place a quote
that sums up where we're about to head:

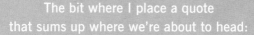

"Each of us is responsible for everything
and to every human being."

DOSTOYEVSKY

(upfront, before I forget)

The bit where I thank those who inspired me to love food more
Mum (always), Michael Pollan, and my first boyfriend, George.

The bit where I thank my crew, the *I Quit Sugar* team.
Especially Jo Foster, who made sure this book didn't veer
into a compost heap.

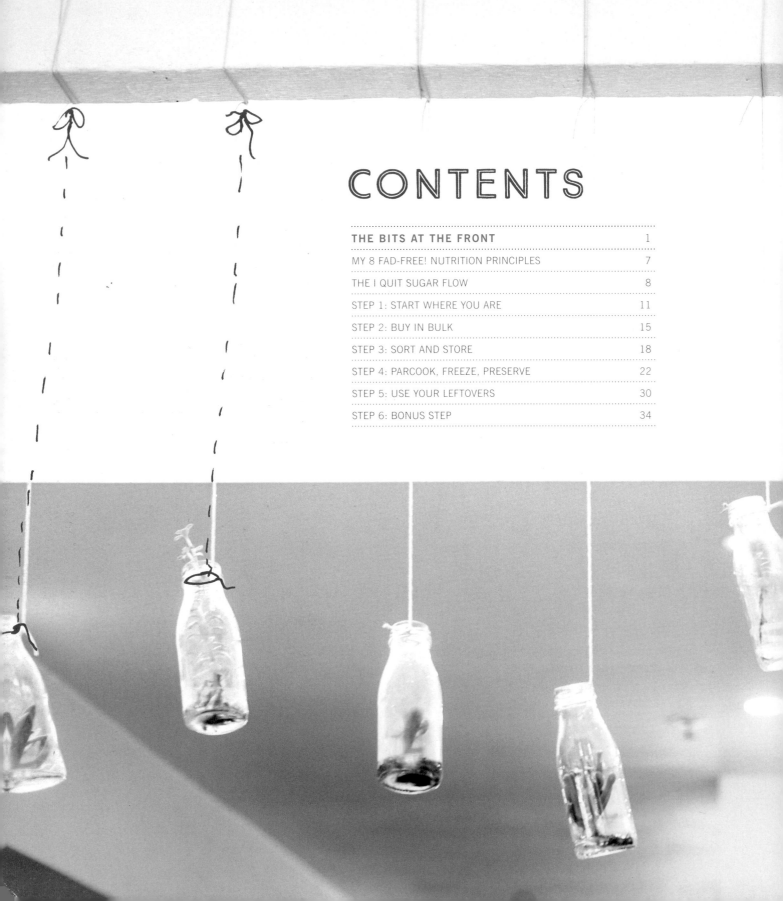

CONTENTS

THE BITS AT THE FRONT   1

MY 8 FAD-FREE! NUTRITION PRINCIPLES   7

THE I QUIT SUGAR FLOW   8

STEP 1: START WHERE YOU ARE   11

STEP 2: BUY IN BULK   15

STEP 3: SORT AND STORE   18

STEP 4: PARCOOK, FREEZE, PRESERVE   22

STEP 5: USE YOUR LEFTOVERS   30

STEP 6: BONUS STEP   34

THE RECIPES 39

THE BASICS 40

AGAINST-THE-GRAIN BREAKFASTS 58

SNACKALICIOUS 90

ABUNDANCE BOWLS 126

A CHAPTER DEDICATED TO GROUND MEAT ... 138

SUSTAINABLE FISH IN A DISH 152

SO I HAVE THIS STACK OF VEGETABLES 168

JUST LIKE GRANDMA USED TO MAKE 192

A BUNCH OF SUNDAY COOK-UPS 210

MIDWEEK ONE-PAN WONDERS 226

MY LEFTOVER MISHMASHES 246

A SMALL CHAPTER OF SHOW-STOPPING TREATS ... 266

A CELEBRATION MENU 300

FERMENTS AND OTHER GUT-HEALING FUNCTIONAL FOODS ... 332

THE BITS AT THE BACK 355

A TIDY LITTLE SHOPPING LIST 356

SUBSTITUTIONS AND FIXES 358

YOUR DEFINITIVE GUIDE TO SUGAR AND SAFE SWEETENERS ... 360

AYURVEDA 101 362

VERY FREQUENTLY ASKED QUESTIONS ALL IN THE ONE SPOT ... 363

TEN DAYS OF DINNER FOR FOUR 364

A MINDFUL LEFTOVERS INDEX 365

GENERAL INDEX 367

ACKNOWLEDGMENTS 376

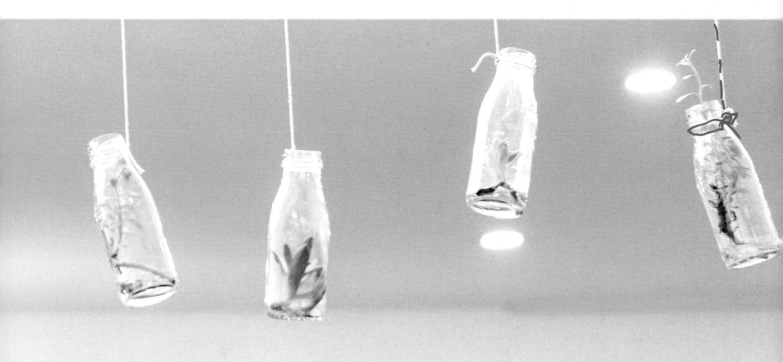

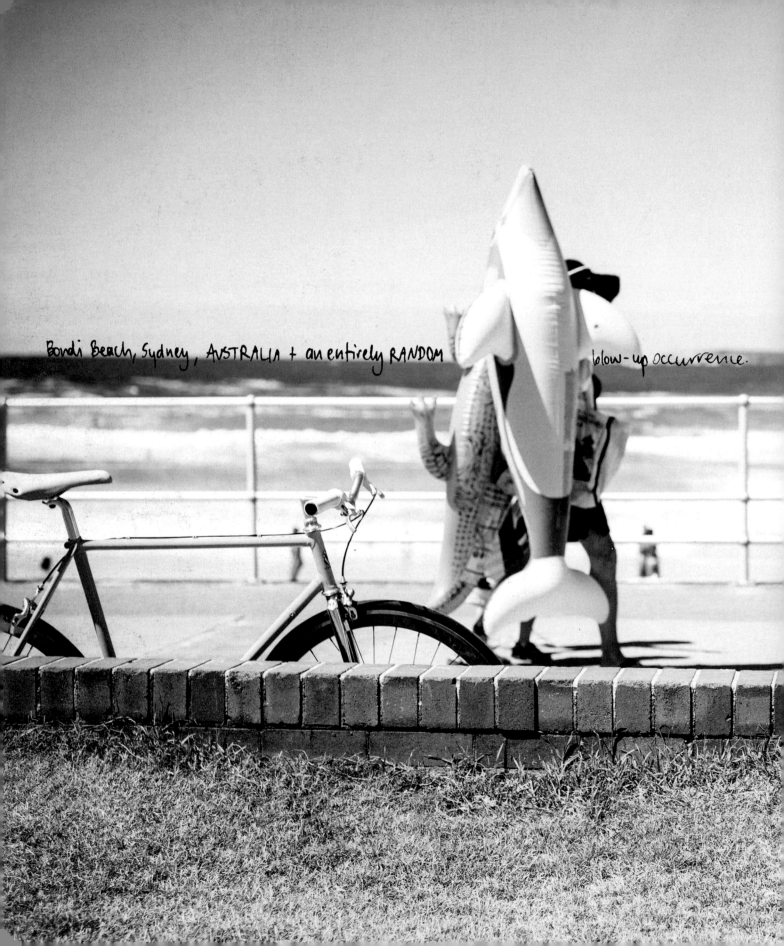

Bondi Beach, Sydney, AUSTRALIA + an entirely RANDOM blow-up occurrence.

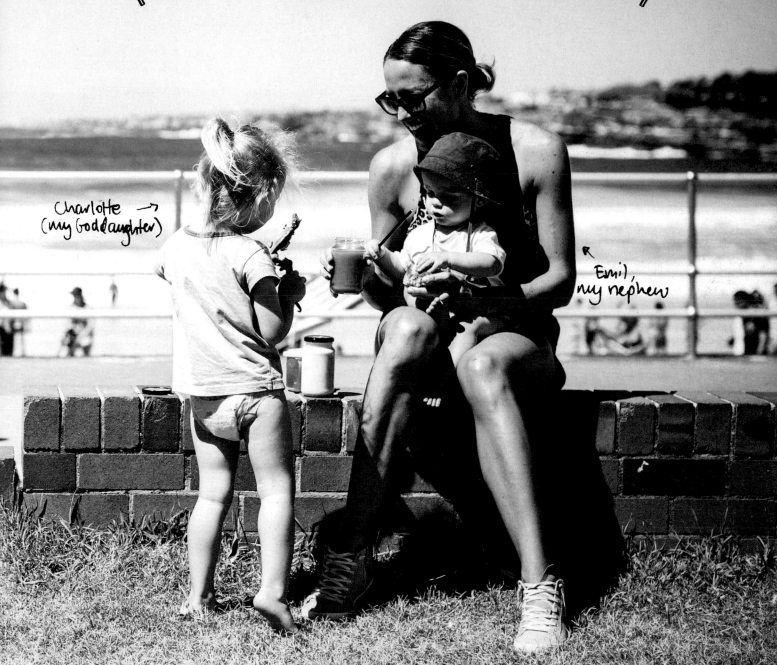

THE BITS AT THE FRONT

Charlotte →
(my Goddaughter)

Emil,
my nephew

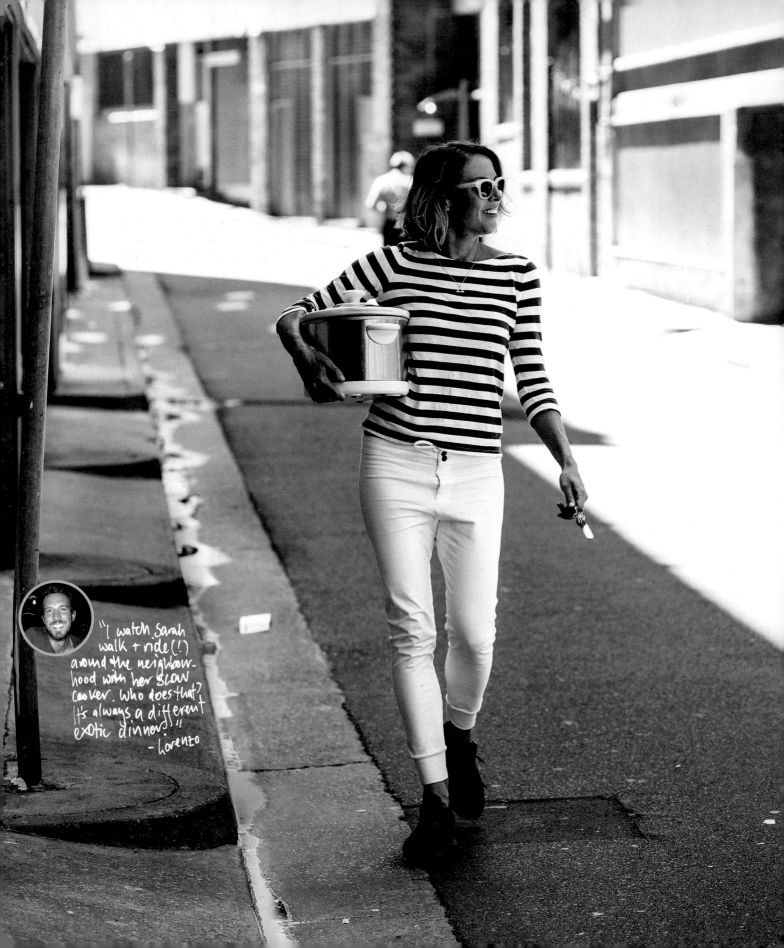

"I watch Sarah walk + ride (!) around the neighbourhood with her slow cooker. Who does that? It's always a different exotic dinner!"
— Lorenzo

Dear Reader.

I'd like to take a few moments to justify the next 373 pages.

As you may or may not know, I first quit sugar back in January 2011 because I had an autoimmune disease that seriously mucked with my ability to enjoy life. I wanted a better life, a richer life, a well life, so I tried going sugar-free. It worked and so I continued with the experiment a little longer. But along the way, several bigger, deeper themes emerged. I realized food waste mattered. More than anything else, actually. I also realized it shouldn't just be the quirky obsession of earnest types with black-framed glasses, farmers' market satchels and single-speed bikes. *Ha! Hello!*

You see, it goes like this: the biggest source of CO_2 emissions on the planet is food waste (not cars, not factories). The biggest food wasters are consumers (us!), not farmers or Big Food. Indeed, we toss out up to 50 percent of our groceries every week. *— must*

I'll say it straight—this is unconscionable, and the change we seek so deeply in life (to the planet, to our being) can come from each of us. Each of us is responsible. For everything. And to every human being.

When you quit sugar, you essentially quit processed food and all its associated nasty additives. Which means you benefit not only from the absence of sugar, but also from eliminating a stack of other toxic chemicals, crappy fats and low-brow carbs. Quitting sugar, by necessity, steers you to the right outcome.

Plus, when you quit processed food you're left with real, whole food only—which you have to cook, right? This means you're motivated (forced?) to cook, which means you save money and time, plus your health improves with exponential flourish. Which in turn means you stick to this way of eating and living because it feels so good. And on and on the sustainable vibe flows.

I've always eaten the whole apple, core and all. My tiny apartment kitchen is littered with recycled jars filled with the drippings from last night's chops (which I use to sweat my veggies, thus adding the right fats for absorbing the essential vitamins), the water from steaming my chard (perfect for padding out soup) and the olive oil from the marinated feta my friend was going to chuck when I was at her place for lunch last weekend (ready-made salad dressing, people!).

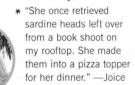

sustainable

Other Things I Do (as collated by my oft-bewildered friends and family):

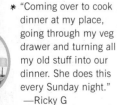

* "She once retrieved sardine heads left over from a book shoot on my rooftop. She made them into a pizza topper for her dinner." —Joice

* "Coming over to cook dinner at my place, going through my veg drawer and turning all my old stuff into our dinner. She does this every Sunday night." —Ricky G

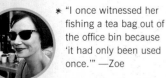

* "I once witnessed her fishing a tea bag out of the office bin because 'it had only been used once.'" —Zoe

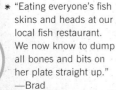

* "Eating everyone's fish skins and heads at our local fish restaurant. We now know to dump all bones and bits on her plate straight up." —Brad

Friends tell me they don't cook because it's too complicated and time consuming. But I've conducted tests, I have timed friends as they got takeout while I cooked my beef stew for myself (with six portions of leftovers). My friends took *37 minutes* (finding car keys, driving there, waiting in line, reheating each dish separately) while I took *11 minutes*. Divide that by six and, well . . . you can work it out.

versus

My fridge is a rainbow of fermented vegetables made from the "ugly" veggies my local markets can't sell. My freezer boasts a plastic bucket containing three fish carcasses that I retrieved from guests' plates at a friend's dinner party a few weeks back. They'll be turned into fish stock shortly, a quart of which I'll send back to said friend as a thank-you gift. And I should mention the carcass haul came *after* I'd been through my friend's garbage and pulled out a bag of still-sprightly celery leaves and asked if I could keep them . . . for making my Leftovers Pesto (page 55).

If she's lucky she'll get a batch of that, too.

I should also mention I've been known to ask strangers at the restaurant table next to me if I can take home their leftovers (well, they had no intention of doing so themselves); they acquiesced and I turned their indulgent Angus beef strips into a Vietnamese soup. Aren't you just glad you only know me from a distance?

All of which I share here to explain why I've decided to write the ultimate sugar-free cookbook about how to eat your scraps. Sustainability has always been at the guts of my books, albeit camouflaged behind pretty recipes and shiny, smiley pictures of myself. My recipes use leftovers and secondary cuts of meat. I've used my sugar-free platform to promote doggie bags and, um, cauliflower, to the masses.

And BTW, recycling and composting don't cut it. Not buying and wasting it in the first place does. That is, using what we have, cooking our leftovers, eating the whole food—pith, peel, stalks, stems, leaves, bones, brine, fat, skin and all. This is the future, my dear friends.

I soon realized that buying, cooking and eating this way made life better. Because when you learn to eat your scraps and consume less, life begins to flow. Things become simpler, more elegant; everything falls into place and makes sustainable sense. You don't have to worry whether local or organic or egg-yolk-free is better, or whether your dinner classifies as a superfood. Nope, you simply find yourself flowing to the "right" outcome. Without the palaver.

Slow cookers use less power than a light bulb! And they never break . . . which is why you don't see them advertised!

Another benefit:
When you eat secondary cuts of meat you save money (they're much cheaper), plus you tick ethical and environmental boxes, too, as you're contributing to more of the beast being eaten (or less of it being wasted). Secondary cuts are best slow-cooked, which requires less electricity (saving you even more), and they are more densely nutritious—even more so when cooked slowly. Plus, as the slow-cooked flavor is richer, you can use less meat, saving money and the environment and . . . oh, you get the point! Needless to say, this book celebrates the secondary cut.

Slow-and-low cooking preserves the meat's enzymes and also releases wonderful gut-healing gelatin and minerals.

True story! It's also why you always find them in mint condition at every garage sale around town.

And one more:
Ever gone to make a recipe, realized you're missing an ingredient or two so improvised with what you've got . . . and found it tasted better? My favorite meals are the ones I've made when camping and I've used leftover trail mix to flavor the evening stew. Or when I've created a fridge surprise (check out my creations on Instagram at #fridgesurprise) from a dearth of talent in my crisper.

I believe we like to fend, to create from what we have. We actually *like* living without. We are most creative in these situations. Also, we like it when we don't have corner cupboards bulging with waffle-makers. Or moldy lettuce at the bottom of the crisper.

So. We cook with what we've got, with scraps and leftovers, and we become happier and more creative. We also stop going to the shops as often to pick up a lone endive or carton of cream or whatever, which saves time, gas and money, and prevents processed-food temptation at the checkout. All of which sees us get happier and scrappier. And on we flow.

This book helps you quit sugar for good by elevating leftovers to the main attraction, saving you money, time, nutrients, scraps, energy, pans, dishwashing and all those random ingredients that usually sit at the back of the pantry after a single use.

I don't start and finish with a recipe. A meal never should. It should keep going and going—a perpetual recipe—the juices, scraps and leftovers all repurposed into other meals. The recipes in this book, right from the get-go, are orchestrated to work to a magnificent, elegant flow where we take an ingredient and use every last bit of it. A chicken can spread to 13 meals, 3 pounds of cheap stewing steak to 14.

I cheat, take shortcuts and do stuff my culinary peers no doubt frown upon. I use my fingers to test the readiness of food, skip pointless steps, toss salads with my hands and feature fridge dregs in my ingredients lists. I improvise, fend, get loose, get responsible . . . and I encourage you all to do the same.

This is the new sugar-free lifestyle. This is what makes life better.

Where's the proof?
I haven't bogged this book down in data. However, all claims, factlets, etc., are backed with science or my own research, and a simple search on **iquitsugar.com** or **sarahwilson.com** will deliver the data you're after. Also head to **sarahwilson.com** and click on **The Kit**, where much background guff will be housed for your deeper reading pleasure.

Sarah xxxxxxxxxxx

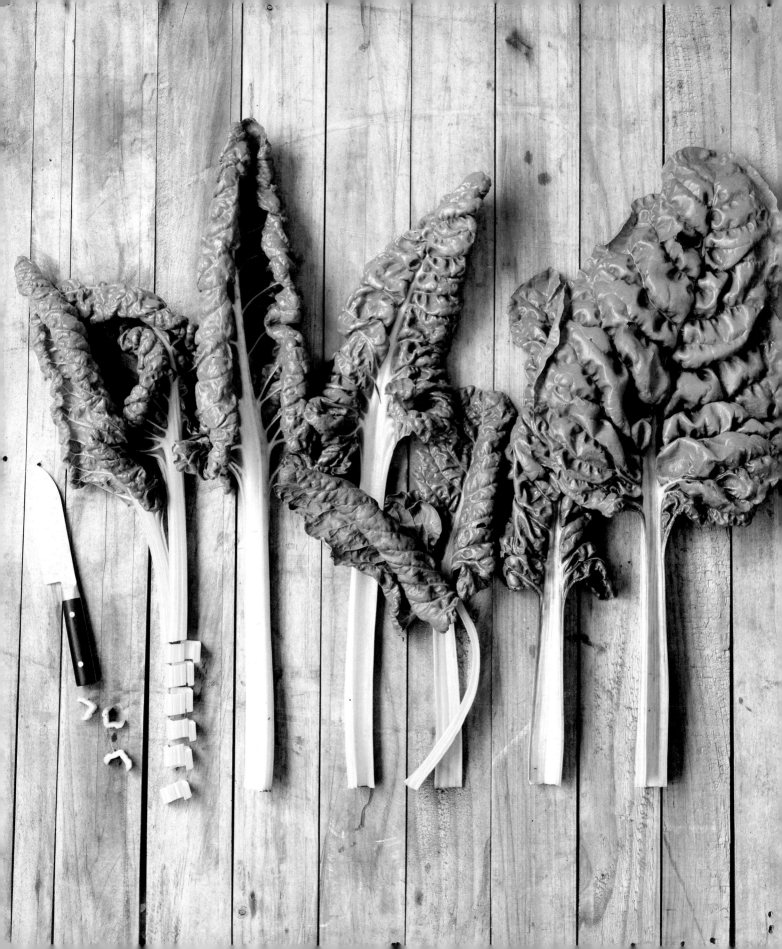

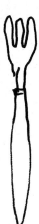

MY 8 FAD-FREE!! NUTRITION PRINCIPLES

For the past 50 years we've made a clusterfork of our dinner. "Nutritionism" has complicated things to the point where most of us have no idea what we're meant to eat. In this book I avoid referring to superfoods and have left off vegan and paleo considerations (many recipes will suit both, as well as those with lactose, nut and dairy intolerances) because I want to keep my message "simplicious." That said, there are a few mantras I work to:

1. Eat for gut health

The gut is where it's at. More than one-third of us have an inflammation-related disease (including obesity, arthritis, fatty liver, allergies and high cholesterol), stemming from poor bacteria in the large intestine. I focus on food-prep techniques that assist in building the gut microbiome and aid digestion, primarily fermenting, sprouting, preserving enzymes and minimizing toxins.

2. Opt for the most nutrient-dense option

And steer away from toxins. Where possible. My recipes include carbs and legumes and soy, which contain anti-nutrients. But rather than eliminating these foods, I focus on preparing them properly and veering toward more nutritious options.

3. Eat like your grandmother (or great-grandmother) used to

Sixty years ago we ate an appropriate amount of sugar and metabolic diseases were almost unheard of. My offal recipes are a homage to All of the Nanas. 'Cos they had it going on.

4. Less is more

Partly for gut health reasons, having too many ingredients in a dish causes unnecessary angst.

5. The French are right to be arrogant

About food, that is. After spending time in France over the past few years, I've come to admire the Francophile way of eating. They eat proper meals and don't snack; they eat like they mean it. They've also made an art of using leftovers. Lots of my recipes draw on their techniques.

6. Go slow and low

Cook slow and at a low temperature to preserve enzymes and maximize nutrients. Eat slow to maintain mindfulness and elegance and good gut health.

7. Try some Ayurvedic balance

I have a lot of time for this Indian approach to wellness. It's about (among many things) using food to maintain balance. Which is not quite the same as using food as medicine. According to Ayurveda, we don't need to fix or reverse anything; we balance disease or wobbliness using certain foods. For more, see page 362.

8. And, yes, JERF

Just Eat Real Food, people.

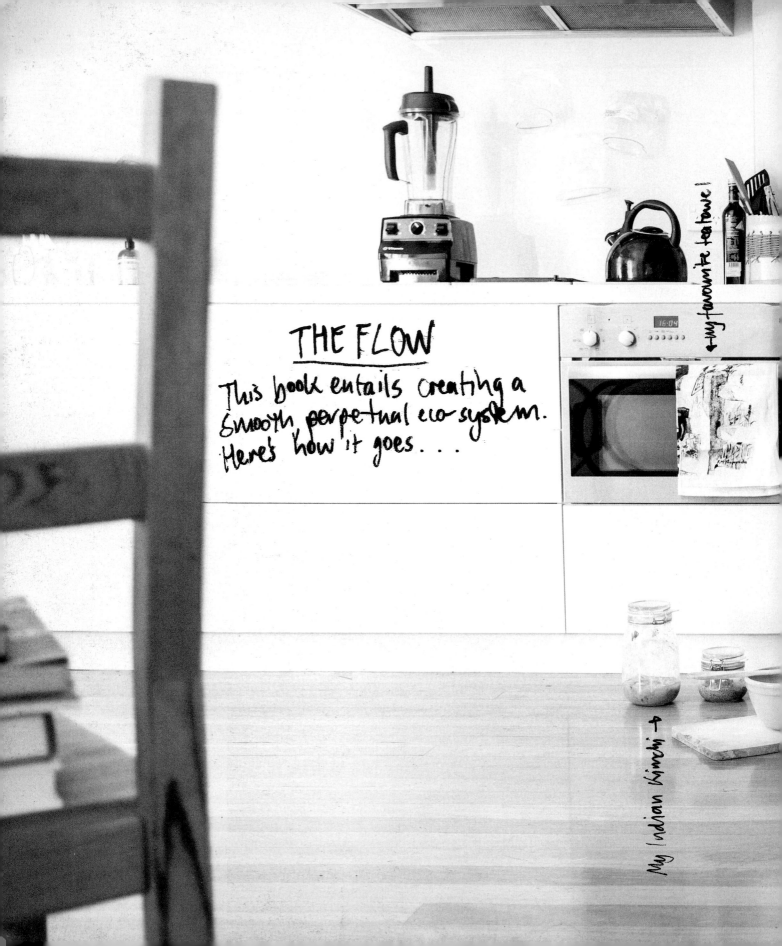

THE FLOW

This book entails creating a smooth perpetual eco-system. Here's how it goes. . . .

← my favourite teatowe!

My Indian kimchi →

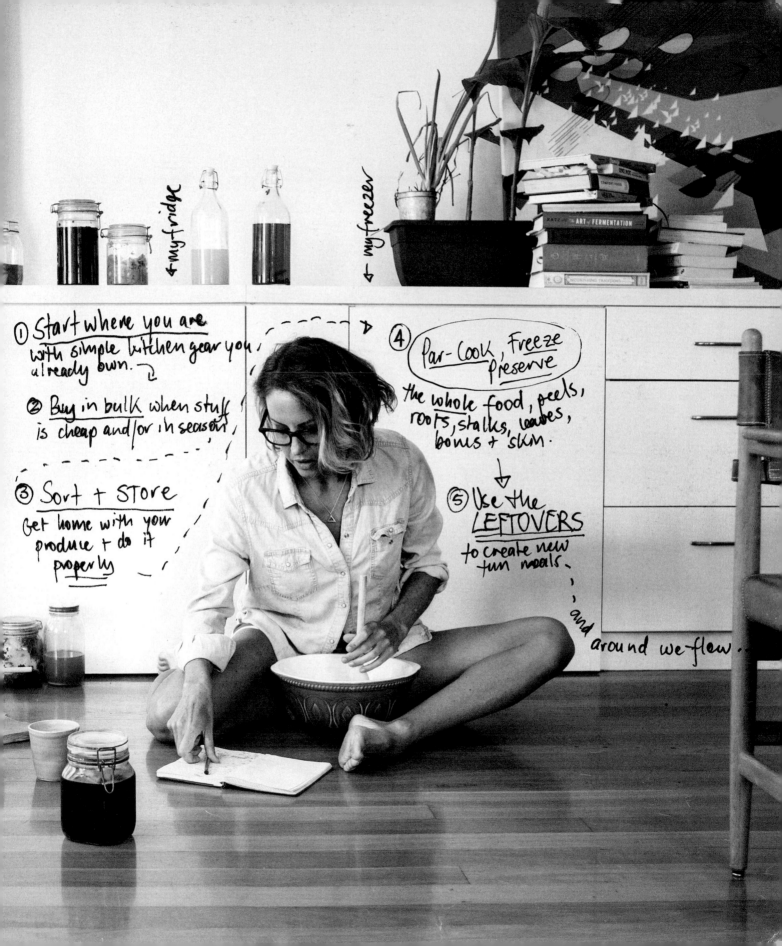

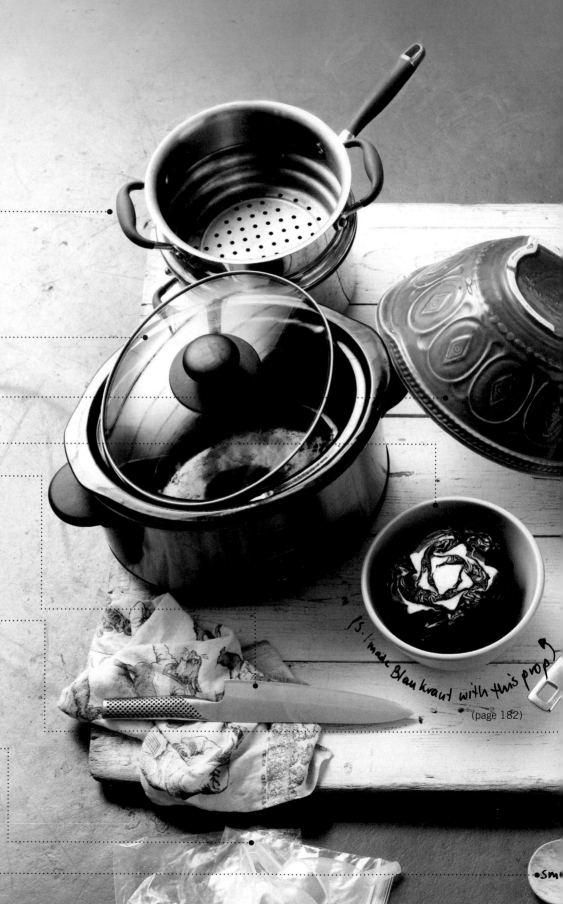

Double steamer: A 2–3-quart one is best. I boil my starchy veg down below, steam my greens up top.

4½-quart slow cooker: These one-pot wonders cook your dinner while you're at work, are cheap, use less electricity than a light bulb, and cook slow and low, preserving minerals and enzymes, thus making your food more digestible. There is really little discussion to be had here. P.S. An oval shape is best and if I had to do it over, I'd get one with a timer.

Big mixing bowl: The old ones are best: nice lips! I got this at a garage sale after a walk in the woods.

Little mixing bowl: Inherited from Grandma with this tea towel from the 1950s.

One big (chef's) knife: I've had mine for a decade. Go to a good knife shop and ask for their help.

Two paring knives: Knife blocks just take up too much room and I've never needed a bread knife in my life.

Immersion blender: Also called a stick blender or handheld blender. Again, cheap. Takes up no room. Allows you to blend stuff in the pot it was cooked in. Even better: you might like to buy yours as part of a multi-function processor kit (with grater, chopper, etc.). I did. I use most of the said kit, especially the grating and mandoline blades.

Zip-lock bags: Worth the plastic investment if you wash and re-use. To dry, slap them to your kitchen window or backsplash. When they're dry, they'll drop off. I use them daily but have only ever bought three packs in four years.

Wooden spoons: Generally inherited with character built-in.

P.S. I made Blaukraut with this prop (page 182)

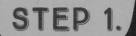

STEP 1.

START WHERE YOU ARE

The best cooks improvise. The worst kitchens are those with unused waffle-makers in the corner cabinet. The worst cookbooks are those with long lists at the front telling you what you should go and stock up on from scratch. This is not one of those lists. It's an illustration of what I use and why.

Large frying pan with lid: 13-inch should be large enough to serve 6. (This way I have a smallish skillet for meals to serve 1–3, and a bigger pan for dinner parties or cook-ups.)

Cast-iron skillet: 10-inch is best for most things.

Cast-iron vs. non-stick vs. stainless steel frying pans

Cast-iron: This is my pick. It gives you even heat and a really anchored cooking experience, and will last a lifetime. Cast-iron pans are also best for one-pot cooking (you can brown food on the stove, then plonk in the oven or under a broiler without transferring between pans). They're also naturally non-stick, if you care for them properly. Google "How to season a cast-iron skillet." If possible, buy one second-hand or nab Grandma's old one and Google "How to bring cast iron back to life."

Non-stick: Cheap and convenient, but only buy non-Teflon varieties. Drawbacks: You can't work up a hearty reduction or put them over super-high heat to get crusts and crispy bits. Also, they don't last long—they scratch and dent.

Stainless steel: Expensive but good for pots and bigger pans. Invest in triple layers (aluminum between two layers of steel) and riveted handles.

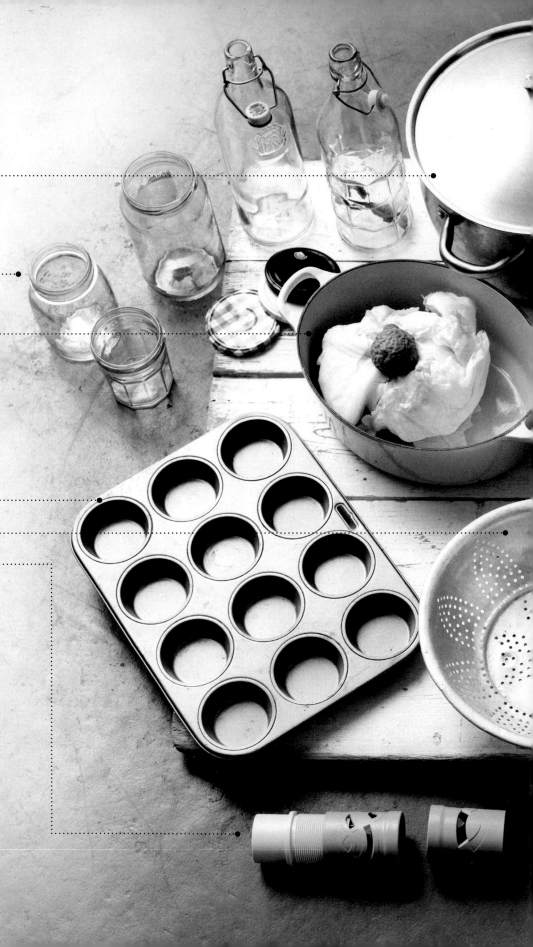

Big stockpot: About 8 quarts is fine. No need to invest; no need for special features.

Glass jars and dishes: No need to buy fancy mason jars or plasticware. Most things can go in a jar instead. Added bonus—you can see what you've stored.

Enameled cast-iron Dutch oven: I got this 3-quart one for my birthday years ago from Mum and Dad. It's about perfect to serve 6.

Baking pans and dishes: My kit contains a 9 × 5-inch loaf pan, a 9-inch springform cake pan, and a couple of muffin pans. I've inherited most of these from people who had too many in their corner cupboard. A 9 × 13-inch glass, stoneware or enamel baking dish can be used not only for roasting veggies and baking pies and slices, but also for baking casseroles, etc. One with a lid is great; it becomes a container afterward.

Old colander with no legs: From Grandma.

Spiralizer: Great for novelty veggie noodles (I'd grab one if I had kids).

Microwave: Yes, I use one.

Are microwaves okay?
The science says they don't kill nutrients any more than boiling. Indeed, some studies show they retain more nutrients than other cooking methods. Nor do they radiate you. They use a form of non-ionizing radiation (it can't directly break up atoms or molecules). Just stand back a little (3 feet) when it's in use to avoid the EMFs (electromagnetic fields) and don't put plastic in there. Use glass or ceramic containers instead.

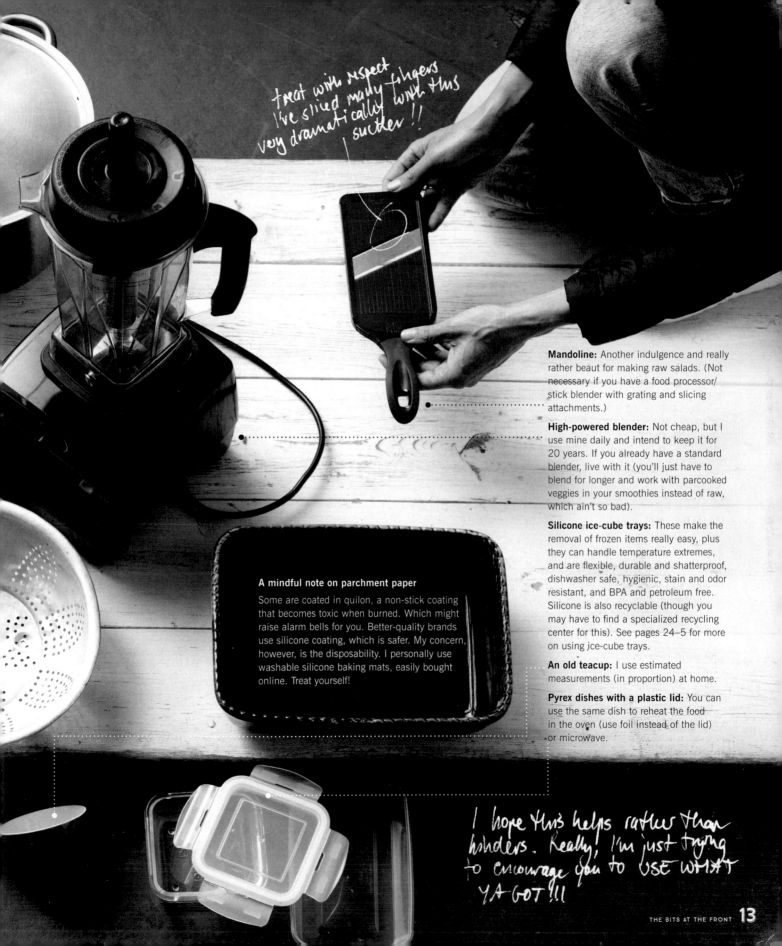

treat with respect I've sliced many fingers very dramatically with this sucker!!

Mandoline: Another indulgence and really rather beaut for making raw salads. (Not necessary if you have a food processor/ stick blender with grating and slicing attachments.)

High-powered blender: Not cheap, but I use mine daily and intend to keep it for 20 years. If you already have a standard blender, live with it (you'll just have to blend for longer and work with parcooked veggies in your smoothies instead of raw, which ain't so bad).

Silicone ice-cube trays: These make the removal of frozen items really easy, plus they can handle temperature extremes, and are flexible, durable and shatterproof, dishwasher safe, hygienic, stain and odor resistant, and BPA and petroleum free. Silicone is also recyclable (though you may have to find a specialized recycling center for this). See pages 24–5 for more on using ice-cube trays.

An old teacup: I use estimated measurements (in proportion) at home.

Pyrex dishes with a plastic lid: You can use the same dish to reheat the food in the oven (use foil instead of the lid) or microwave.

A mindful note on parchment paper

Some are coated in quilon, a non-stick coating that becomes toxic when burned. Which might raise alarm bells for you. Better-quality brands use silicone coating, which is safer. My concern, however, is the disposability. I personally use washable silicone baking mats, easily bought online. Treat yourself!

I hope this helps rather than hinders. Really, I'm just trying to encourage you to USE WHAT YA GOT !!!

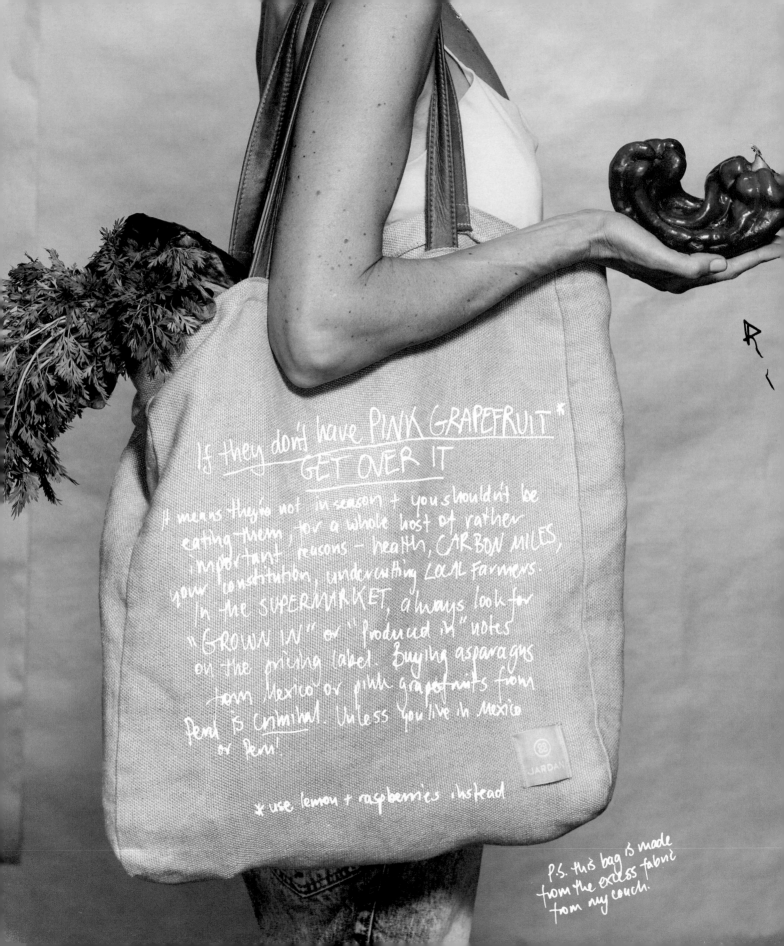

BUY IN BULK

This really doesn't have to be complicated. And you don't have to be particularly organized—just fired up! Local produce markets are the best option. Not just for the free samples and overwhelming earnestness (and fewer carbon miles), but because you'll be buying stuff that's in season and therefore the best food for your Ayurvedic constitution (see page 362). Yeah, we call it flow. (The greengrocer or supermarket is just fine, however.)

SAVE AT THE SUPERMARKET WITHOUT TRYING

This is how I cut corners, save coin and generally win.

Buy stuff in season: I'll say it again. This is the easiest way to save money (and the planet).

Buy discount meats and hard cheeses: Perishable items are often discounted a few days before their "best before" date. If I'm going to eat something straight away or I can freeze it (or it's a food that improves with age anyway), I buy up. Ground meat is a great one to buy discounted. Turn it into meatballs (see pages 144–45) and freeze immediately, thus rendering the use-by date redundant.

Buy secondary cuts of meat: These are the less popular and therefore cheaper cuts. They tend to be more muscly, leaner cuts, yet they have more flavor and nutrient density. Go for:

* **Chicken wings and legs**—not breasts (wings and legs are often half the price, plus dark meat contains more minerals than the white).
* **Lamb and pork shoulder, rump roast, topside or leg cuts**— not loin chops, cutlets or tenderloin filets.
* **Beef osso bucco, silverside, topside, gravy, chuck and brisket**— not rib eye, tenderloin, rump or T-bone.
* **Fish offcuts**—if you're making soup or curry, why do you need a full fillet?

Look for imperfect veggies: Most supermarkets now stock these deformed "rejects" at a portion of the price of the pretty picks. If you're not using your veg as props for an oil painting, always choose the rejects.

Grab some meat bones: My butcher gives them to me for free. Most will charge a few dollars for a big bag that will yield several quarts of life-giving, joint-soothing, gut-calming bone broth/stock (see page 42).

Buy scruffy roots 'n' shoots: Turnips, parsnips, sweet potatoes, cauliflower, cabbage . . . they're mostly available year-round and are generally cheaper than chips. Accordingly, I use them a lot in this book.

CHEAT, SOMETIMES WITH PACKAGED VERSIONS

I always prefer to buy fresh or make my own to avoid packaging. But sometimes the processed or packaged version is good (okay, better).

Frozen peas and corn: Freezing stops the starch in these little veggies from breaking down into sugars, helping them retain vitamins, fiber and minerals, and making the frozen versions "fresher" than the, um, fresh ones.

Bags of slaw: They cost a few dollars and are dead nifty at times. Forgivable.

Roast chicken: If you can find a place that roasts organic chickens, then don't lose a second's sleep over buying a precooked one. It will probably be more energy efficient this way anyway, seeing as they roast stacks at once. Remember to boil up the bones to make stock afterward (page 42).

Frozen berries: Just make sure they're organic and not from China or Canada (carbon miles). Even during berry season frozen berries are usually a fraction of the price of fresh ones. Plus, even the non-organic frozen berries contain less chemicals than fresh.

Curry paste: Yes, yes, yes. Grinding your own spices fresh is fab. And yes, yes, yes, most pastes use vegetable oil in the mix. But many don't contain sugar or other added nasties and can deliver a sound result, without having to keep 23,473,276 herbs and spices on hand. I tend to add Fermented Turmeric Paste (page 340) or kaffir lime leaves (which I keep in the freezer) to store-bought paste for some extra oomph.

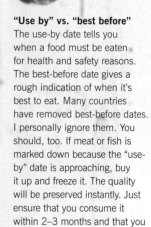

"Use by" vs. "best before"
The use-by date tells you when a food must be eaten for health and safety reasons. The best-before date gives a rough indication of when it's best to eat. Many countries have removed best-before dates. I personally ignore them. You should, too. If meat or fish is marked down because the "use-by" date is approaching, buy it up and freeze it. The quality will be preserved instantly. Just ensure that you consume it within 2–3 months and that you don't refreeze it once thawed.

Ugly veggies make pretty

FOODS YOU SHOULD REALLY BUY ORGANIC

You might not be flush enough to buy your whole market haul from the organic section, but the following stuff is worth the investment. I've tried to keep this simple.

Almonds: Many toxic pesticides and herbicides are used on almond trees. Due to almonds' high fat content, the chemicals are easily retained.

Beef: Non-organic beef can be treated with growth-promoting hormones—regardless of whether it's grass fed or not. Interestingly, Australia deems these hormones unfit for chickens but okay for cows.

USDA data shows 52 different pesticide residues on a fresh blueberry compared to 21 on a frozen blueberry.

Berries: These are more contaminated than any other fruit and have some of the highest levels of pesticide contamination recorded for any produce. If you can't find local, organic ones, it might be better to buy them frozen. Why? Berries farmed to be frozen are sprayed way less than those destined to be sold fresh since fresh ones need more chemicals to maintain shelf life.

Chicken and eggs: Organic is the ONLY way to eat chicken. Free-range birds might be able to move outside a cage but they can still be fed nasty chemical-laden feed and supplements. Most consumer authorities say it's worth investing in organic chicken products. This is especially important if you're eating the whole chicken (which we do in this book); you don't want chemicals leaching from bones. Or into the eggs.

Coffee: Not just a hipster affectation! Coffee can be a significant source of pesticides as coffee beans are heavily sprayed.

Dairy products: The high fat content in dairy retains any chemicals ingested by the cow.

Peanut butter: Peanut shells are super-porous and any chemical or pesticide is easily absorbed into the meat of the nut. The high fat content of peanuts also allows for easy absorption (and retention) of these chemicals. However, be careful with the organic stuff, too. Peanuts easily attract fungus and mold, the most problematic being aflatoxins, which have carcinogenic and liver-damaging effects. If you buy organic, be sure to refrigerate it.

Thin-skinned fruit: Soft fruits with fine skin (including stone fruit, apples and pears) absorb and retain more pesticides than fruits with thicker skin like bananas and melons. Scrubbing and even peeling doesn't eliminate the residue completely.

Veggies that can't be peeled: Especially thin-skinned veggies like bell peppers and celery. And leafy greens. With veggies that have no protective skin, it's almost impossible to wash off the chemicals. The leafiness of leafy greens and herbs means the chemicals permeate the plant's structure. Rosemary and spinach in particular have been shown to retain high levels of chemical residues.

SORT AND STORE

Once you get your shopping home, you need to sort it and store it. You might think, *Really!? I have to do annoying prep stuff after enduring the shops?* Yeah, you do. It doesn't take long and it will save you time down the track. P.S. I do my unpacking, storing, and the next bit—parcooking, freezing and preserving (see page 22)—all in one hit.

HOW TO STORE YOUR FRESH STUFF

Most vegetables are best in the fridge. Onions and potatoes are outliers. Leave them in a cabinet or pantry, alone in the dark, away from the other vegetables and each other.

Cucumber, tomatoes, bell peppers, pumpkin, eggplant and zucchini: Don't wash these until you need them. Leave at room temperature (if your house is cool—i.e., 54–68°F—and you're eating them within 2–3 days) or in the fridge in paper bags (but off the bottom shelf, which is usually the coldest part).

Lemons: Keep in a *sealed* bag—they'll last up to a month this way. Yep.

Carrots: Trim off the green tops (they will draw nutrients and flavor from the roots) and store them as you would herbs (see opposite). Place the carrots in the fridge in a covered container filled with water.

If you've cut open an unripe avo, sprinkle the flesh with lemon juice, place back together, cover with plastic wrap and return to the fridge. It'll soften up without browning.

Avocado: Store unripe avos in a paper bag on the counter with a banana or apple—they'll ripen within 5 days.

Beets: Remove the leaves and store them as you would herbs (see opposite). Don't wash the beets—the dirt helps them hold moisture. Keep beets in the crisper, in a bag if you like.

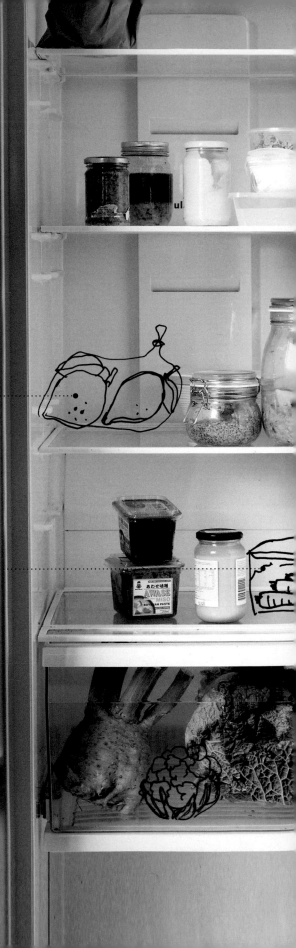

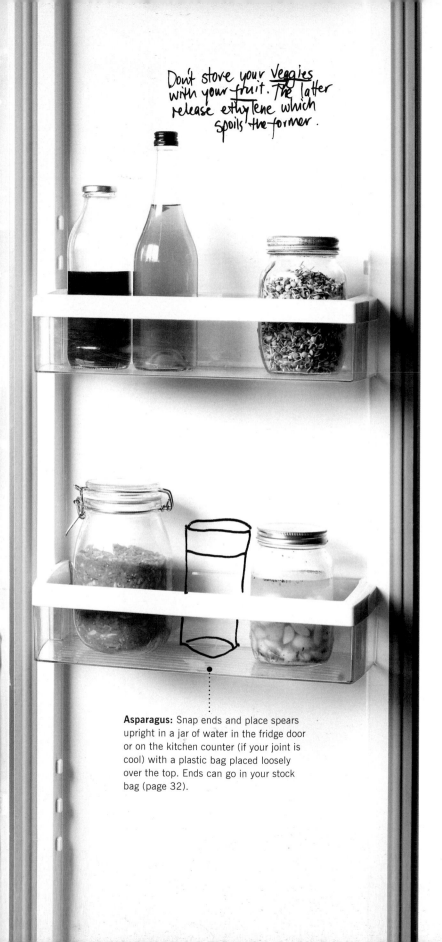

Don't store your veggies with your fruit. The latter release ethylene which spoils the former.

Green onions (scallions): Plant the whole bunch in a pot of soil or in your garden, removing a whole stem as you need it. Or place in a jar, glass or clear vase of water on the windowsill and cut off the green tops as you need them.

Meat: Store in the meat compartment in your fridge if you're going to cook it in the next 3 days; otherwise freeze in meal-sized batches.

Kale and other greens: To be honest, it's best to cook and eat these ASAP, but if you want to store them, do it the same way as you do lettuce (see below). Put the stalks in your stock bag (see page 32).

Lettuce: Cut away the stalk, pull apart the leaves, wash in a sink of cold water, then dry and store as per the herbs, below.

Or use the bath towel trick: lay the leaves on an old towel and roll up into a log. You then unroll as required, revealing a few leaves at a time!

Herbs: Wrap in dishtowels or re-usable cloth (paper towel if you must), stacked together in a big container with a lid or in a large zip-lock bag. Or you can trim the roots and place in a jar or glass with water and stick a plastic bag loosely over the top. Both work well.

I use hospital gauze you can get from the pharmacy.

Watercress: Wash immediately in a sink of water, dry really well (see below) and store as you would herbs.

Asparagus: Snap ends and place spears upright in a jar of water in the fridge door or on the kitchen counter (if your joint is cool) with a plastic bag placed loosely over the top. Ends can go in your stock bag (page 32).

How to dry watercress (and other leafy greens)
Place your washed greens inside a clean pillowcase or washing bag. Go outside and swing the bag around madly. Or place the bag in the washing machine on the spin cycle for 20 seconds. I'm serious. Cress will last more than a week this way.

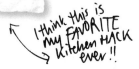

I think this is my FAVORITE kitchen HACK ever!!

THINGS YOU CAN PUT STRAIGHT INTO THE FREEZER

As a general rule, proteins and fruit are best frozen raw, while most veggies are best frozen parcooked. Freezing food that is as fresh as possible ensures the quality is maintained, as it slows the normal breakdown of foods by bacteria. Here are my tips for freezing your haul:

Always keep your freezer full.
It's more energy efficient than an empty one, as solids freeze at a lower temperature than air.

Wash them in soapy water, rinse, turn inside out and stick to your backsplash or window to dry.

If you use zip-lock bags:
Divide cooled veggies and meat into "per serve" portions (½ cup) and line them up like books to save space and to generally be An Organized Person. (You can wash and re-use your bags.)

Avoid using plastic containers if you can.
But don't go out and buy new containers: use recycled jars as often as possible. Or invest in quality Pyrex baking dishes that can be used for cooking as well.

Always leave a good 1 inch free at the top.
Liquid expands when frozen, so this will ensure the container doesn't crack.

RAW BUCKWHEAT

SQUASH OR
SWEET POTATO
PURÉE
(see page 23)

PARCOOKED 'N'
FROZEN VEGGIES
(see page 22)

other things people put in their freezer:
* credit cards (in a cup of water, frozen) — Ingrid
* ex-boyfriends' names written on a bit of paper
* jeans (instead of washing them; avoids fading)

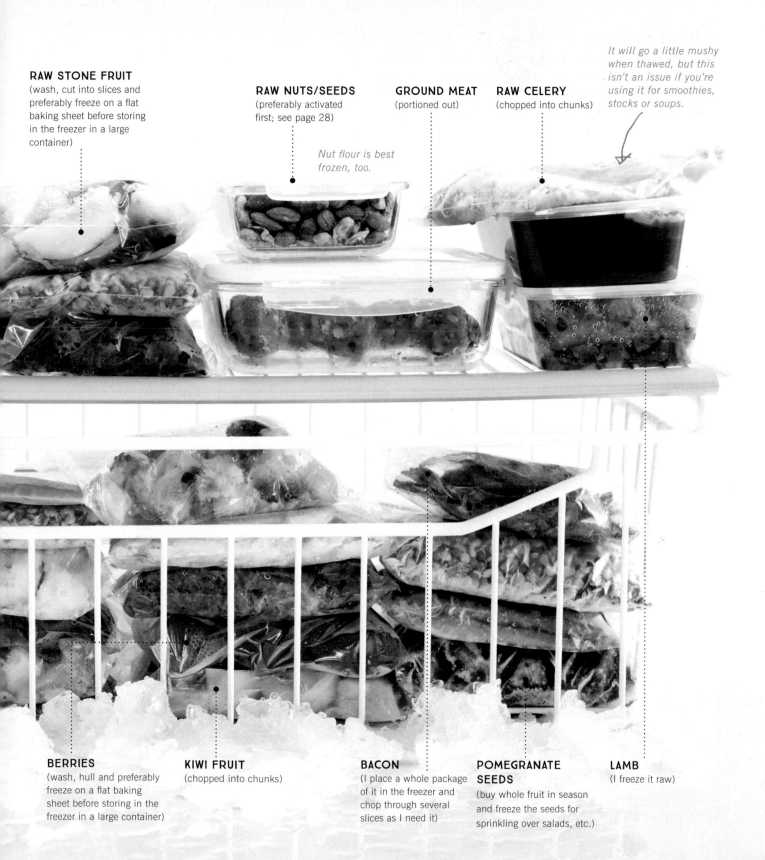

RAW STONE FRUIT
(wash, cut into slices and
preferably freeze on a flat
baking sheet before storing
in the freezer in a large
container)

RAW NUTS/SEEDS
(preferably activated
first; see page 28)

*Nut flour is best
frozen, too.*

GROUND MEAT
(portioned out)

RAW CELERY
(chopped into chunks)

*It will go a little mushy
when thawed, but this
isn't an issue if you're
using it for smoothies,
stocks or soups.*

BERRIES
(wash, hull and preferably
freeze on a flat baking
sheet before storing in the
freezer in a large container)

KIWI FRUIT
(chopped into chunks)

BACON
(I place a whole package
of it in the freezer and
chop through several
slices as I need it)

**POMEGRANATE
SEEDS**
(buy whole fruit in season
and freeze the seeds for
sprinkling over salads, etc.)

LAMB
(I freeze it raw)

PARCOOK, FREEZE, PRESERVE

Next, you cook up your shopping haul, in bulk, a lot of which you freeze. Excess bits you preserve (see pages 332–53 for ferments, pickles and tonics). This puts you in front on three fronts: you snap in the nutrients of your food, you free up space in the fridge and you have food ready to go for months. I parcook most veggies; otherwise the enzymes will continue to age them, even when frozen. This technique, done weekly or twice a month, is possibly the most ingenious part of my flow.

PARCOOKED 'N' FROZEN VEGGIES

Try any firm, non-salad-y veggies, but these are my staples:

broccoli and cauliflower, chopped into small florets

any leafy greens (spinach, kale, beet leaves),
cut into ½-inch-wide strips (including stalks/stems)

string beans, trimmed

Use a saucepan with a steamer and steam one variety at a time, using the same water, over and over, topping it up as you go. Steam each batch for 1–2 minutes or until they're about 60% done, then rinse in cold water to stop the cooking process.

I divide my parcooked veggies into per-serving portions and place them in containers or zip-lock bags. Or you can pre-freeze them all on a baking sheet first and then place them in one large container, breaking off what you need as you go, as you would frozen peas.

USE THE LEFTOVER BOILING WATER:
This makes a good vegetable stock.

CAULIFLOWER OR BROCCOLI RICE

MAKES 4–6 CUPS

1 head cauliflower or 1 large head broccoli,
roughly chopped (including the stalk)

Pulse in a food processor until it resembles rice. Divide into 1-cup portions and freeze for up to 3 months.

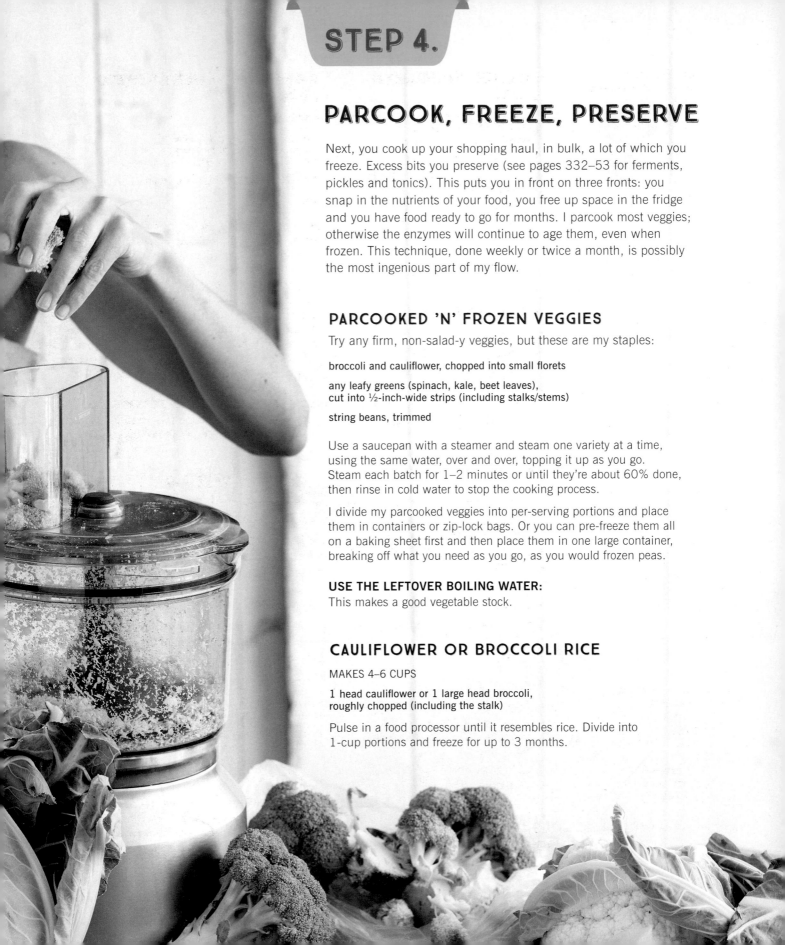

**Got constipation?
Eat cold roots and beans!**
The latest movement
for, um, helping with
lack of movement is
resistant starch, which
travels undigested to the
small intestine, where
it feeds good bacteria.
This, in turn, can get
things humming along
healthily. One of the most
easily accessible ways to
consume resistant starch
is with a good serving of
cooked and cooled potato,
sweet potato or legumes
that is then reheated.

**While you have the
oven on at 350°F...**
Make some Carrot
"Bacon" (page 115),
Vegan "Ground Meat"
(page 186), Celery
Leaf Salt (page 265) or
The Whole Brassicus
Hummus (page 187).

COOKED 'N' FROZEN BEETS

4–5 beets (reserve the leaves
for Leftovers Pesto; page 55),
trimmed, scrubbed and pricked
with a fork (don't peel them!)

Preheat the oven to 350°F. Place
the beets on a baking sheet (no
oil, no salt, no parchment paper)
and cook for 30 minutes until just
tender. Cool and peel (I don't as I
like the texture of the skin), then
place in the freezer.

ROASTED ROOTS

Roasted vegetables taste better
after a few days. Use them in
Leftover Mishmashes (pages
246–65) and Abundance Bowls
(pages 126–37). Depending on the
season, you might choose from:

1 pumpkin (any kind), peeled, seeded
(use a big spoon to scrape them out)
and chopped into 1½-inch chunks

2–3 sweet potatoes, scrubbed
and chopped into 1½-inch chunks

4–5 parsnips, carrots and/or turnips,
cut into 1½-inch chunks

brussels sprouts, trimmed (halve
them if they're particularly large)

a few sprigs of rosemary

1–2 heads of garlic, tops trimmed

butter, ghee or coconut oil, melted,
for drizzling

sea salt

Preheat the oven to 350°F.

Place the veggies on a large baking
sheet with the rosemary and garlic.
Drizzle over the butter, ghee or oil
and salt and toss with your hands.
Place on the middle shelf in the
oven and roast for 40–60 minutes.
Squeeze out the garlic cloves and
pull the rosemary leaves from the
charred twig. Once cool, store the
veg in the fridge for 3–4 days.

SQUASH OR SWEET POTATO PURÉE

MAKES 4–6 CUPS

1 large squash (about 4–6 pounds),
cut into 4 big wedges, or 4 large
sweet potatoes, scrubbed and left whole

2 tablespoons butter, ghee or coconut oil

pinch of sea salt

Preheat the oven to 350°F. Scoop out and discard
the pumpkin seeds and pulp. Place the squash or
sweet potato on a baking sheet and rub with the
butter, ghee or oil and salt. Bake on the middle
oven rack until tender—about 1 hour. (If you're
pressed for time, cut the squash or spuds into
smaller chunks and bake for 30 minutes.) Scoop
out the squash flesh (or slip off the sweet potato
skins when they've cooled) and purée using an
immersion blender or a potato masher. Once cool,
freeze in 1 cup batches or ice-cube trays.

USE THE LEFTOVER SWEET POTATO SKINS:
Pan-fry in coconut oil or bacon lard over a high
heat with a big sprinkle of salt to make chips.

MASSAGED KALE OR BEET GREENS

Don't laugh! There is seriously such a thing.
Kale and beet greens are fibrous and, when
eaten raw, are hard on the guts and quite
bitter. "Kneading" or "massaging" the stuff with
some dressing with oil and acid softens it and
pre-digests it for us. The leaves will darken,
shrink in size and become silky in texture and
sweeter in taste. Plus, a robustly massaged
kale or beet salad will keep for up to a week in
the fridge.

1 bunch kale, stems removed, leaves torn
(or 1 bunch beets, leaves torn)

⅓ cup Powerhouse Dressing (page 53),
or 2 tablespoons each of olive oil and
lemon juice

1 teaspoon sea salt

In a bowl combine all the ingredients and
massage the leaves—like, a deep-tissue one,
squeezing and kneading—for 5 minutes or until
soft and wilted. Eat as is or use in a salad.

TWO PAGES OF THINGS I LIKE TO DO WITH MY ICE-CUBE TRAY

Here's how it works, for cooking flow:

1. Freeze leftover bits 'n' bobs in tray
2. Once frozen, pop your leftovers cube out + place in a freezer-proof container (thus freeing up your tray)
3. Label your bags
4. Use your cubes to deglaze, add liquid, bulk or flavor stuff.

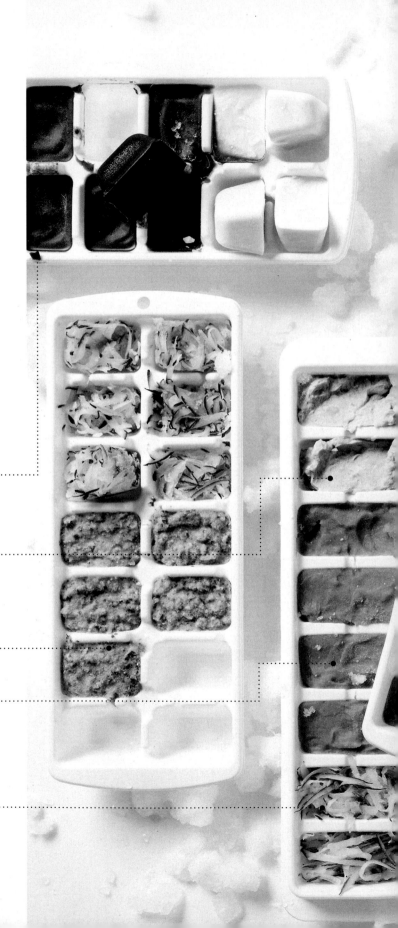

Basic Raw Chocolate (page 56): Instant hot chocolate recipe: drop a cube into a cup of simmering milk. Imbibe. Or for an instant treat, melt a cube and drizzle over ice cream.

Leftover avocado: Purée with coconut water or coconut cream and/or a little lime juice. Perfect for making Misomite (page 54), Green Minx Dressing (page 54), smoothies, and Leftovers Pesto (page 55).

Pesto and dressings: A cube is the perfect size for a single serve. Use with pasta, Abundance Bowls (pages 126–37), salad, fish, meat.

Squash or Sweet Potato Purée (page 23): Add to casseroles, pasta and anything that needs a mock-tomato hit. Or toss into smoothies, hot chocolate, muffins or slices in place of sweetener (just add some chia seeds to soak up liquid if used in baking).

Grated raw zucchini: Smoothie fodder.

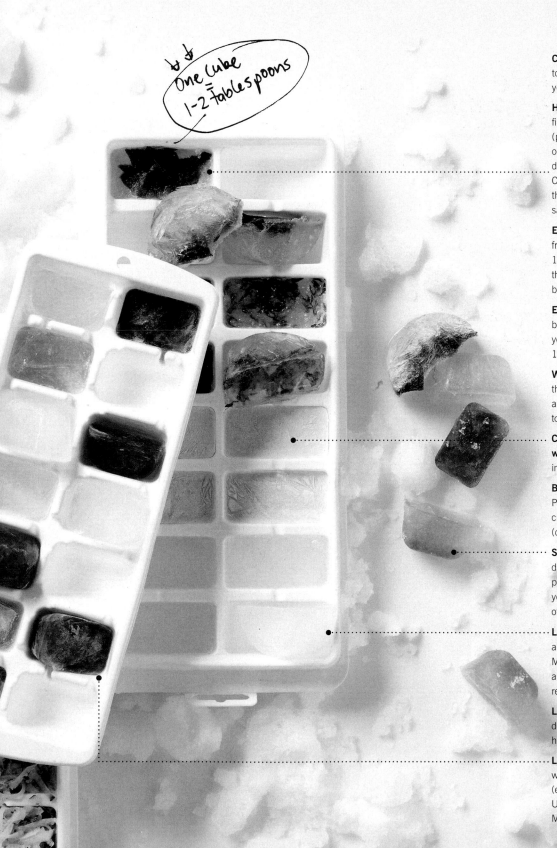

One cube ≠
1-2 Tablespoons

Cooked greens: Purée and freeze—great to toss into smoothies, sauces or wherever you feel the need to up the nutrient ante.

Herbs in oil, wine or stock: One-third fill each cube with chopped fresh herbs (parsley, thyme, rosemary, sage and oregano work best) and top with the dregs of a wine bottle, stock or olive oil. Chuck into casseroles and soups, or use them to sweat your veggies instead of sautéing them in oil.

Egg whites: Transfer the cubes to a sealed freezer-proof container and use them within 12 months (really!). And make sure you thaw them completely before using—they'll beat better at room temperature.

Egg yolks: So that they don't turn to jelly, beat in ⅛ teaspoon salt for every 3 large yolks. When using in cooking, substitute 1 tablespoon thawed egg yolk for 1 fresh yolk.

Whole eggs: If you're worried you won't use the whole carton before they go bad, whisk a few eggs and pour into a tray ready to add to omelettes.

Coconut milk, coconut cream, coconut water: Ready to toss into smoothies, or to use in recipes when you need small amounts.

Berries with coconut cream: Pop a few berries in and top with cream or yogurt to eat as a sweet treat (or for smoothies).

Stock: Great for using up the stock that didn't fit into the bigger containers (see pages 42–43 for recipes). Use to deglaze your pan, or to sweat your veggies instead of sautéing in oil.

Lemon and lime juice: Citrus juice is a pain to prepare a tablespoon at a time. Make in bulk in your blender (or juicer) and freeze in 1–2 tablespoon serves ready to go.

Lard and drippings: Use cubes to braise, deglaze or sauté your veggies. Or pour over herbs and freeze in cubes (see above).

Leftover sauces and stew liquid: A great way to keep the dregs of a delicious sauce (e.g., Watercress Sauce; page 176) or stew. Use for braising, deglazing and Leftover Mishmashes (pages 246–65).

BEANS, GRAINS, NUTS AND SEEDS

You might know the toxin drill surrounding BGNSs by now.
No? It goes like this:

* Most of the little devils contain anti-nutrients—chiefly enzyme inhibitors that make them difficult to digest—and phytic acid, which binds to minerals and prevents their full absorption.

* This doesn't mean BGNSs should be banned from your diet. It just means choosing the least toxic varieties, preparing them right—soaking and fermenting (as our grandmothers did)—and eating them in moderation.

* Soaking and sprouting or fermenting BGNSs breaks down the phytic acid so you don't get the mineral-leaching thing going on; helps to release beneficial nutrients, making them more bioavailable (more easily digested); *and* creates enzymes that further assist digestion of the proteins and fibers. Triple boon!

COOKED QUINOA

Before cooking, quinoa must be rinsed well—twice—to remove the toxic but naturally occurring coating saponin.

MAKES 4 CUPS

1 cup quinoa, rinsed
and drained twice

2 cups water

Place the quinoa in a saucepan and pour in the water. Cover and bring to a boil. Reduce the heat and simmer, covered, for 15 minutes or until all the water has been absorbed. Remove the pan from the heat and let it stand for 5 minutes, covered. Fluff the quinoa with a fork. Divide into 1-cup portions and freeze for up to 6 months (or store in the fridge for 4–5 days).

MAKE IT EVEN MORE NUTRITIOUS:
Activate your quinoa first.
Cover 1 heaped cup of
well-rinsed quinoa with
water and add 2 tablespoons
of acid (apple cider vinegar,
lemon juice or whey). Cover
with a dishtowel and leave
for 12–24 hours before
cooking.

RAW QUINOA

ACTIVATED AND
COOKED QUINOA

Buckwheat can get awfully confusing

Buckwheat groats are the raw seeds that look like little light-tan/green pyramids. You cook and eat these like you would quinoa or rice, and you can sprout them for salads. Activated groaties (also called buckinis) are soaked and then dried at a low temperature. They are ready to eat as is, as soup toppers or a crunchy cereal or in desserts. They can also be cooked as you would raw groats, but take less time. Kasha is the name for raw groats that have been toasted. Got it?

Buckwheat vs. quinoa

* Both are high in protein, containing all the essential amino acids. Buckwheat comes out slightly on top. (I'm not concerned about vitamin and mineral content—you'll get bigger doses from veggies and meat.)
* Both are gluten-free and relatively low in toxins, if prepared correctly.
* But buckwheat is much higher in antioxidants than quinoa.
* And buckwheat is more ethically sound. The popularity of quinoa in the West has left traditional South American communities starving as they can no longer afford the stuff.
* Also, buckwheat is often grown as a rotation crop to prime the soil for grains. It's a leftover before it even gets to the package!
* Finally, buckwheat is faster to cook (less electricity!) and I personally love the toasty, caramel-y flavor and texture of activated groaties.

COOKED BUCKWHEAT

MAKES 8 CUPS

2 cups raw buckwheat groats

3 cups Homemade Stock (page 42) or water

½ teaspoon sea salt

I put mine on to soak just as I go to bed

Soak the buckwheat overnight in plenty of water (buckwheat is thirsty stuff). The next day, rinse well, drain and plonk in a saucepan with the stock or water, and the salt.

Bring to the boil, then reduce to a simmer and cook for about 8 minutes, until all the water is absorbed. When done, allow to sit for 5 minutes with the lid on and then fluff with a fork. Divide into ½-cup servings and freeze for up to 3 months.

MAKE IT FASTER:

Instead of soaking, you can also reduce some of the phytic acid by toasting the groats in a dry frying pan (no oil) over medium-low heat for 5 minutes before adding the water. Cook for 15 minutes.

Buckwheat is relatively high in phytase (the good enzyme that breaks down phytic acid), so keep the soak time to 7–8 hours max, or it will become too mushy. Bear in mind a bit of mushiness is normal, though.

ACTIVATED GROATIES

MAKES 4–6 CUPS

2 cups raw buckwheat groats, soaked overnight, rinsed and drained well

Spread the buckwheat on a large baking sheet. Dry in the oven on the lowest temperature possible (no more than 125°F) for about 8 hours, until crispy. Store in an airtight container in the pantry for 3 months.

MAKE THEM EVEN MORE NUTRITIOUS:

Sprout your buckwheat first by soaking the raw groats for 1–2 hours, then put them in a fine-meshed sieve over a bowl (or in a big jar with a muslin cloth secured over the top) and wash and drain twice a day for 1–2 days, until tiny little tails form (see page 352 for more info about sprouting). Then dry in the oven as above.

MAKE THEM SWEET SPICE GROATIES:

Combine soaked or sprouted buckwheat with 3 teaspoons of Pumpkin Spice Mix (page 45) or 2 teaspoons of ground cinnamon and 1 teaspoon of ground nutmeg.

MAKE THEM SALTED CARAMEL GROATIES:

Combine soaked or sprouted buckwheat with 2 teaspoons of maca, 1 teaspoon of sea salt and 1 teaspoon of ground cinnamon.

MAKE THEM MIDDLE EASTERN GROATIES:

Combine soaked or sprouted buckwheat with 3 teaspoons of Ras el Hanout Mix (page 45) and 1 teaspoon of sea salt.

SPROUTED BUCKWHEAT

ACTIVATED GROATIES

RAW BUCKWHEAT GROATS

A few things about beans and legumes

* Avoid canned (unless you can find organic)—they're not prepared properly. Plus there's the carbon footprint (and BPA issues) from the can.
* Brown lentils are your most nutritious option. And are also the quickest to cook. They're featured a bit in this book.
* Soak most of them for 24 hours if you can. This will eliminate 20–50% of the phytic acid.
* Store your beans in their cooking stock. They keep better (in both fridge and freezer) and can be used together for most dishes.

Optional, but it will break down the phytic acid even more.

COOKED BEANS AND LEGUMES

MAKES 3 CUPS

I'm not a paid-up fan of legumes (oh, the bloat), but when prepared and cooked properly they're a reasonably nutritious addition to the diet and an economical way to pad out a dish. Most books at this point feature a highly complex chart of different soaking and cooking times for the myriad beans and legumes out there. A waste of paper and your sweet time! I assure you it can be as flow-y as this:

I soak my lentils for 7 hours, even though most people don't.

1 cup dried beans (any type, even lentils or mung beans)

3 cups hot water

3 teaspoons whey, apple cider vinegar or lemon juice

Place all of the ingredients in a bowl and leave to soak overnight. The next morning, drain and transfer to a saucepan. Cover with water and bring to the boil over medium heat. Boil for 10 minutes, then reduce the heat and simmer until the beans are soft (up to 1 hour).

Cool and divide into 1-cup portions (½ cup of beans and ½ cup of their cooking liquid). Beans and stock will keep in the fridge for 3–4 days like this. Or you can freeze for up to 6 months.

ACTIVATED NUTS AND SEEDS

Activating brings digestive benefits as well as producing a crunchier, slightly toasty version of the original nut or seed. Worth the stigma!

1 package of raw nuts or seeds (e.g., almonds, pepitas, walnuts)

pinch of sea salt

Place the nuts or seeds in a bowl with plenty of water. Add the salt, cover and leave to soak overnight.

The next morning, drain the nuts/ seeds. Spread them out on a baking sheet (no oil, no parchment paper) and dry in the oven for 12–24 hours at the lowest temperature possible (less than 150°F for gas ovens, on the pilot light). When cool, store in a sealed container in the freezer.

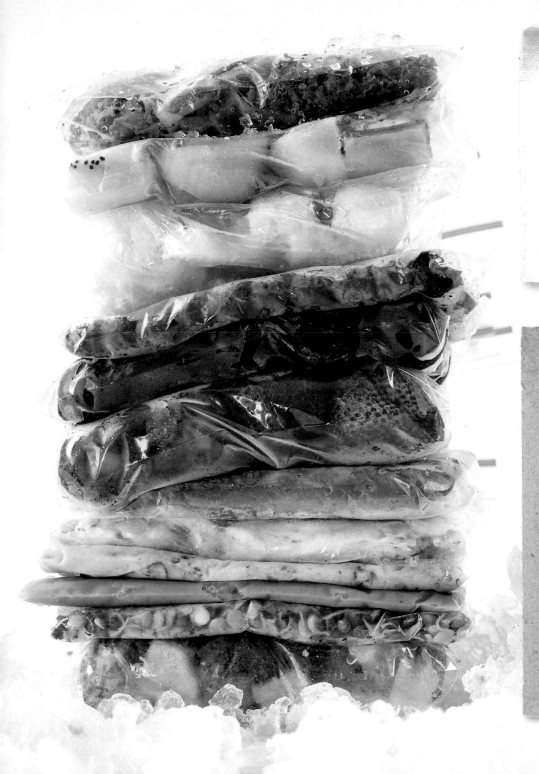

HOW LONG IN THE FREEZER?

You can actually freeze food indefinitely (from a safety POV) but for parcooked and frozen veggies, a 3-month storage is best for optimal texture and flavor. As for other foods, here are some recommended freezing times:

Fish (cooked)—1 month

Meat soup—2 months

Meat (cooked)—2 months

Beans, grains, nuts and seeds (cooked)—3 months

HOW TO FREEZE AND THAW STUFF PROPERLY

Always cool food first so it freezes fast; a slow freeze will cause the water cells to expand, which ruptures the food and denatures it.

Defrost food slowly in the fridge (over a day or two is best), though some ingredients can be tossed into your smoothie, stew, soup, pasta sauce, etc., frozen.

You can refreeze food that's been thawing in the fridge, if you realize you're not going to eat it . . . so long as it's still *very* cold or partially frozen.

Let meat, poultry and seafood thaw in the fridge (don't leave it out on the counter for more than 2 hours). Stew meat, poultry and seafood should stay good for about 2 days, while red meat cuts (such as beef, pork or lamb roasts, chops and steaks) are good for 3–5 days after thawing.

USE YOUR LEFTOVERS

This is not really a separate step in my cooking flow, but sort of happens along the way, both when I sort, store and precook produce, and when I do cook-ups and make meals for friends. I've just put it in one spot so you can see how it fits in.

Please note that it would make me immensely happy if you were to regard this bit of the book and my Leftovers recipe chapter as the most important and interesting parts. Stick on a Post-it, pull out a highlighter, if you must. I will hug you if I see evidence of this when you greet me at a book signing down the road. Promise!

FIRST, USE YOUR LEFTOVER SUGAR

Let's walk the leftovers talk from the get-go. Don't toss your sugar when you quit the stuff. Put it to good use.

1. MAKE AN AYURVEDIC FACE SCRUB

1 cup sugar

⅓ cup coconut oil, softened
(or use olive oil)

1 teaspoon pure vanilla extract (or make your own; see page 45) and/or one of the oils or spices below

Combine all of the ingredients in a glass jar with a lid. It will keep in your bathroom for 2 months.

To use, take 1 tablespoon and apply to a very slightly moistened, clean face (you don't want it too wet, or the scrub will dissolve). Massage in circles. Rinse with warm water.

CHOOSE YOUR OWN SPICE ADVENTURE

For Kaphas (or during winter):
Replace ½ cup of sugar with ½ cup of salt and add some dried sage or rosemary and 5 drops of eucalyptus oil.

For Vatas (or when it's windy):
Replace some of the sugar with honey and add 1 teaspoon of Pumpkin Spice Mix (page 45), or 1 teaspoon of ground nutmeg, cinnamon or cardamom, or 5–10 drops of lavender, rose, sandalwood or geranium oil.

For Pittas (or during summer):
Add 1 teaspoon of ground turmeric or rose water or 5–10 drops of jasmine or rose oil.

2. KEEP YOUR FLOWERS ALIVE

Dissolve 3 teaspoons of sugar in 2 tablespoons of white vinegar and add the syrup to a vase of water. The simple carbs in the sugar will help the flowers stay strong and the vinegar will kill bacteria and keep bugs away from the vase.

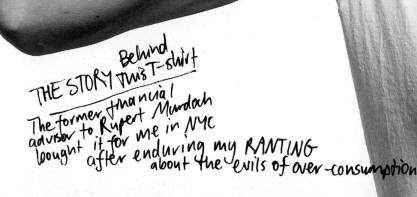

THE STORY Behind THIS T-shirt
The former financial advisor to Rupert Murdoch bought it for me in NYC after enduring my RANTING about the evils of over-consumption

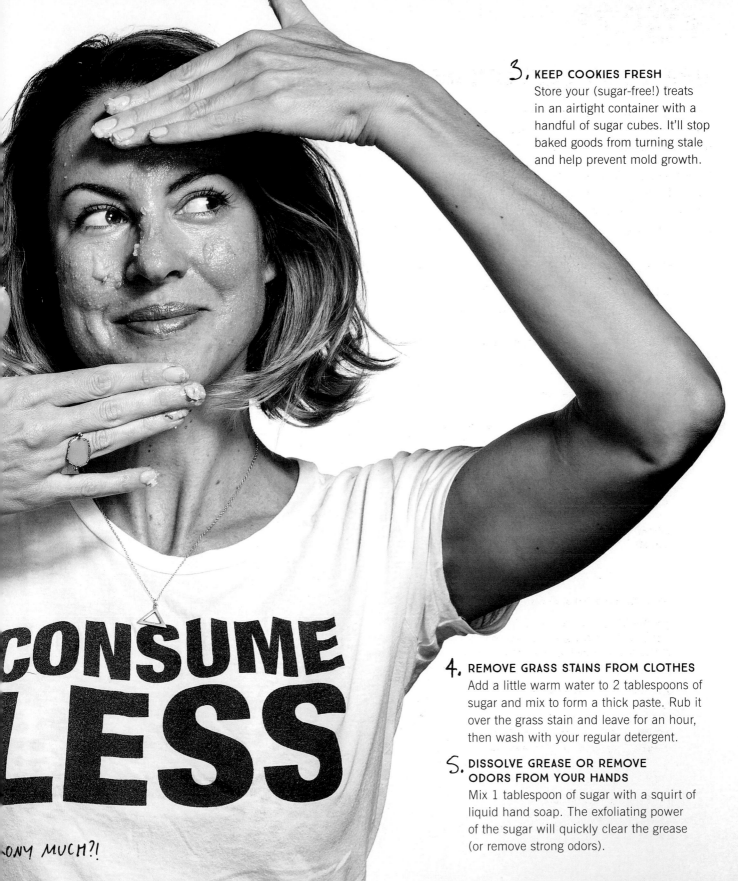

3. **KEEP COOKIES FRESH**
Store your (sugar-free!) treats in an airtight container with a handful of sugar cubes. It'll stop baked goods from turning stale and help prevent mold growth.

4. **REMOVE GRASS STAINS FROM CLOTHES**
Add a little warm water to 2 tablespoons of sugar and mix to form a thick paste. Rub it over the grass stain and leave for an hour, then wash with your regular detergent.

5. **DISSOLVE GREASE OR REMOVE ODORS FROM YOUR HANDS**
Mix 1 tablespoon of sugar with a squirt of liquid hand soap. The exfoliating power of the sugar will quickly clear the grease (or remove strong odors).

PACK UP YOUR SCRAPS AS YOU GO

I keep all the peels, leaves, stalks, offcuts, bones and other leftovers in bags or containers, ready to turn into stocks, smoothies and pestos. If I don't have time to make something straight away, I throw the bags in the freezer.

CREATE A VEGETABLE STOCK BAG

Place onion and carrot tops, celery bits, herb stalks, Parmesan rinds, etc. in a freezer-proof bag in the freezer ready to make veggie stocks or to add to meat stocks or to cooked beans. Don't save the following for stocks (they're too overpowering): cabbage, brussels sprouts, broccoli, cauliflower, turnips or artichokes.

You'll need about 4 cups of leftover veggies to make 2 quarts of stock.

I keep a separate bag for asparagus stock (page 43).

CREATE A CHICKEN OR BEEF BONES STOCK BAG

Reserve raw bones or cooked bones from chicken or beef, literally off people's plates after they've eaten, until you have about 2–4 pounds (see Homemade Stock, page 42).

CREATE A FISH STOCK BAG

You need a good couple of carcasses to make fish stock (see page 42). Collect them over time. Add leek and fennel offcuts to this bag.

CREATE A LEFTOVERS PESTO BAG

Put aside stems, stalks and excess leaves from your kale, beets, mint, parsley, coriander, leafy greens, carrot tops, etc. The pesto works best if you use no more than 2–3 different herbs or greens in one batch (see page 55).

CREATE A SMOOTHIE BAG

Grated zucchini, celery offcuts, herbs, leftover cooked greens, and fruit offcuts go into this one.

HOW I USE CONDIMENT LEFTOVERS TO MAKE FLAVOR BOMBS

* **THE BRINE OR OIL FROM OLIVES** goes into dressings.

* **THE OLIVE OIL FROM ANCHOVIES** goes into dressings.

* **THE OLIVE OIL AND HERBS FROM MARINATED FETA** go into dressings or are used for cooking.

* **THE BRINE OR SPRING WATER FROM TUNA** is used to sauté or deglaze.

* **THE SALT FROM CAPERS** seasons dishes.

* **THE JAR CONTAINING DRIED MUSTARD DREGS** becomes my salad-dressing shaking jar.

REGROW YOUR BUTT

Oh, the joy of taking a root and shooting it, watching it grow and eating it all over again. Oh, and in the meantime, using the budding beauty as a room decoration. Here are my favorite regrowth projects:

Perpetual green onions: Either plonk a bunch directly into a pot of soil, or sprout the white root ends in a glass jar filled with water, and leave in a sunny position. Within days it will shoot and you can use new shoots as required, leaving the white root in (fresh) water to keep growing.

Cilantro and lemongrass: As above, using the white root in water method.

Bok choy, celery and romaine: As above, regrow the white root, but in a shallow bowl of water—enough to cover the roots but not the top of the cutting. Place in a sunny position, topping up the water as required. After a few days, roots and leaves will appear. After a week, transplant it into soil with just the leaves showing above the soil. The plant will continue to grow, and within a few weeks it will sprout a whole new head.

Ginger and turmeric: You know how they sprout if you leave them on the counter too long? Simply place in a pot of soil with the newest buds facing upward, leave in a filtered-light position and water regularly. It will grow a big indoor-plant-like frond within days (rather handsome). After a few weeks, pull up the whole plant, roots and all. Remove a piece of the root (to eat), and re-plant it to repeat the process.

Pineapple: I don't actually eat the stuff (it's pretty high in fructose), but I inherited two recently and (a) gave one to my parents; (b) cut the fronds off the other to regrow a pineapple for fun and decorative purposes (it takes 2 years for the thing to reach edible stage); and (c) froze the fruit, in pieces, to use sparingly in smoothies.

To regrow, grab the fronds and give them a hefty twist to remove them neatly from the fruit bit. Cut away any bits of fruit attached (if any). Pull off enough leaves to expose 1 inch of stalk. Then carefully shave off small slices from the bottom of the stalk until you reveal root buds (small brown dots on the flat base of the stalk). Place in a jar of water in the sun for a week. Once roots shoot, pot in soil and enjoy its hipster, pot-planty effect for the next few years.

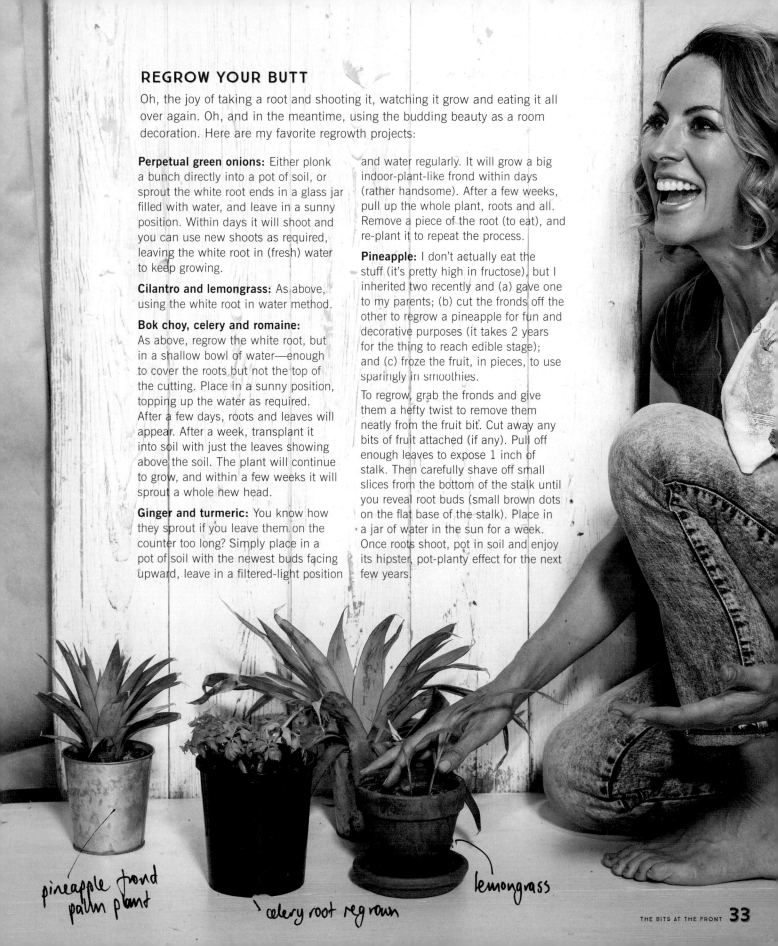

pineapple frond palm plant

celery root regrown

lemongrass

→ *Bonus step!*

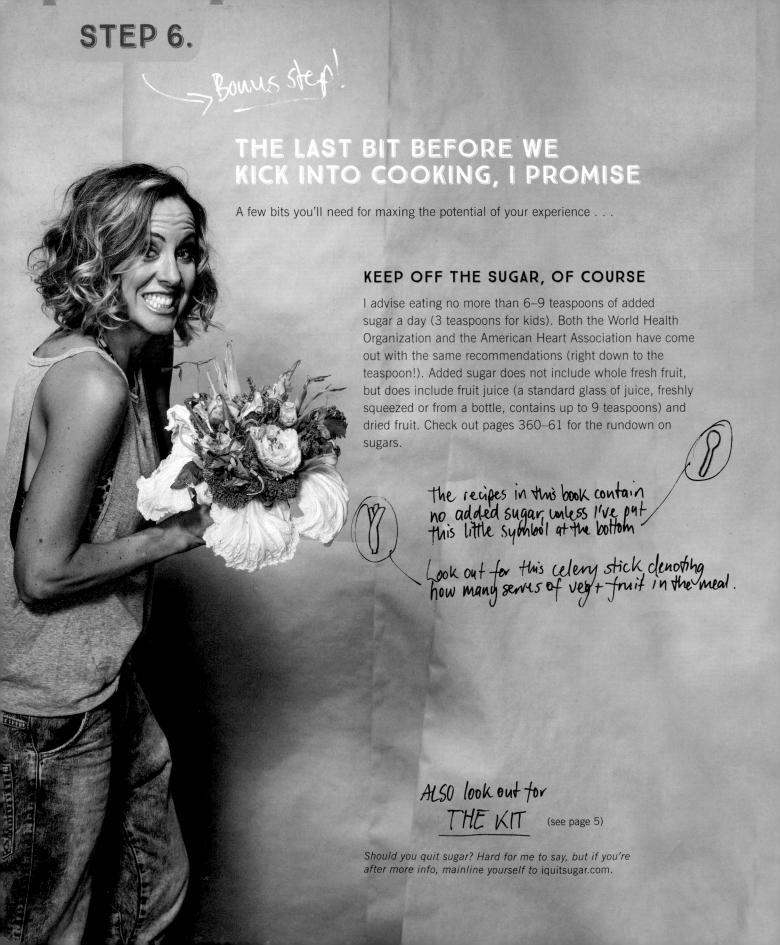

THE LAST BIT BEFORE WE KICK INTO COOKING, I PROMISE

A few bits you'll need for maxing the potential of your experience . . .

KEEP OFF THE SUGAR, OF COURSE

I advise eating no more than 6–9 teaspoons of added sugar a day (3 teaspoons for kids). Both the World Health Organization and the American Heart Association have come out with the same recommendations (right down to the teaspoon!). Added sugar does not include whole fresh fruit, but does include fruit juice (a standard glass of juice, freshly squeezed or from a bottle, contains up to 9 teaspoons) and dried fruit. Check out pages 360–61 for the rundown on sugars.

the recipes in this book contain no added sugar, unless I've put this little symbol at the bottom

Look out for this celery stick denoting how many serves of veg + fruit in the meal.

ALSO look out for
THE KIT (see page 5)

Should you quit sugar? Hard for me to say, but if you're after more info, mainline yourself to iquitsugar.com.

There's a substitutions list on pages 358–59 if you want to be more certain about your creative license.

What counts as "1 serving"?

Leafy greens (raw) = **1 cup**

All other vegetables (raw) = **½ cup**

Red meat and pork = **2 ounces cooked (3–3½ ounces uncooked)**

Fish = **3½ ounces cooked (4 ounces uncooked)**

Eggs = **2 large ones**

Beans = **1 cup**

Nuts = **1 ounce**

Yogurt = **½ cup**

Milk = **1 cup**

Cheese = **1½ ounces**

What are the daily requirements?

I work to standard dietary guidelines but up the ante on the nutrients.

Vegetables: 6–8 servings per day; 5 for kids

Protein: 3 servings

GET LOOSE AND BREAK THE RULES

This is an invitation, not an instruction. Don't peel your vegetables, don't bother browning meat to make stocks and slow-cooked casseroles. When making soup, toss the ingredients in without browning them in oil first. When you make a roast, shred or pull the meat rather than carve it. It generally tastes better and is more appropriate for a secondary cut. Use spice mixes that approximate the combo in a recipe. Go on! Use a microwave if it helps you get a nutritious meal on the table.

BUILD YOUR MEALS RIGHT

This is how I go about making my meals. Every meal should aim to work to these proportions.

1. **Start with 2–3 servings of vegetables.** Even at breakfast. "Eat mostly plants" is a good way to operate.

2. **Add a bit of starch or bulk if you need it.** A starch/carb-free diet isn't sustainable for many. My preferred starches/carbs are sweet potato, buckwheat and frozen peas. Use these ingredients to provide sweetness, too.

3. **Toss in some protein.** I use meat to flavor and boost a meal, rather than focusing on it as the starting point.

4. **Add fat.** Generally about 1–2 tablespoons per person, in the form of oil, avocado, dressing, cheese or nuts, and even butter. This is partly for nutrient absorption, partly for flavor and partly for appetite control.

5. **Amp things with some ferment or bitters.** I try to do this at one meal a day. Two tablespoons of sauerkraut or kimchi or 3 tablespoons of tonic or kombucha is enough.

Remember, fat doesn't make us fat, sugar does. The most recent respected science shows there is no link between the consumption of saturated fat and cholesterol in food and cholesterol problems or heart disease.

Look out for this bit in my recipes, it's pivotal to sustainable cooking.

USE THE LEFTOVER EGG YOLKS:
Make an omelette or frittata.
Or freeze them.

EMBRACE THE SUNDAY COOK-UP

This concept is a big part of the I Quit Sugar program. It entails bulk-cooking and freezing your veggies, but also bulk-cooking a dish that provides leftovers that can be frozen for meals down the road—as well as fun projects that will stock your kitchen with clever condiments (and can be used as gifts, too).

CREATE YOUR OWN FLOWS

Feel free to devise or create your own flows, then share with me on social media. It's an art, a sport.

Create challenges for yourself. I do. Like:

* Making a meal from frozen bits and fridge-door condiments only.

* Just when you think you need to go to the store, see if you can leave it one extra meal. And then another. And another. Until the fridge is truly bare.

* If a meal needs something extra, will frozen peas, a handful of ferment, a portion of frozen sweet potato purée cut it?

* Collect your scraps from preparing a meal. Be deeply satisfied when they can fit into half a fistful. Social-media it! I'll look out for your post.

SHARE, BRAG, CONNECT

I'm not just saying it; I do love to see your achievements and creations and flows and ideas on social media.

INSTAGRAM: @_sarahwilson_ and @iquitsugar

FACEBOOK: SarahWilson and IQuitSugar

TWITTER: @_sarahwilson_ and @iquitsugar

Hashtags: #iqscookbook (or #sarahwilsoneats for leftovers bragging and mishmash meals)

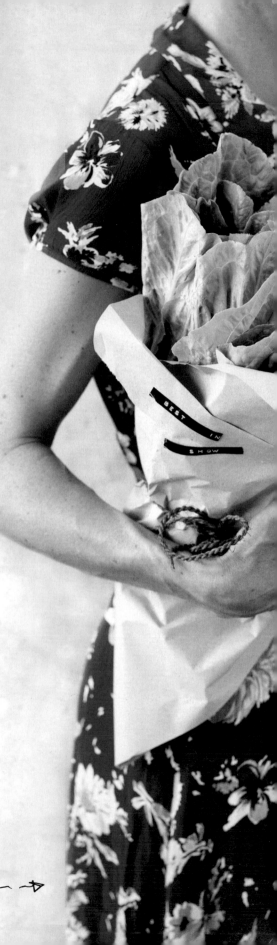

HERE'S ONE OF MY FLOWS

I set aside an hour or two (max) to bulk-cook and prepare a bunch of things. I keep the oven on and my steamer boiling away and off I go.

* Preheat the oven to 200°F. Roast 8 heads of garlic.
* Meanwhile, fill the sink with water and dunk the watercress and lettuce. Remove and drain the greens (keep the sink water), then spin and store (see page 19).
* Snap asparagus ends and place in stock bag (see page 32); store the stems (see page 19).
* Load up the slow cooker with veg and stewing steak for my Cheapest Stew Ever (page 212).
* Remove the garlic from the oven and set aside.
* Turn the oven up to 350°F. Scrub a few roots in the sink water: 2 sweet potatoes; 1 bunch beets and 1 bunch baby carrots. Pop in the oven for 40–60 minutes. Mcanwhilc, wash and dry the beet greens and carrot tops, and 1 bunch chard.
* Boil water in the double steamer and cook a bunch of eggs, then use the same water to steam the beet greens, followed by the chard. In the bottom, blanch the carrot tops.
* Use the sink water to cool the eggs and store (page 44).
* Make Leftovers Pesto (page 55) with carrot tops and Parmesan. Add the rind to the asparagus stock bag.
* Make Sweet Potato Purée (page 23) with the sweet spud. Pop the carrots and beets into containers and leave in the fridge for salads during the week.
* Place all veggie scraps in a vegetable stock bag (page 32).
* Make Good for Your Guts Garlic (page 340) with the roasted cloves, using whey from last week's Homemade Cream Cheese.

And so on I flow . . .

Time taken: 2¼ hours (including doing a load of washing)
Fridge/freezer items created: 12
Meals created: 6–8 (plus heaps more when the stew is cooked)

ENOUGH RUN–UP, LET'S GET TO IT!

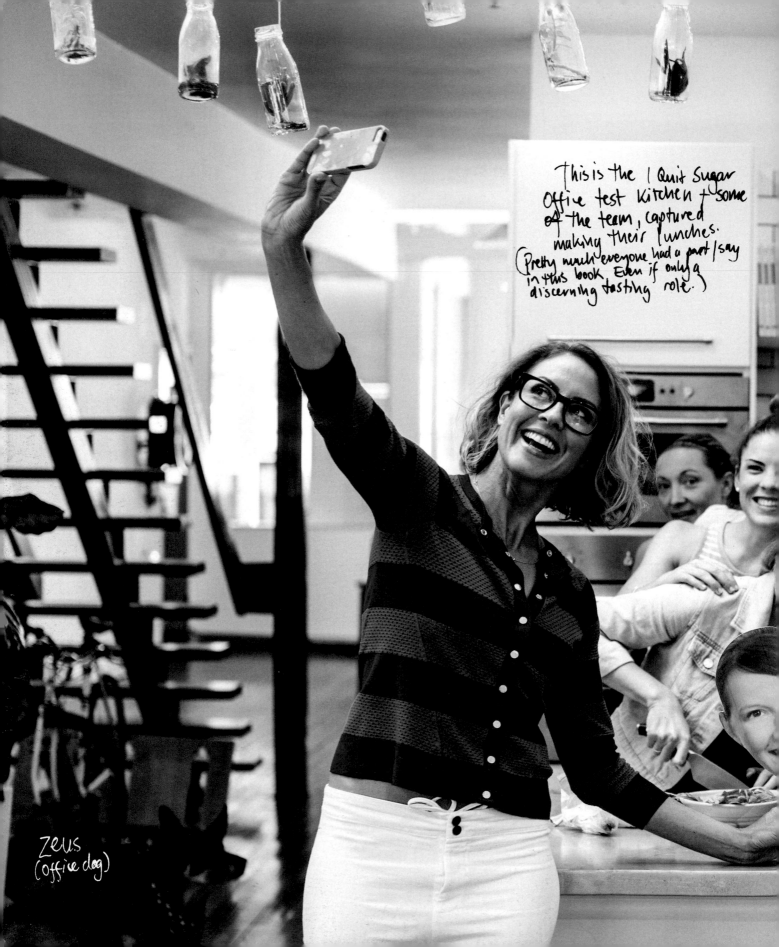

This is the I Quit Sugar office test kitchen + some of the team, captured making their lunches. (Pretty much everyone had a part/say in this book. Even if only a discerning tasting role.)

Zeus (office dog)

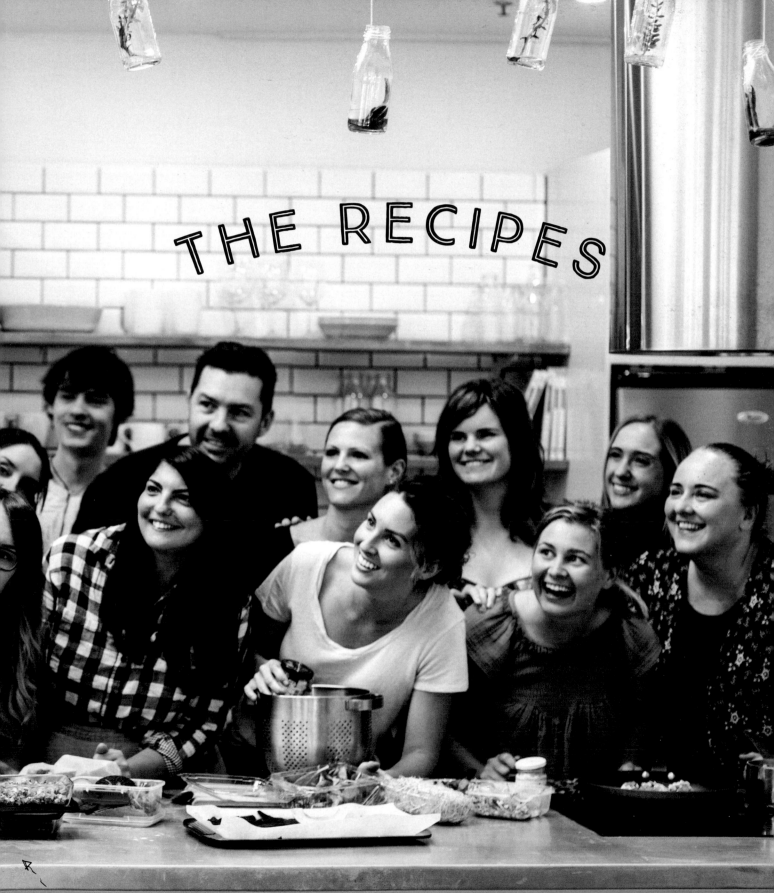

THE RECIPES

This, here, is Zoe my great mate + IQS general manager. On a stick.

THE
BASICS

really rather SIMPLE dressings,
sauces,
JAMS
fermented CHEESES
STOCKS

with which to fill
your pantry,
fridge and
FREEZER...

ingenious Pestos,
101 MAYO,
and other clever
FLAVOR BOMBS

... so you're 100% sorted + can just get on with cooking......

HOMEMADE STOCK

MAKES ABOUT 3 QUARTS

Stock is the ultimate leftover foodstuff. I have jars of it in the fridge and freezer at all times. Later on I'll share how to make stock as you prepare meals, but here's how to make stock from scraps. Bone broth or stock is made with cheap bones or carcasses you can get from your butcher, and is simmered for a super-long time. Work to the amounts below, filling your pot with enough water to clear the contents by 2 inches but still leaving 1 inch of room at the top of the pot. Each batch you make will come out differently, so don't fret too much about getting it "right."

Be aware: food fad cynics hate it when stock is called "broth." Thus, I call it stock. Its the same stuff.

FOR BEEF STOCK:

My butcher gives them to me cheap.

2–4 pounds beef bones (marrow, knuckle, ribs, neck)

FOR CHICKEN STOCK:

1–2 leftover (cooked or uncooked) chicken carcasses plus extra bony chicken bits if you have them (wings, necks, feet)

FOR FISH STOCK:

2 pounds fish carcasses (heads, tailbones or offcuts of white-fleshed fish—don't use oily fish!)

2 tablespoons apple cider vinegar (or just plain white will do)

I include the skin, but some people don't because they reckon it makes the stock bitter.

1 onion, coarsely chopped

2 cups veggie scraps, including peels, coarsely chopped

Whatever you've got—carrot and celery are best. Avoid cabbage, turnips and bitter greens, as they'll make it bitter.

1 bay leaf or several sprigs of fresh thyme

½ teaspoon dried green or black peppercorns

Sourcing fish carcasses
Next time you're at the fishmonger, ask for a bag of fish carcasses. Even better: when buying fillets for a dish, ask your monger to fillet it fresh and let you keep the carcass. Then you know it's fresh and you have a longer chat with your monger. Which I think is nice.

Place the bones in a very large stockpot with the vinegar and cover with cold water. (For beef stock, soak the bones for 30 minutes before cooking. You can also roast the meatier bones in a 400°F oven for 10 minutes first to make a browner broth. I rarely bother.) Add enough water to cover the bones, but the liquid should come no higher than within 1 inch of the rim of the pot, as the volume expands slightly during cooking. (The water should be cold—slow heating helps bring out the flavors.)

Bring to the boil. Reduce the heat and add the veggie scraps, herbs and peppercorns, then simmer:

Beef: 12–72 hours
Chicken: 4–24 hours
Fish: 1–3 hours

When the stock is cool enough, remove the bones, then strain the liquid into a large bowl. (For beef bones, feel free to do a second batch with the same bones and new veggies. It won't be as "gel-y" or flavorful, but you'll get extra minerals from it.) Refrigerate the stock until cool and then, using tongs or large spoons, remove the layer of congealed fat on top—you can literally pick it up in chunks (like ice over a pond)—and toss it. (Not always pretty.) Divide the remaining liquid into 1-cup portions and freeze for up to 3 months (for fish stock, 1 month).

MAKE IT IN A SLOW COOKER:
Follow the method above, placing everything in your crock and cooking on low for 8–24 hours.

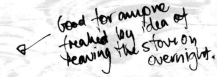
Good for anyone freaked by idea of leaving the stove on overnight.

PROSCIUTTO–PARMESAN STOCK

Combine some prosciutto rinds or ends, a few pieces of Parmesan rind, 2 crushed cloves of garlic and a sprig of fresh rosemary in a saucepan with 1–2 quarts of water. Bring to a boil, reduce the heat and simmer for 1 hour. Strain.

ASPARAGUS STOCK

Boil the woody stems of 2–3 bunches of asparagus (preferably in leftover asparagus steaming water) for 45 minutes until super soft. Remove the stems, purée in a blender or food processor, then return the purée to the cooking water. Pass the lot through a sieve, pressing with the back of a spoon. You will be left with a purée-ish stock.

CORN COB STOCK

don't be scared of the slobber – all bacteria are boiled into oblivion!

Cover 6 corn cobs (pre-gnawed and stripped of kernels) with 1–2 quarts of water. Add a couple of bay leaves and bring to the boil over medium heat. Simmer for 1 hour. Strain.

Why celery in stocks and sauces?
Have you noticed it features with carrots and onions in all the classic bases (soffrito, mirepoix)? There's a reason: Japanese scientists have found that when it's cooked slow and low, a bunch of volatile compounds are released that enhance the perception of sweetness and umami from the other ingredients.

PRECOOKED EGGS AND BACON — true story!

Eggs will keep for a while in the carton, but it's handy to cook a bunch at a time because they keep great when cooked, too. Ditto, bacon.

Eggs poach better when fresh and boil best when they've been sitting around a while—older eggs are easier to peel!

REALLY SIMPLE POACHED EGGS

I cook half a dozen poachies at a time and store them in a bowl of cold water in the fridge for several days.

white vinegar or rice vinegar (optional)

fresh eggs at room temperature

Fill a small, shallow lidded skillet with water (or pour water into a wide saucepan to a depth of 2 inches). Bring to a boil. Add a dash of vinegar if you like—this will help the egg whites to congeal neatly rather than spread out in the water. Break an egg into a teacup, then gently tip the egg from the cup into the water. (You can poach a few eggs at a time, if you like.) Turn off the heat immediately and cover the pan tightly. Leave for 3–4 minutes, then remove each egg with a slotted spoon.

How to perfectly peel a boiled egg
Half-fill a sturdy container with water, pop in your boiled egg, seal the lid tightly and shake. You'll have a very cracked egg, but the shell will fall off flawlessly, all done in less than 10 seconds. Rad.

PERFECT BOILED EGGS

I boil in bulk and store the eggs in their shells for up to a week. Place some older eggs (at room temperature) in a saucepan and cover with plenty of cold water. Bring to a gentle boil, uncovered. Remove from the heat, cover with a lid and set your timer.

Soft-boiled: leave in the pan for 4 minutes.

Medium: leave for 8 minutes.

Hard-boiled: leave for 12 minutes.

Drain, then plunge the eggs into cold water. Store in the fridge for up to a week.

BACON BITS

This entails one of my favorite kitchen hacks—it not only eliminates stinky splattering, but also renders the bacon fat perfectly.

Remove the rind only from 6–10 strips of streaky bacon (keep all the fat on) and cut the bacon into ¾-inch squares. Place in a skillet or large saucepan and add just enough water to cover the bottom of the pan. Cook over medium-high heat until the water has evaporated. Reduce the heat to medium and cook the bacon until crisp (about 10 minutes—no need to turn). This will take longer than frying but is more effective. Remove the bacon and allow to cool on a wire rack over the pan to catch all the juices.

To freeze bacon bits, lay them on a baking sheet and place in the freezer. Once frozen, transfer to a freezer-proof container or zip-lock bag and return to the freezer (this will make it easier to snap off what you need).

USE THE LEFTOVER BACON FAT:
It's great for frying eggs and making popcorn. Just drain the rendered fat into a jar (or leave it in the pan ready to cook your next meal). It will keep for a month in the fridge.

PANTRY FLAVOR BOMBS

I'll be using these time-saving, entirely useful mixes throughout this book. So feel free to make up a batch of each.

RAS EL HANOUT MIX

MAKES ABOUT ½ CUP

2 tablespoons ground coriander seeds

2 tablespoons ground cinnamon

2 tablespoons ground cumin

1 tablespoon cayenne pepper

Put all the ingredients in an airtight jar, seal with the lid and shake. Will keep for 6 months.

SEAWEED DUKKAH

MAKES ABOUT 1½ CUPS

1 cup macadamias

2 teaspoons cumin seeds

1 teaspoon coriander seeds

2 tablespoons white sesame seeds

¼ cup dulse flakes or 4 nori sheets

2 teaspoons dried Greek oregano

sea salt and freshly ground black pepper

Toast the macadamias in a skillet over a medium heat until golden (about 4 minutes). Remove from the pan and leave to cool, then finely chop.

Grind the seeds (and nori if using) finely in a blender (or use a mortar and pestle). Add to the pan and toast until fragrant (about 2 minutes). Cool, then stir in the macadamias, oregano and dulse flakes (if using). Season to taste with salt and pepper. Will keep for 1 month in an airtight container.

PUMPKIN SPICE MIX

MAKES ABOUT ½ CUP

⅓ cup ground cinnamon

1 tablespoon ground ginger

1 tablespoon ground nutmeg

3 teaspoons ground allspice

Put all the ingredients in an airtight jar, seal with the lid and shake. Will keep for 6 months.

NEVER-ENDING VANILLA EXTRACT

I use this stuff a lot so I figured it was time to share a recipe for it. Try to use a long, narrow bottle or jar (an old capers jar—well washed or sterilized—is perfect).

3 vanilla pods

½ cup vodka (or bourbon, brandy or rum)

Split the vanilla pods lengthwise. Place in your bottle or jar (cut them in half to fit if need be) and cover with vodka or whatever booze you're using. Seal, shake and store in the dark. Whenever you see it in your pantry, give it a shake (a few times a week); it will be ready to use in 4 weeks.

Note: it will get stronger the longer you keep it.

MAKE IT BOTTOMLESS:

Simply add more booze as you drain the bottle. Also add another pod or two as the flavor wanes (a great way to use up pods when you've used the seeds for something else).

See also Celery Leaf Salt (page 265) and Kale Flakes (page 179).

A FEW DAIRY THINGS

Which yogurt?
Go for plain (unflavored), organic and full-fat (most low-fat varieties have added sugar). I find the Greek styles are often best. BUT look at the nutrition label. It should contain no more than 4.7 grams of sugar per ½-cup serving. This is the natural lactose contained in dairy foods and is perfectly fine (unless you're lactose intolerant). Anything more than 4.7 grams per ½ cup is added sugar.

HOMEMADE CREAM CHEESE AND WHEY

It's so simple to make your own cream cheese and whey.

32 ounces full-fat organic plain yogurt

Be sure to use full-fat organic yogurt—I've found that this recipe doesn't work well if you use the commercial stuff.

Pour the whole tub of yogurt onto a large handkerchief-sized square of clean cheesecloth or muslin. Bunch the ends together like you're tying a sack and secure with an elastic band or string. Suspend the bag over a large bowl—I attach mine to a wooden spoon placed across the bowl, while others hang theirs from a cabinet knob, or even a chandelier! You're going to be straining out the whey, leaving a beautifully creamy curd in the sack. Drain for 12–24 hours. Store the cream cheese in the fridge for up to 1 month, and use it as you would the commercial stuff (see the Cream Cheese Frosting recipe on page 56).

Transfer the whey into an ice-cube tray. When frozen, store the cubes in a freezer-proof container in the freezer. Use for fermenting or making pesto or mayonnaise.

MARINATED GOAT'S CHEESE

Buy the goat's feta in bulk (feel free to double the quantities below) and make it last 3 months by preserving it in oil.

7 ounces organic soft goat's feta, chilled

½ cup good-quality extra-virgin olive oil

1 clove garlic, peeled

3 sprigs fresh thyme or 2 bay leaves

1 teaspoon fennel seeds, peppercorns or allspice berries

pinch of sea salt

Cut the feta into ½-inch cubes. Place a little olive oil in the bottom of a smallish squat jar. Add half the feta, the garlic clove and half of your chosen herbs and spices. Sprinkle with salt. Add some more oil and the remaining feta, herbs and spices until you've filled the jar. Pour over the rest of the oil, adding more, if necessary, to ensure the feta is completely covered. Seal the jar and refrigerate for 2–3 days to allow the flavors to infuse before eating.

USE THE LEFTOVER HERB-INFUSED OIL:
Combine it with apple cider vinegar or lemon juice in a 2:1 ratio (oil to acid) and use as a dressing.

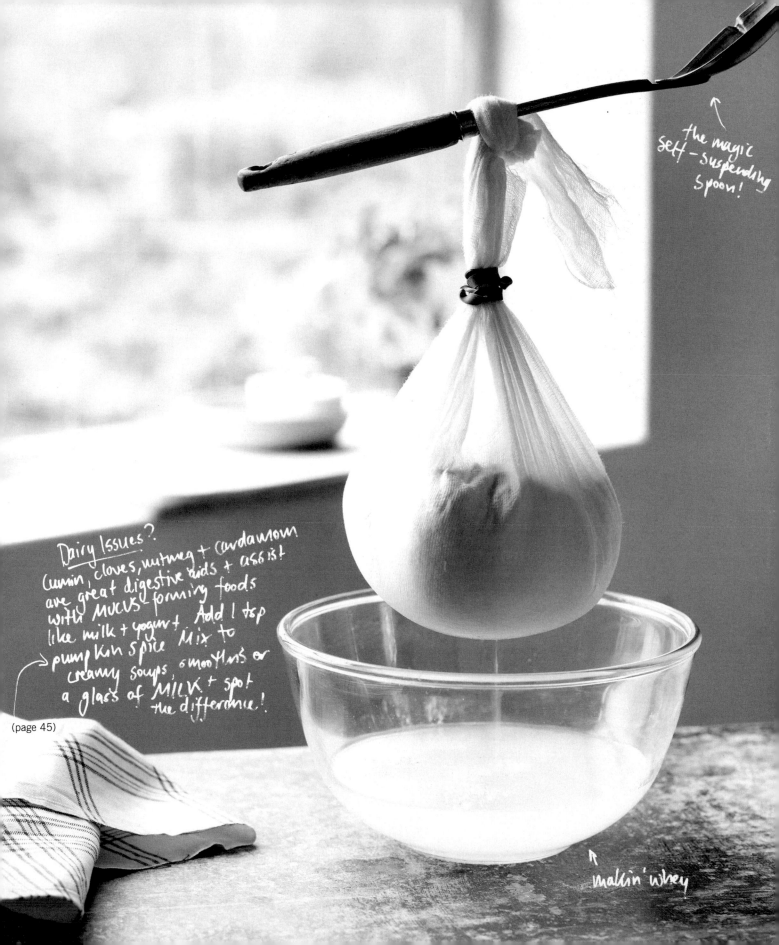

the magic
self-suspending
spoon!

Dairy Issues?.
Cumin, cloves, nutmeg + cardamom
are great digestive aids + assist
with MUCUS forming foods
like milk + yogurt. Add 1 tsp
pumpkin spice Mix to
creamy soups, smoothies or
a glass of MILK + spot
    the difference!

(page 45)

makin' whey

HOMEMADE PANEER

This Indian version of the IQS community's much-loved haloumi is one of the easiest cheeses to make at home. Plus it's also one of the easiest to digest, which I guess is why it features a bit in Ayurvedic recipes (it's chiefly recommended for nourishing and calming Vata and increasing Kapha). It's also often recommended as an Ayurvedic cure for female infertility. There you go!

2 quarts full-fat milk

juice of 4 lemons

1 teaspoon sea salt

Warm the milk in a large saucepan over medium heat until it reaches the "almost boiling" point (around 195°F). If it looks like it might boil over, take it off the heat and blow directly across the rising foam (taking it off the heat won't be enough). Your breath is much cooler than the boiling milk and should get it back down in the pot quickly. When ready, the milk should be foamy and steamy.

(1.)

Stir in the lemon juice really quickly for no more than 5 seconds until the milk curdles. If it doesn't separate properly, then VERY carefully stir through a little more lemon juice, again without disturbing the curd too much, then simmer for a few seconds until the milk curdles.

I Quit Sugar's Marly, also a cheese maker, told me that excessive stirring can break up the curd too much.

Remove from the heat and allow to sit, uncovered and undisturbed for 20 minutes while the curd separates from the whey (which will be yellow and milky).

Line a colander with a piece of cheesecloth or muslin and place over a bowl. Pour in the curdled milk. Tie the corners of the cloth together and squeeze out the excess liquid. Open the "sack," sprinkle over the salt and massage it gently through the cheese. Form the cheese into a square, then re-wrap the cloth around it as you would a book you're giving as a present. Place it on a plate or tray. Place another plate or pan on top with a weight (e.g., a bowl of water or a can of tomatoes) and allow it to flatten and cool for at least 1 hour (3–4 hours is best). Refrigerate before use. It will keep in the fridge for about a week.

2.
3.

4. cut into cubes.

USE THE LEFTOVER WHEY:
Add it to smoothies for a protein hit or use it in place of water in baking recipes. Note: This whey doesn't have fermentable properties, as it's been heated.

Cold paneer is less likely to crumble.

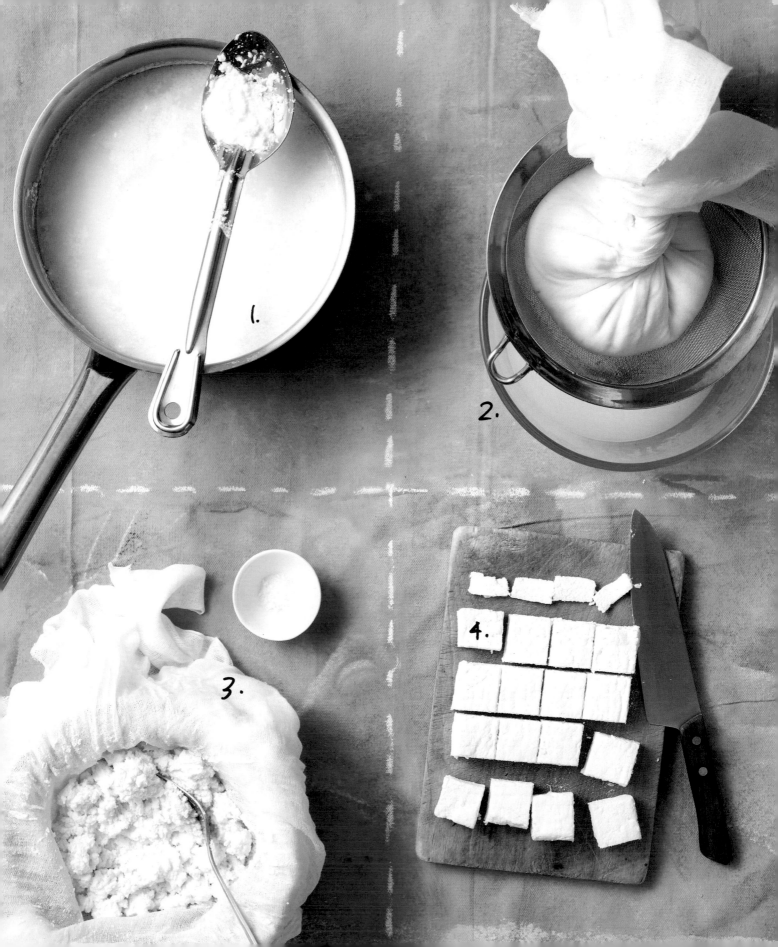

A WHOLE BUNCH OF SAUCES, DRESSINGS AND PESTOS

This is how I do dressings. I make one based on the ingredients I have lying around, then I put it in a jar in the fridge and use it on Abundance Bowls (pages 126–37), Leftover Mishmashes (pages 246–65), pizzas, dosas, etc. As it starts to run low, I make up another sauce or dressing and do the same. This way I have two at a time to choose from and I don't get bored.

The following recipes are designed to last as long as possible. If you're worried they might not keep for the prescribed distance, please do this: pour a portion into an ice-cube tray, freeze, then pop the blocks into a freezer-proof container or zip-lock bag so you can thaw and use one cube at a time.

WHEY-GOOD MAYO

MAKES ABOUT 1½ CUPS

1 egg

1 teaspoon Dijon mustard

1 tablespoon lemon juice

1 tablespoon Homemade Whey (page 46)

big pinch of sea salt

1 cup good-quality extra-virgin olive oil

Blend together all the ingredients except the oil in a food processor on a low speed for 30 seconds. With the motor running (still on low), very slowly drizzle in the oil until the mayo is thick and smooth. (Did I mention drizzling it very slowly? You want it to pour in a very, very fine stream; otherwise it won't form an emulsion.) Cover the mayonnaise and let it sit at room temperature for 8 hours before refrigerating. This activates the enzymes in the whey and means it will last for 3 months in the fridge.

MAKE IT A QUICK MAYO:
To make a mayo you can use straight away, omit the whey, and prepare as above without the fermenting stage. Refrigerate the mayo immediately and use within a week or two.

MAKE IT A HOMEMADE AIOLI:
Make the mayo, then simply stir through 2 cloves of garlic, minced to a paste, at the end. (You might like to divide your batch in half to make one portion of mayo and one portion of aioli; though if you do this, use 1 clove of garlic instead.)

NOMATO SAUCE

MAKES ABOUT 1 QUART

Tomato purée with no 'matoes? No mata … this concoction is infinitely better than any tomato sauce or purée you've tasted. As someone in the office said: "It's liquid pizza!" Make it in big robust batches (I triple the mixture) and freeze as cubes, ½-cup and 1-cup batches.

2 tablespoons extra-virgin olive oil

4 shallots (or 2 white onions),
finely chopped

6 cloves garlic, finely chopped

1 large beet (14 ounces), trimmed, scrubbed
and coarsely grated

2 celery stalks, coarsely grated

3 carrots, coarsely grated

1 teaspoon sea salt

1 tablespoon finely chopped fresh oregano

2 cups Homemade Stock (page 42), or water

¼ cup pitted black olives, such as kalamata
(for the umami flavor)

2 tablespoons lemon juice

Heat the oil in a saucepan over medium-low heat. Cook the shallots, garlic, beet, celery and carrots for 10 minutes or until the shallot is translucent. Add the salt, then the oregano and stock or water and bring to a boil. Reduce the heat to a simmer and cook for 15 minutes or until the vegetables are tender. Transfer the mixture to a blender with the olives and lemon juice and process until smooth. Store in a sealed container in the fridge for 1 week or in the freezer for up to 6 months.

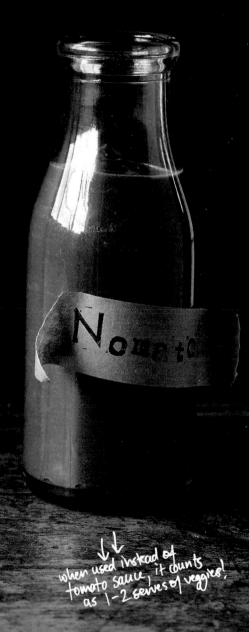

when used instead of
tomato sauce, it counts
as 1–2 serves of veggies!

2 SERVINGS VEG + FRUIT PER SERVING

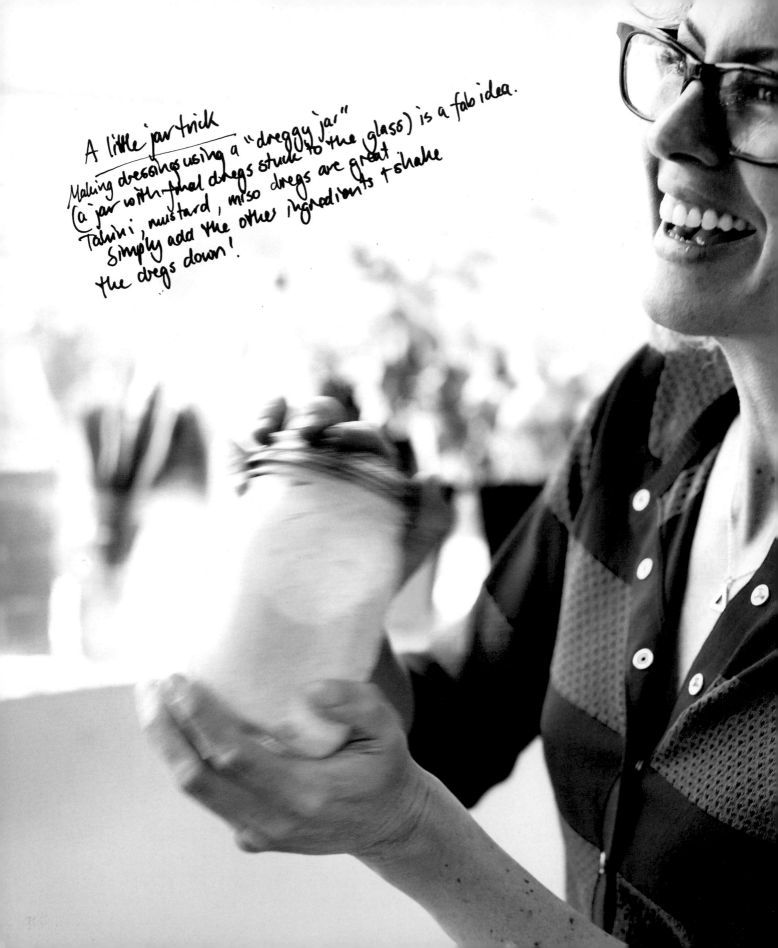

A little jar trick

Making dressings using a "dreggy jar" (a jar with final dregs stuck to the glass) is a fab idea. Tahini, mustard, miso dregs are great. Simply add the other ingredients + shake the dregs down!

TMT DRESSING
(TAHINI MISO TURMERIC)

MAKES 1½ CUPS

¾ cup tahini

½ cup hot water

3 tablespoons red miso paste
(or ½ cup white miso paste)

1 tablespoon Fermented Turmeric Paste
(page 340) or a 1-inch piece of turmeric,
finely minced (or 1 teaspoon ground turmeric)

1 tablespoon finely minced Good for Your
Guts Garlic (page 340), or 2 cloves of garlic, minced

3 tablespoons lemon juice, apple cider vinegar
or ferment brine (see page 334)

*If you're using fresh
turmeric and garlic, throw
them in the blender whole
(saves the mincing drama).*

Place all the ingredients in a blender and process until
lovely and smooth. Transfer to an airtight container or
jar and keep in the fridge for up to 1 week, adding a
little extra water and shaking before each use.

Tahini vs. peanut butter
In this book I play with the
former quite a bit, in part
because so many are allergic
to the latter, but also ...

✳ Tahini is an excellent
   source of calcium and
   is higher in protein than
   most nuts.

✳ It's high in vitamin E and
   B vitamins (B^1, B^2, B^3,
   B^5 and B^{15}) that promote
   healthy cell growth and
   function.

✳ It's rich in magnesium,
   lecithin, potassium and
   iron.

✳ It's also a great source
   of methionine, which
   aids liver detoxification.

✳ It's easier to digest than
   peanut butter due to
   its high alkaline mineral
   content.

✳ And it is high in good
   (unsaturated) fat.

POWERHOUSE DRESSING

MAKES ABOUT 1½ CUPS

Choose your own adventure with this one and
create your family or group-house special flavor.

⅓ cup good acid (kombucha,
apple cider vinegar, lemon juice,
or some excess brine from one
of your ferments)

1 cup oil (olive, avocado or walnut)

1 teaspoon sea salt

1 clove garlic, minced

1 tablespoon finely chopped fresh soft herbs
such as basil, tarragon or chives and/or
1 teaspoon Dijon mustard, ground allspice
or ground cloves

*I make mine with kombucha dregs
(the stuff at the end of a batch that's
gone sour).*

Place all the ingredients in a large jar, seal with a tight-fitting
lid and shake until well combined. Keep in the fridge for
1–3 weeks.

*If you use a brine or
kombucha it will last longer.*

GREEN MINX DRESSING

MAKES ABOUT 2 CUPS

There are 101 Green Goddess dressings out there these days. They're based on a dressing created in the 1920s as a nod to the play by the same name (and here I was thinking it was Just Another Instagram Fad). With my version, I undress things with a little saucy thrift and voluptuous nutrition.

1 large avocado or 1 cup Whey-Good Mayo (page 50)

1 large handful of fresh cilantro, including stalks (or you can use parsley, chives or basil, or a combo)

1 large handful of chopped lettuce

1 small zucchini (or ½ cup Parcooked 'n' Frozen zucchini; page 22)

2 cloves garlic (preferably fermented; see page 340)

2 tablespoons apple cider vinegar, ferment brine (see page 334) or lemon juice

¼ teaspoon each of sea salt and freshly ground black pepper

Process all the ingredients in a blender or use an immersion blender and a large mixing bowl. Thin, if required, with a little water.

If you use avocado, this will keep for 3–4 days in the fridge, or it can be frozen for 1–2 months in a freezer-proof airtight container, as long as the dressing is totally puréed (lumps make the dressing icy). To use, simply thaw in your refrigerator or in a bowl of cold water. Whisk to bring everything back together and serve cold!

MAKE IT LAST LONGER:
If you use Whey-Good Mayo instead of avo, it will last for up to a month in the fridge.

MISOMITE

MAKES ABOUT 1 CUP

Yep, a yeast-free, sugar-free salty fermented spread in, like, two ingredients flat.

1 avocado

½–1 tablespoon red miso

Blend together with a fork. Done. Will keep in the fridge for 1–3 days. Use as a dip or spread.

See also 'Bucha Mustard (page 336) and my other ferments (pages 337–40)

1 SERVING VEG + FRUIT PER SERVING

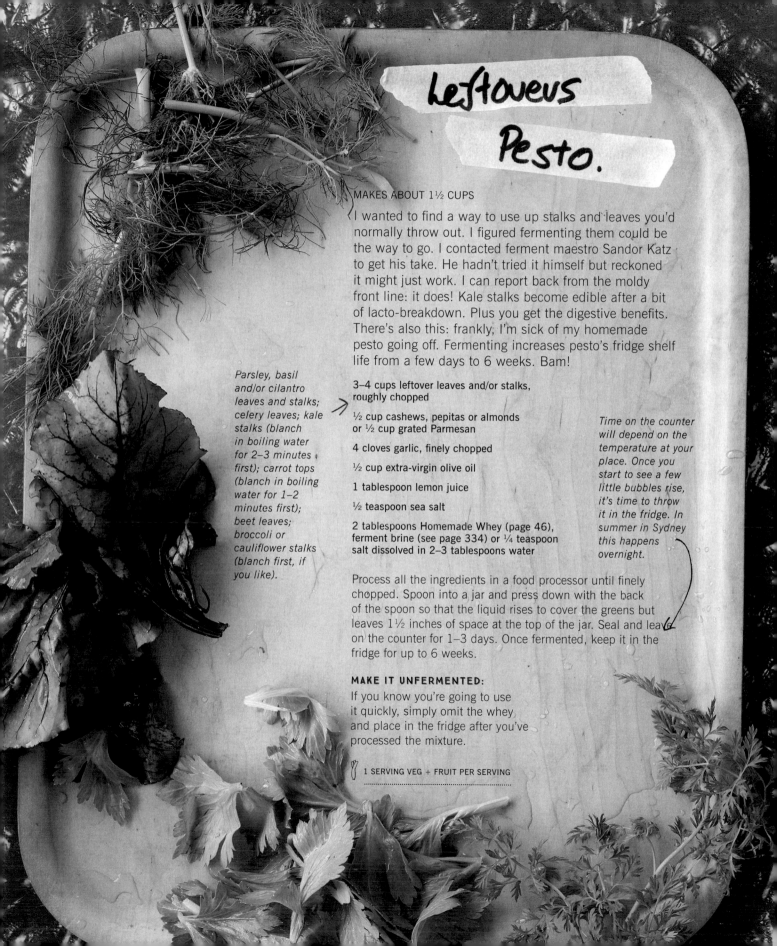

Leftovers Pesto.

MAKES ABOUT 1½ CUPS

I wanted to find a way to use up stalks and leaves you'd normally throw out. I figured fermenting them could be the way to go. I contacted ferment maestro Sandor Katz to get his take. He hadn't tried it himself but reckoned it might just work. I can report back from the moldy front line: it does! Kale stalks become edible after a bit of lacto-breakdown. Plus you get the digestive benefits. There's also this: frankly, I'm sick of my homemade pesto going off. Fermenting increases pesto's fridge shelf life from a few days to 6 weeks. Bam!

Parsley, basil and/or cilantro leaves and stalks; celery leaves; kale stalks (blanch in boiling water for 2–3 minutes first); carrot tops (blanch in boiling water for 1–2 minutes first); beet leaves; broccoli or cauliflower stalks (blanch first, if you like).

3–4 cups leftover leaves and/or stalks, roughly chopped

½ cup cashews, pepitas or almonds or **½ cup grated Parmesan**

4 cloves garlic, finely chopped

½ cup extra-virgin olive oil

1 tablespoon lemon juice

½ teaspoon sea salt

2 tablespoons Homemade Whey (page 46), ferment brine (see page 334) or **¼ teaspoon salt dissolved in 2–3 tablespoons water**

Time on the counter will depend on the temperature at your place. Once you start to see a few little bubbles rise, it's time to throw it in the fridge. In summer in Sydney this happens overnight.

Process all the ingredients in a food processor until finely chopped. Spoon into a jar and press down with the back of the spoon so that the liquid rises to cover the greens but leaves 1½ inches of space at the top of the jar. Seal and leave on the counter for 1–3 days. Once fermented, keep it in the fridge for up to 6 weeks.

MAKE IT UNFERMENTED:
If you know you're going to use it quickly, simply omit the whey and place in the fridge after you've processed the mixture.

1 SERVING VEG + FRUIT PER SERVING

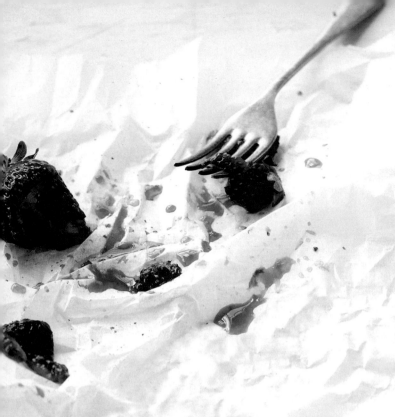

WHIPPED COCONUT FROSTING

MAKES ABOUT 1½ CUPS

14-ounce can full-fat coconut cream, refrigerated upside down

1–2 tablespoons brown rice syrup or ½–1 teaspoon granulated stevia

Open the can the right way up without shaking it. Spoon out the top layer of liquid and freeze it for smoothies or other recipes requiring coconut milk or coconut water.

dish-saving trick ←

Leave the rest of the firm cream in the can, add the syrup or stevia and then blend with an immersion blender until creamy. (If you don't have an immersion blender, remove the cream from the can and place in a blender.)

MAKE IT SUPERCHARGED COCONUT FROSTING:

Make as above, but blend in a small bowl, adding 2 tablespoons of powdered gelatin in a thin, steady stream before you add the sweetener. Continue mixing until soft peaks form. Use immediately or store in the fridge and use within 4–5 days.

½ TEASPOON ADDED SUGAR PER SERVING

A FEW FROSTINGS, TOPPINGS AND JAMS

These can be frozen in ice-cube trays and stored in the freezer ready for making or decorating muffins or cakes as required.

CREAM CHEESE FROSTING

MAKES ABOUT 1½ CUPS

9 ounces Homemade Cream Cheese (page 46)

1–2 tablespoons brown rice syrup or ½–1 teaspoon granulated stevia

zest of 1 lemon (optional)

3 tablespoons coconut cream or unsalted butter

Blend the cheese in a high-speed blender along with the syrup and zest (if using). Slowly add the coconut cream or butter until the mixture is nice and thick. If needed, add more coconut cream or butter. This will last for up to 1 month in the fridge.

½ TEASPOON ADDED SUGAR PER SERVING

BASIC RAW CHOCOLATE

MAKES ABOUT 1⅓ CUPS

1 cup coconut oil, softened

⅓ cup raw cacao powder

1 tablespoon brown rice syrup or 1 teaspoon granulated stevia, to taste

2 pinches of sea salt

Blend all the ingredients in a blender until smooth (or mix by hand). Use immediately in recipes, or pour into small silicone molds or ice-cube trays and keep in the freezer for up to 3 months.

Snack trick: Pop out a cube to eat as a choc treat. Or melt + use as a chocolate drizzle on fruit etc.

½ TEASPOON ADDED SUGAR PER SERVING

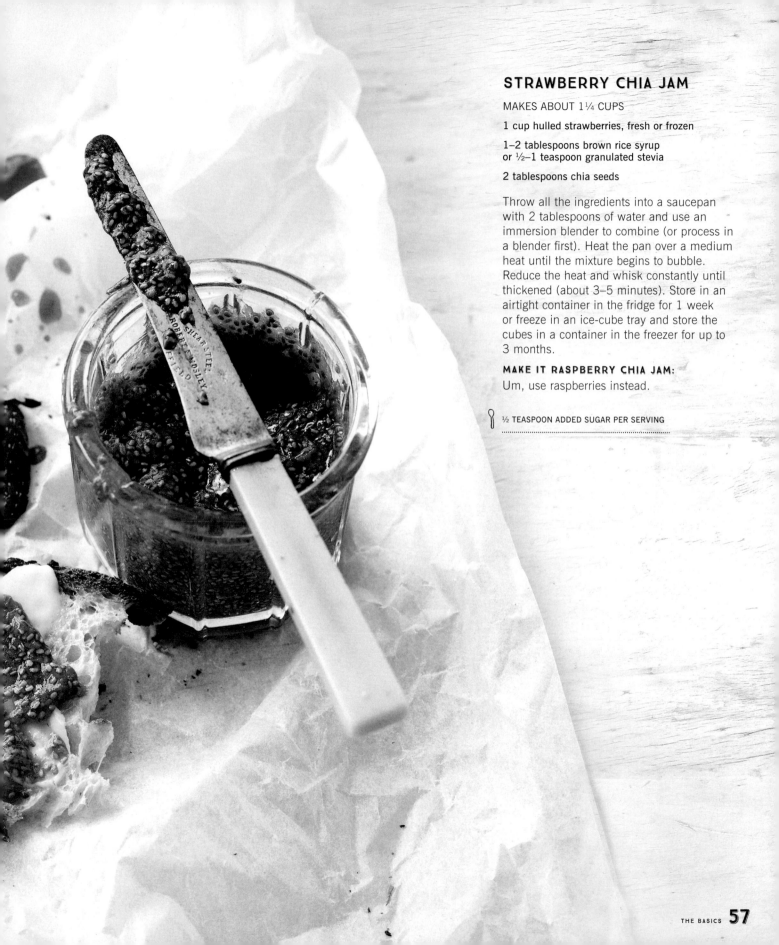

STRAWBERRY CHIA JAM

MAKES ABOUT 1¼ CUPS

1 cup hulled strawberries, fresh or frozen

1–2 tablespoons brown rice syrup
or ½–1 teaspoon granulated stevia

2 tablespoons chia seeds

Throw all the ingredients into a saucepan with 2 tablespoons of water and use an immersion blender to combine (or process in a blender first). Heat the pan over a medium heat until the mixture begins to bubble. Reduce the heat and whisk constantly until thickened (about 3–5 minutes). Store in an airtight container in the fridge for 1 week or freeze in an ice-cube tray and store the cubes in a container in the freezer for up to 3 months.

MAKE IT RASPBERRY CHIA JAM:
Um, use raspberries instead.

½ TEASPOON ADDED SUGAR PER SERVING

AGAINST-THE-GRAIN
BREAKFASTS

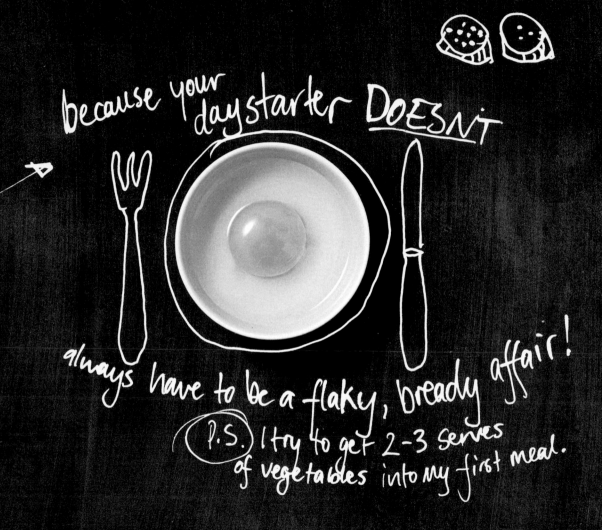

because your daystarter DOESN'T

always have to be a flaky, bready affair!

(P.S.) I try to get 2-3 serves of vegetables into my first meal.

"PIZZA" MUGGINS

MAKES 2 MUGS

Kids totally get the hands-on, cut-the-guff, intuitive approach. The ingredients in these mini-muffins-in-a-mug are just to give you some ideas—use leftovers and whatever you have on hand.

olive oil, coconut oil or butter, for greasing

some red things: cherry tomatoes, halved; diced red pepper

some green things: Parcooked 'n' Frozen broccoli (page 22) or tiny florets of raw broccoli

some sweetness: frozen peas, 1–2 cubes frozen Squash or Sweet Potato Purée (page 23)

some pizza flavor: 1–2 olives, pitted and chopped

some meat: Bacon Bits (page 44) or a small portion of chopped Pulled Beef (page 223) or Shredded Chicken (page 214)

2 eggs

grated cheese or crumbled feta

Rub the insides of two mugs with a little oil or butter. Hand them over to the kids and invite them to add whatever ingredients they like until the mug is half-full. Cover the mug (I use a saucer or small plate) and heat in the microwave for about 45 seconds.

Now get the kids to crack an egg into their cup(s) and sprinkle over the cheese. They can then stir the lot with a fork. Microwave again for another 30–60 seconds.

MAKE IT WITHOUT A MICROWAVE:
The kids can assemble all the ingredients in a ramekin and then crack an egg over the top and sprinkle with some cheese. Bake in an oven preheated to 350°F for 15 minutes.

MAKE IT FOR THE LUNCHBOX:
Make the muggins in a microwave-safe container and, once cooled, top with the lid.

½ SERVING VEG + FRUIT PER SERVING

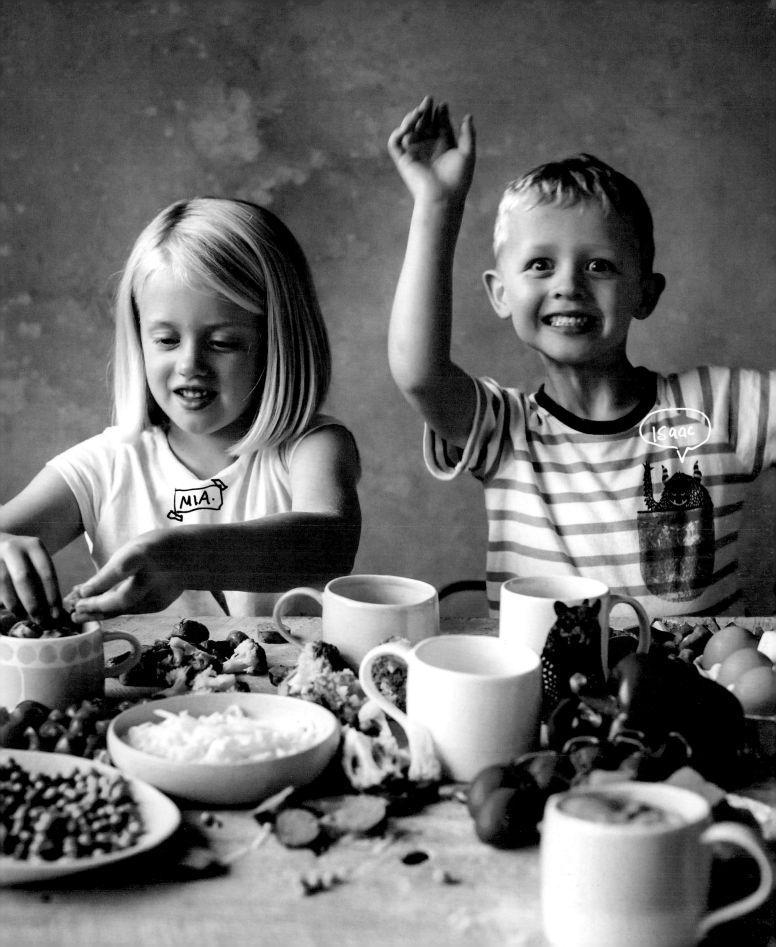

SLOW-COOKER ZUCCHINI AND PUMPKIN SPICE BREAKFAST PUDDING

SERVES 6

If you have a slow cooker with a timer, work things so the pudding greets you with a warm cinnamon vibe as you rise. Equally, this works really well made in advance, divvied up into lunch containers to be heated in the office microwave and served with a big splodge of yogurt.

coconut oil, butter or ghee, for greasing

½ cup butter, softened

¼ cup brown rice syrup

2 eggs

1 cup Squash or Sweet Potato Purée (page 23) or 2 cups grated raw pumpkin or sweet potato

1½ cups grated zucchini

2 tablespoons milk (any kind)

2 teaspoons pure vanilla extract (or make your own; see page 45)

2 cups almond meal

1 cup plain flour (gluten-free if you prefer)

1 teaspoon baking soda

1 teaspoon sea salt

2½ teaspoons Pumpkin Spice Mix (page 45) or 2 teaspoons ground cinnamon and ½ teaspoon ground nutmeg

¼ cup chia seeds

½ cup pecans, lightly toasted and roughly chopped

Lightly grease the slow-cooker insert with coconut oil, butter or ghee and line with parchment paper so that it reaches quite high up the inside of the pot.

Using an immersion blender, beat the butter and brown rice syrup together in a large bowl. Add the eggs, one at a time, beating after each addition. On low speed, beat in the squash or sweet potato, zucchini, milk and vanilla. Using a wooden spoon, stir in the almond meal, flour, baking soda, salt, spices and chia seeds and mix until well combined.

Pour the batter into the slow-cooker insert and sprinkle the pecans over the top. Cover and cook on low for 4–5 hours, or on high for 2–3 hours. Check the pudding by inserting a toothpick in the center—it should come out clean. If not, continue cooking on high with the lid off.

2 TEASPOONS ADDED SUGAR PER SERVING ← !! (feel free to reduce the sweetener – I do!)

1 SERVING VEG + FRUIT PER SERVING

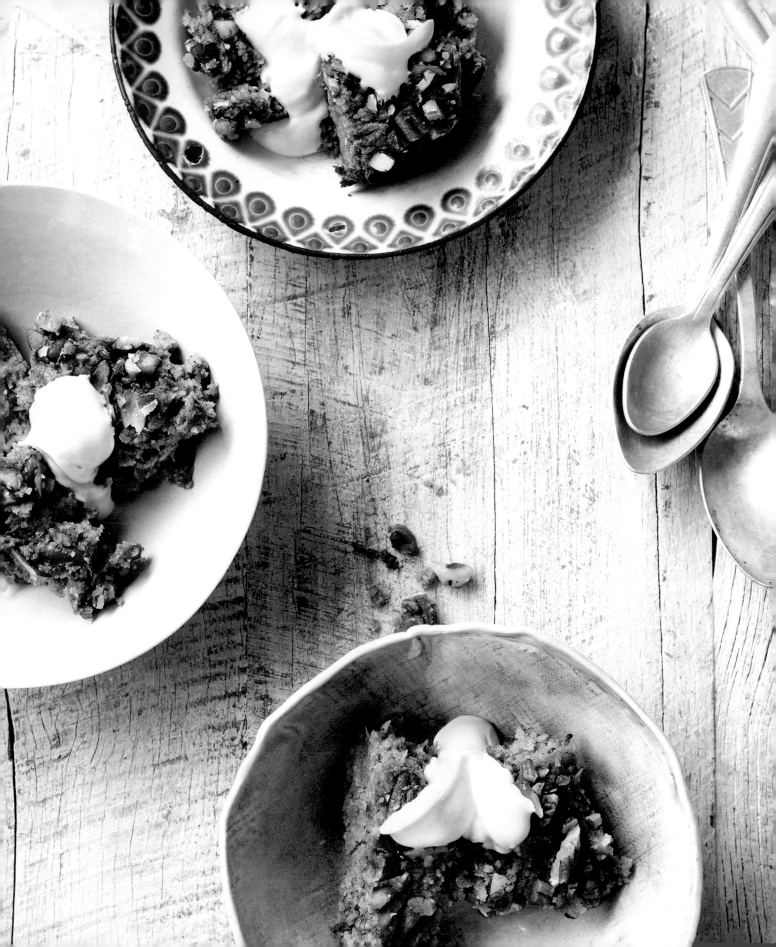

MUSHROOM, THYME AND HAZELNUT OATMEAL

SERVES 2 —

Savory oatmeal. For real. And it will probably change your life.

1 teaspoon butter or olive oil

1 small onion, chopped

1 cup sliced button mushrooms

1 teaspoon dried thyme or 1 tablespoon thyme leaves, plus extra to serve

1 cup whole rolled oats, Cooked Quinoa (page 26) or Cooked Buckwheat (page 27)

¾ cup Homemade Stock (a veggie variation; page 43) mixed with ½ cup water

2 ounces goat's feta

¼ cup hazelnuts, toasted and chopped

Heat the butter or olive oil in a saucepan over medium heat and sauté the onion until translucent (about 3 minutes). Add the mushrooms and thyme and cook until soft. Add your chosen "grain," the stock and water and, if using oats, also add an extra 1¼ cups of water. Stir and cook for 6–8 minutes or until the liquid has been absorbed. Remove from the heat and stir in half of the feta and half of the hazelnuts.

Divide the oatmeal between two bowls and serve topped with the remaining feta and hazelnuts and a sprinkle of thyme.

2 SERVINGS VEG + FRUIT PER SERVING

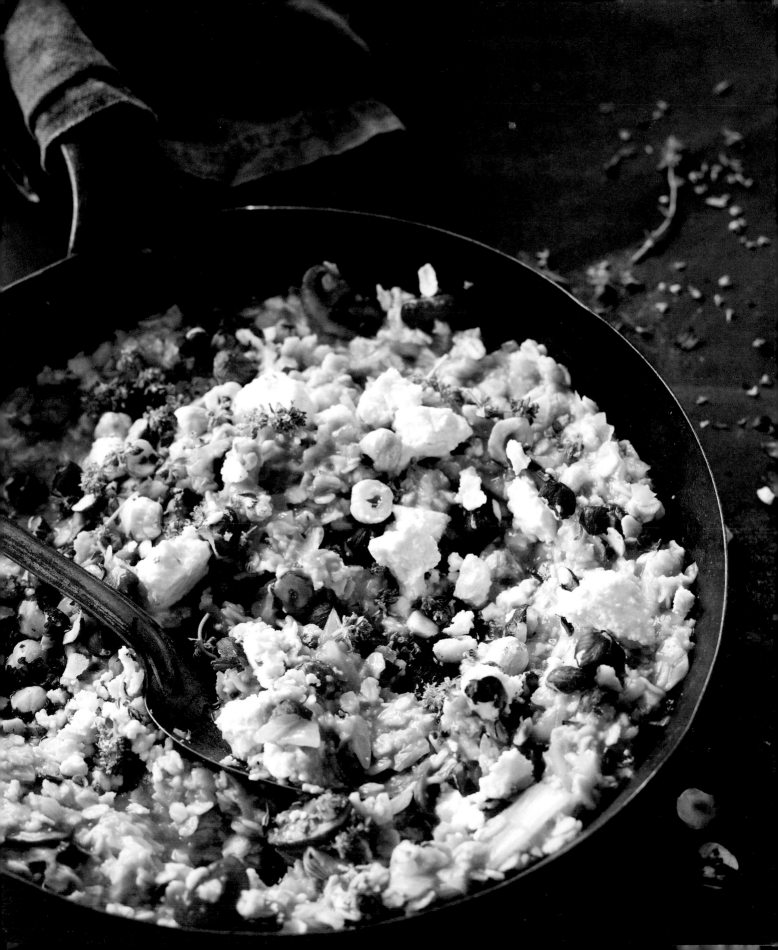

BACON 'N' EGG OATMEAL

Another talking-point savory oatmeal for you.

2 teaspoons coconut oil, olive oil, butter or ghee

1 small onion, chopped

1 cup whole rolled oats, Cooked Quinoa (page 26) or Cooked Buckwheat (page 27)

¾ cup Homemade Chicken Stock (page 42) or any stock

½ cup Bacon Bits (page 44), or 4 slices bacon, chopped and fried

2 tablespoons grated cheddar

2 soft-boiled eggs, halved

sea salt and freshly ground black pepper

fennel fronds, to serve (optional)

Heat the oil, butter or ghee in a saucepan over a medium heat and sauté the onion until translucent (about 3 minutes). Add your chosen "grain," stock, and if using oats also add 1¼ cups of water. Stir and cook for 6–8 minutes until the liquid has been absorbed.

Take the oatmeal off the heat. Stir through half of the bacon and all of the cheese. Divide the oatmeal between two bowls, top with the egg halves and remaining bacon, and season to taste with salt and pepper. Garnish with fennel fronds if you like.

You can also toss in 1 tablespoon of chia seeds and an extra ¼ cup of water or stock to the soaking bowl, if you like, to really bulk things out.

MAKE IT ACTIVATED OVERNIGHT OATMEAL:
Soak ¾ cup of whole rolled oats (or ½ cup of raw quinoa or buckwheat groats) in 1½ cups of stock overnight. Add this to the sautéed onions to heat through, along with a little stock or water to stop the "grains" from catching, then continue with the rest of the recipe.

½ SERVING VEG + FRUIT PER SERVING

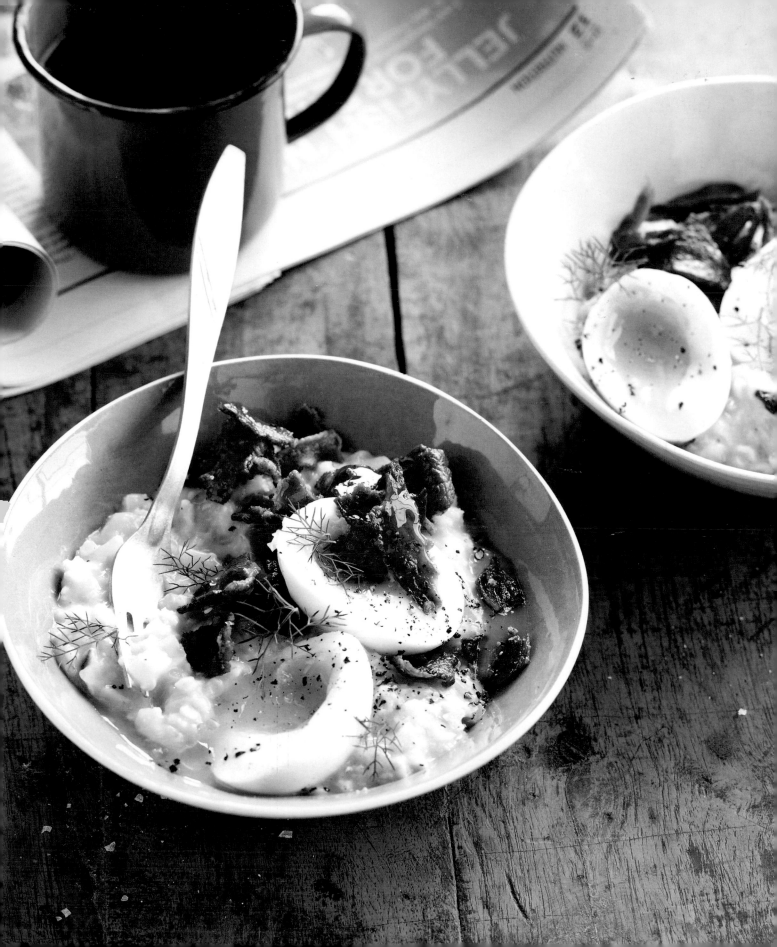

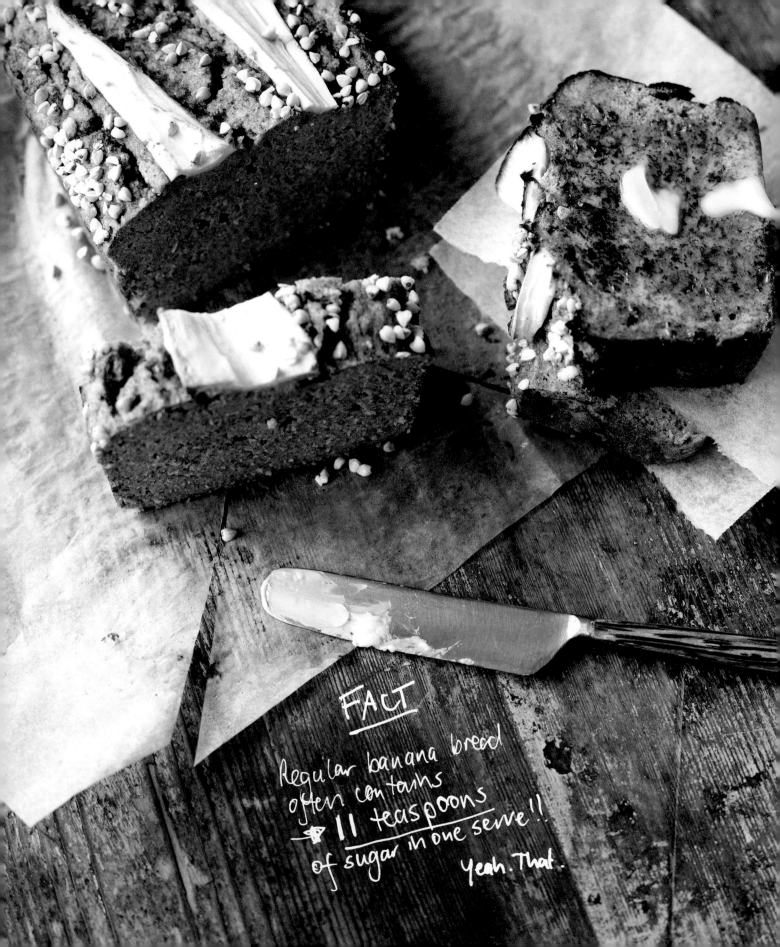

FACT

Regular banana bread often contains 11 teaspoons of sugar in one serve!! Yeah. That.

NOT QUITE
BANANA BREAD

This fake banana trick is a really good one for anyone wanting to up the nutritional count of their breakfast and cut back on fructose. It's great as is. Better toasted under a broiler, in a sandwich press or in a skillet with a dash of coconut oil (or butter if you don't mind dairy).

A bit of history for you
During World War II, bananas were scarce. So housewives of the era used parsnips—boiled and mashed with spices—as mock bananas. Ha!

2 large, very ripe bananas

1 cup grated parsnip
(about 5–6 ounces or 2 parsnips)

4 eggs

⅓ cup coconut oil

2 tablespoons (or 1–2 frozen cubes) full-fat coconut milk

2 teaspoons Pumpkin Spice Mix (page 45) or 1½ teaspoons ground cinnamon and ½ teaspoon ground nutmeg

½ teaspoon ground cardamom

1 teaspoon pure vanilla extract
(or make your own; see page 45)

2 tablespoons chia seeds stirred into 1 cup water and soaked for 10 minutes

½ cup coconut flour, sifted

¼ cup buckwheat or quinoa flour, sifted

1½ teaspoons baking powder

pinch of sea salt

TO GARNISH (OPTIONAL)

1 small, thin parsnip, halved lengthwise

Activated Groaties (page 27) or shredded coconut

Preheat the oven to 350°F. Grease and line a 9 × 5-inch loaf pan with parchment paper.

Place the bananas, grated parsnip, eggs, coconut oil, coconut milk, spices and vanilla in a food processor and process until smooth. Add the chia seed "goo" and pulse to combine. Transfer the mixture to a large bowl and fold through the flours, baking powder and salt until just combined. Transfer to the prepared pan and top with garnishes that float your boat. Bake for 1 hour or until cooked—a skewer inserted in the middle should come out clean. Check after 45 minutes, and if the top is browning too quickly, cover with foil.

Let the loaf sit for 5 minutes then transfer to a wire rack to cool. Slice, and serve.

Store the cooled bread in the fridge for up to 5 days, or freeze (place individual slices between parchment paper) for up to 3 months.

MAKE IT BLUEBERRY BANANA BREAD (BBB):
Add an extra ¼ cup of chia seeds to the chia seed "goo" and 1 cup of blueberries to the main mixture.

THREE SMOOTHIE BOWLS: something between a smoothie, a sou and a porridge.

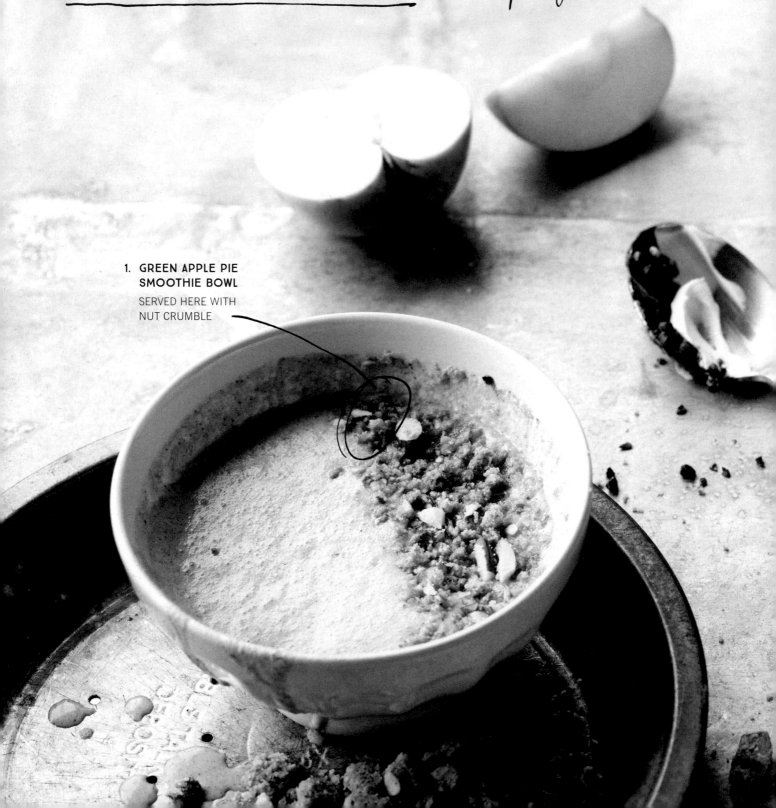

1. GREEN APPLE PIE SMOOTHIE BOWL

SERVED HERE WITH NUT CRUMBLE

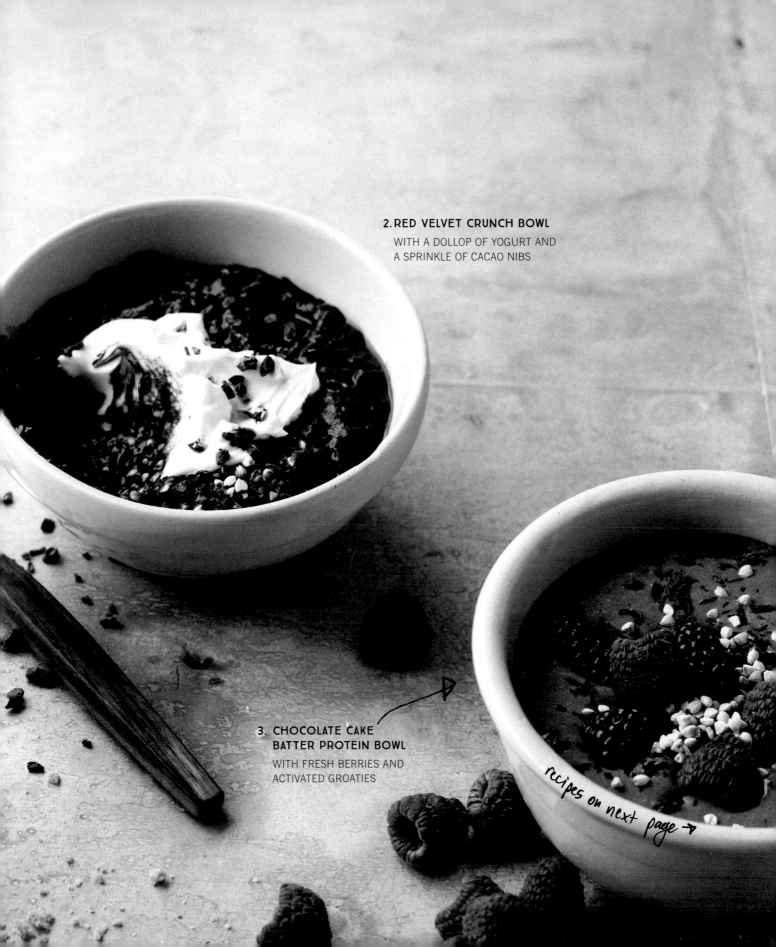

2. RED VELVET CRUNCH BOWL
WITH A DOLLOP OF YOGURT AND
A SPRINKLE OF CACAO NIBS

**3. CHOCOLATE CAKE
BATTER PROTEIN BOWL**
WITH FRESH BERRIES AND
ACTIVATED GROATIES

recipes on next page →

1. GREEN APPLE PIE SMOOTHIE BOWL

SERVES 2

1 green apple, roughly chopped

1½ cups full-fat coconut milk

1½ cups baby spinach leaves

¼ cup vanilla protein powder (optional)

3 teaspoons Pumpkin Spice Mix (page 45) or 2¼ teaspoons ground cinnamon and ¾ teaspoon ground nutmeg

2 tablespoons nut butter (any kind; almond is probably best)

½ cup ice cubes

Nut Crumble (see below), to serve

Put all the ingredients in a blender and process until smooth. Pour into two bowls and top with some nut crumble.

 1½ SERVINGS VEG + FRUIT PER SERVING

NUT CRUMBLE

¼ cup roughly chopped activated almonds (see page 28)

2 tablespoons desiccated coconut

1 teaspoon brown rice syrup

2 teaspoons coconut oil, melted

Combine the lot in a small bowl, spread out on a lined baking sheet and cook for 5 minutes at 350°F until golden. Feel free to make in bulk and store in an airtight container in the fridge for 2 weeks.

 ½ TEASPOON ADDED SUGAR PER SERVING

2. RED VELVET CRUNCH BOWL

SERVES 2

1 frozen (or fresh) banana

1 cup Cooked 'n' Frozen Beets (page 23) or 2 small beets, trimmed, scrubbed and grated

1 cup unsweetened almond milk (or regular milk if you prefer)

⅔ cup frozen raspberries

¼ cup raw cacao powder

1 cup Activated Groaties (page 27) or coconut flakes

Whipped Coconut Frosting (page 56) or full-fat organic plain yogurt, to serve

raw cacao nibs, to serve

Place the banana, beets, milk, raspberries and cacao powder in a blender and process until smooth. Add the groaties to the blender jug and stir through (or if you use coconut, blend briefly). Pour into two bowls. Serve with a dollop of coconut frosting or yogurt and a sprinkle of cacao nibs.

 2 SERVINGS VEG + FRUIT PER SERVING

MAKE IT A BIT FANCY:
Swap the cacao nibs for a few basil and mint leaves.

3. CHOCOLATE CAKE BATTER PROTEIN BOWL

SERVES 2

½ cup coconut cream or full-fat organic plain yogurt

¼ cup vanilla protein powder

1 frozen (or fresh) banana

1½ cups unsweetened almond milk (or any milk)

¼ cup raw cacao powder

¼ cup chopped activated almonds (see page 28) or ¼ cup almond meal

½ cup buckwheat groats or whole rolled oats (or a combo)

Activated Groaties (page 27), berries, nuts, coconut flakes or raw cacao nibs, to serve

Dump all the ingredients except the buckwheat and/or oats into a blender and blend until smooth. Add the buckwheat and/or oats, stir and pour into two bowls. Cover and place in the fridge overnight.

The next morning, scatter with your chosen toppings and serve.

 1 SERVING VEG + FRUIT PER SERVING

SALTED CARAMEL CARDAMOM COFFEE

FOR THOSE OF US WHO "SHOULDN'T REALLY BE DRINKING COFFEE"

SERVES 1

This is actually a recipe for folks trying to cut back on coffee, or who love the coffee but not the adrenaline spike. How so? Coconut oil lengthens and softens out the caffeine hit and cardamom neutralizes the overstimulating effects.

2 cardamom pods, crushed

1 serving of ground coffee

1 tablespoon coconut oil

pinch of sea salt

¼ teaspoon pure vanilla extract (or make your own; see page 45) or pinch of pure vanilla powder

pinch of granulated stevia

Add the cardamom to the ground coffee in your French press, filter or stovetop coffee maker and make 1 cup.

Place all the ingredients in a blender and process until well combined and frothy. (Or use an immersion blender in a beaker.)

I have a friend who takes a shaker of ground cardamom to cafés and sprinkles it over her coffee at the table.

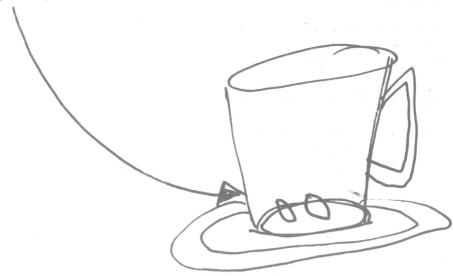

THREE SAVORY YOGURTS

Yep, it's a thing!

I came across this concept—yogurt as a meal with savory toppings—in New York at the Chelsea Market.

1. THE REAL GREEK YOGURT

SERVES 2

10 ounces Greek-style full-fat organic plain yogurt

8 cherry tomatoes, halved

1 small cucumber, cubed

8 pitted kalamata olives, halved

¼ red onion, thinly sliced

small handful of basil leaves and/or mint leaves

2 tablespoons pine nuts, lightly toasted

2 tablespoons extra-virgin olive oil

1 tablespoon lemon juice

sea salt and freshly ground black pepper

Divide the yogurt between two bowls and top each with half of the tomatoes, cucumber, olives, onion, herbs and pine nuts. Drizzle over the olive oil and lemon juice. Season to taste.

1 SERVING VEG + FRUIT PER SERVING

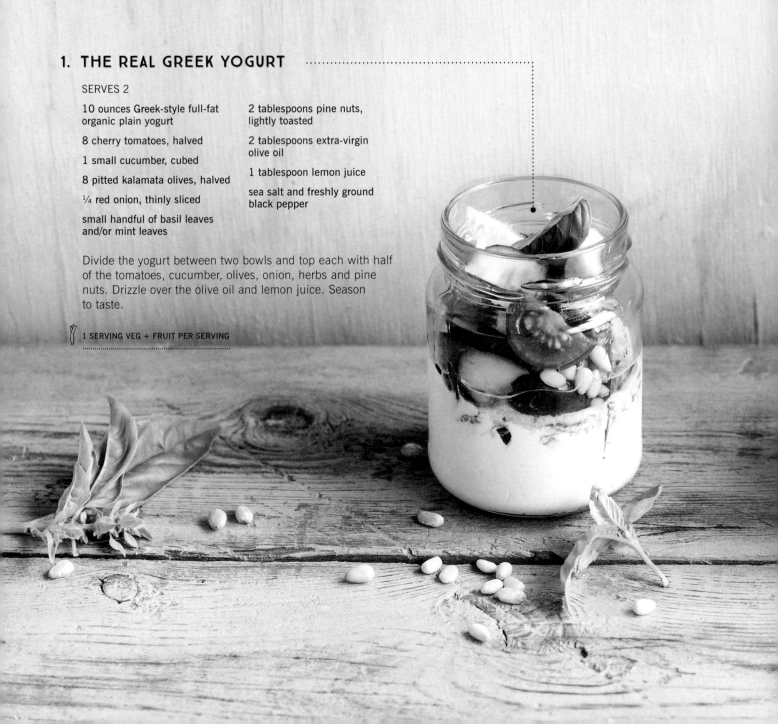

2. WALDORF SMASH-UP

SERVES 2

10 ounces Greek-style full-fat organic plain yogurt

1 celery stalk, finely chopped

3 ounces vintage cheddar, crumbled

¼ cup walnuts, chopped and toasted

½ pear, thinly sliced

sea salt and freshly ground black pepper

Divide the yogurt between two bowls and top each with half of the celery, cheddar, walnuts and pear. Season to taste.

Combining cheese and yogurt might seem odd. But then so is beet on a burger. Give this a try. You'll get it.

3. THE BLAT *(Bacon, Leaves, Avocado, Tomato)*

SERVES 2

10 ounces Greek-style full-fat organic plain yogurt

small handful of watercress (or arugula or basil leaves)

1 avocado, cubed

8 cherry tomatoes, halved

2 slices streaky bacon, chopped and fried (or ¼ cup Bacon Bits; page 44)

2 tablespoons extra-virgin olive oil

sea salt and freshly ground black pepper

Divide the yogurt between two bowls and top each with half of the leaves, avocado, tomatoes and bacon. Finish with a drizzle of olive oil and season to taste.

3 SERVINGS VEG + FRUIT PER SERVING

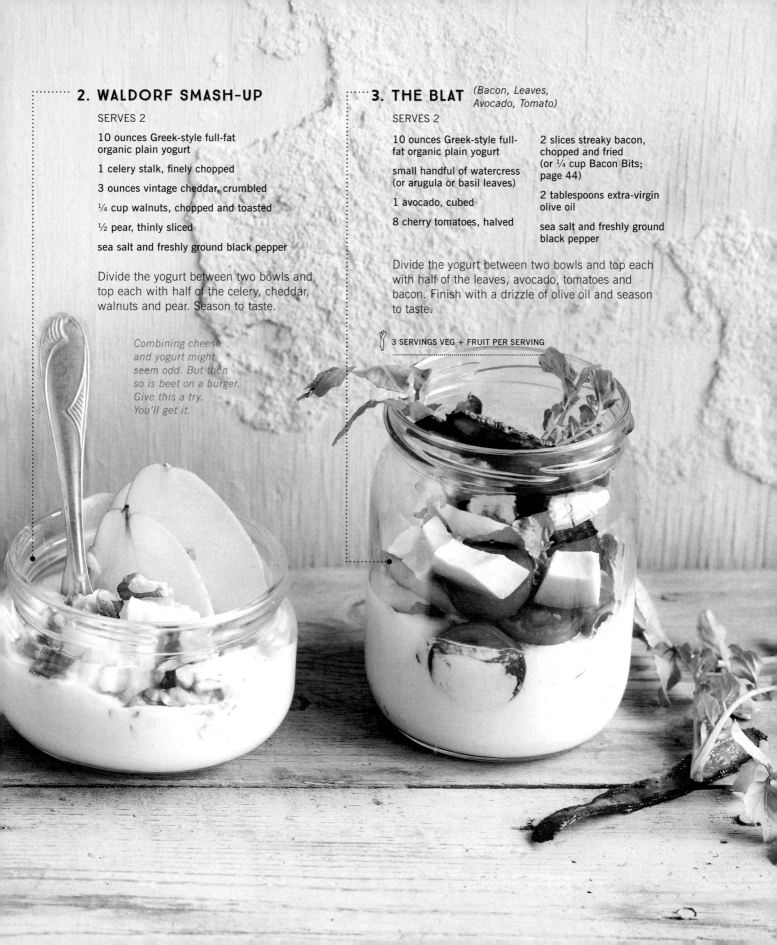

SPROUTED CACAO POPS

MAKES 6 CUPS ————————————————————————————————————

If you've already made up some Activated Groaties (page 27), feel free to use those instead of sprouting from scratch. Here, I'm going the full distance—soaking *and* sprouting the buckwheat before I roast it.

3 cups buckwheat groats

⅓ cup coconut oil

¼ cup brown rice syrup

⅓ cup raw cacao powder

Rinse the buckwheat and place in a large bowl. Add plenty of water (more than enough to cover) and leave to soak overnight.

The next day, rinse the groats really well (they can sometimes get a little slimy), transfer to a large sieve over a bowl and cover with a cloth (or put them in a sprouting jar or pan). Leave the buckwheat for 1–3 days until it starts to sprout, rinsing a few times a day.

Once you see small sprouts appear, preheat the oven to 250°F (or lower if possible) and line a baking sheet with parchment paper.

Melt the coconut oil and brown rice syrup in a large bowl. Mix in the cacao powder, then add the sprouted groats and stir gently to coat.

Plonk the lot onto the lined baking sheet, spreading it out to a thin layer (you may need to use two sheets). Bake for 1–2 hours, depending on how low you can get your oven to go. Stir frequently (every 20 minutes or so) and make sure they don't burn.

Cool, then serve with milk.

Make it just like a chocolate milkshake, only crunchy: add ¼ cup of tahini or natural peanut butter (melted) to the coconut oil mixture.

MAKE IT QUICKER:
Use 3 cups of Activated Groaties (page 27) instead of soaking and sprouting raw buckwheat. Halve the ingredients for the cacao mixture, then coat as above. Bake for 10–15 minutes in a preheated 350°F oven, stirring a couple of times to break up any clusters.

½ TEASPOON ADDED SUGAR PER SERVING

Sarah

Robbie

Robbie + Sarah have been sugar-free since reading my first book, I Quit Sugar

Three WINTER SPICE breakfast ideas

To make these beauties you'll need to whip up a batch of Pumpkin Spice Mix (page 45).

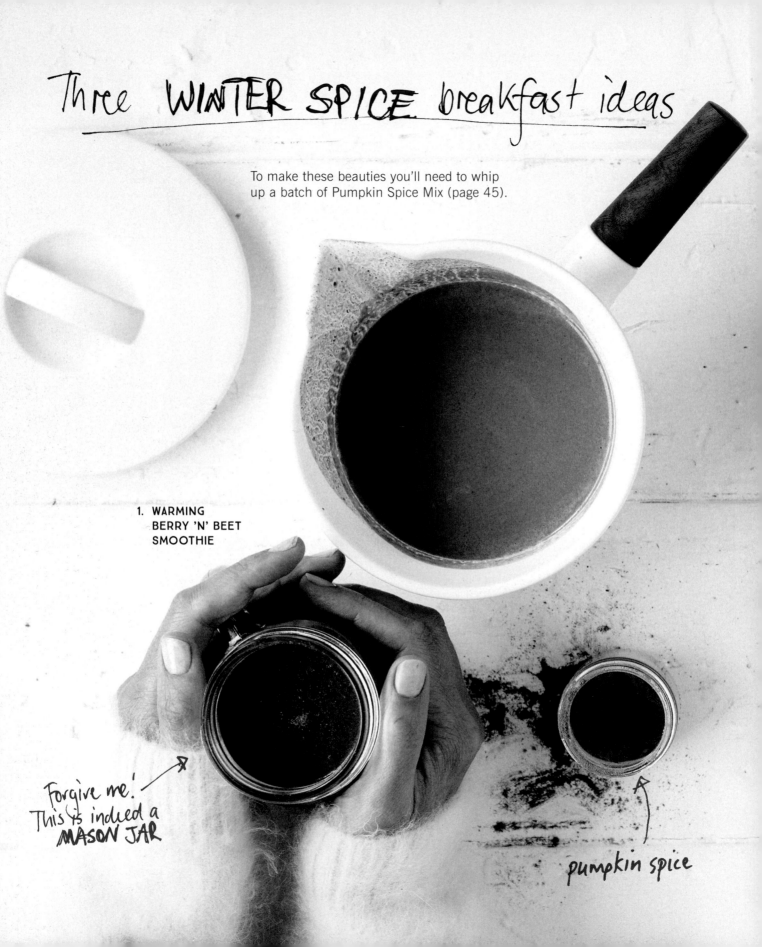

1. WARMING BERRY 'N' BEET SMOOTHIE

Forgive me! This is indeed a MASON JAR

pumpkin spice

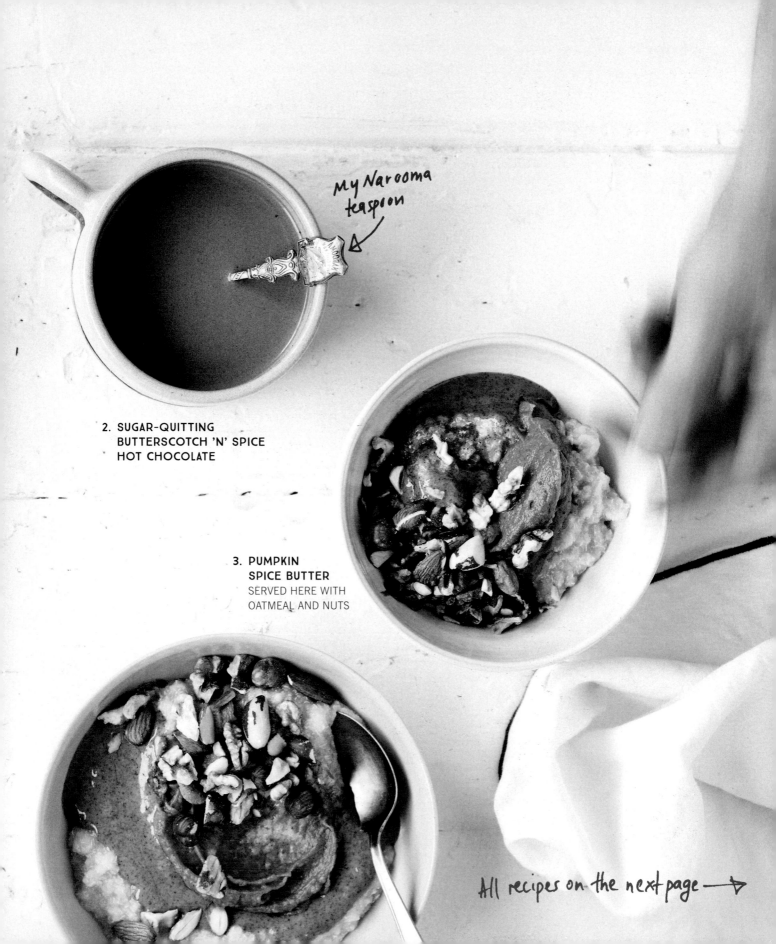

My Narooma teaspoon

2. SUGAR-QUITTING
BUTTERSCOTCH 'N' SPICE
HOT CHOCOLATE

3. PUMPKIN
SPICE BUTTER
SERVED HERE WITH
OATMEAL AND NUTS

All recipes on the next page →

1. WARMING BERRY 'N' BEET SMOOTHIE

SERVES 2

I have a real issue with folks drinking cold smoothies outside of summer. It ain't good for our anxious little souls to be cooled when we need some cozy comfort. The antidote is this nutrient-rich concoction.

2 cups full-fat milk

1 tablespoon chia seeds

2 teaspoons Pumpkin Spice Mix (page 45), plus extra to serve

1 cup fresh or thawed frozen mixed berries (raspberries, blueberries and blackberries work best)

1 beet, trimmed, scrubbed and grated (or ½–1 cup Cooked 'n' Frozen Beets, thawed; page 23)

½ banana

1 tablespoon coconut oil

1 tablespoon aloe vera (optional)

Activated Groaties (page 27), to serve

Or use plums or peaches instead, which are also Vata-pacifying

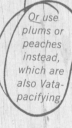

Combine all of the ingredients in a blender and process until smooth. Pour into a small saucepan and heat gently. Serve with groaties and a sprinkling of spice mix.

🥄 1½ SERVINGS VEG + FRUIT PER SERVING

Don't have Pumpkin Spice? Combine cinnamon + nutmeg in a 3:1 ratio.

2. SUGAR-QUITTING BUTTERSCOTCH 'N' SPICE HOT CHOCOLATE

SERVES 2

14-ounce can full-fat coconut milk (or milk of your choice)

2 tablespoons raw cacao powder

1 tablespoon coconut oil

2 teaspoons maca powder (optional, but great)

1½ teaspoons Pumpkin Spice Mix (page 45)

½ teaspoon ground white pepper

pinch of sea salt

pinch of granulated stevia, to taste

Maca helps with cravings, increases metabolism, balances thyroid and improves glucose tolerance.

Place all the ingredients in a saucepan and bring to a boil. Reduce the heat to low and simmer for several minutes while whisking to remove any lumps. Pour into two mugs and sip away.

White pepper helps lower blood sugar levels and has antibacterial, antioxidant and antispasmodic properties.

3. PUMPKIN SPICE BUTTER

MAKES ABOUT 2½ CUPS

3 cups Squash Purée (page 23)

1 tablespoon Pumpkin Spice Mix (page 45)

¼ cup apple cider vinegar or lemon juice

1 teaspoon granulated stevia

Place all the ingredients in a medium-sized saucepan, stir well and bring to the boil over medium heat. Reduce the heat and simmer for 15 minutes, uncovered, stirring often, until the mixture thickens. Cool, then store in an airtight container in the fridge for up to 3 weeks, or freeze for up to 6 months.

MAKE IT IN A SLOW COOKER:
Simply cook on low for 5–6 hours until it's thickened.

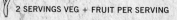

🥄 2 SERVINGS VEG + FRUIT PER SERVING

WARMING GOLDEN MILK

SERVES 1 ──

A cup of Vata-calming goodness for your cockles. You can
add a little stevia or brown rice syrup to taste, if you like.

1 cup milk (coconut or almond milk is best)

¼–½ teaspoon Fermented Turmeric Paste
(page 340)

1 teaspoon coconut oil

generous sprinkle each of pure vanilla
powder and ground cinnamon

Heat all the ingredients in a saucepan over medium heat, stirring constantly.
Serve warm.

MAKE IT A GOLDEN MILKSHAKE:
Place all the ingredients in a blender
and process until foamy.

**FIVE WAYS TO USE
PUMPKIN SPICE BUTTER:**

1. Spread over pancakes, dosas
   and toast.

2. Swirl into yogurt, ice cream,
   oatmeal and smoothie bowls.

3. Make a Pumpkin Spice Butter,
   Walnut and Sauerkraut Toastie
   (page 84).

4. Try an Apple and Peanut Butter
   with Pumpkin Spice Butter
   Snack (page 120).

5. Make Socettes with Nomato
   Sauce and Pumpkin Spice
   Butter (page 106).

"BUT THE KITCHEN SINK" BREAKFAST HASH

SERVES 6

I've been waiting for this moment for years. Yep, I'm finally including a recipe from Jo, my right-hand friend who's supported me in the writing of all my books. Not a massive fan of a pan and a set of hotplates, she arrived in the I Quit Sugar office one day with what she calls "My Chop Suey." Mercifully it doesn't contain packaged chicken noodle soup or pineapple. She eats it naked (the meal, that is!), but you could serve it with a fried egg or poachie.

Which bread is best?

Industrially produced bread generally uses a high-gluten flour (gluten makes bread fluffy) and can contain a lot of sugar. Gluten-free versions generally contain even more sugar. The best options are:

* My Allergy-Free Bread (page 113).

* A sprouted bread—sprouting breaks down the gluten.

* Sourdough—the cultures in the sourdough partially break down gluten and slow our absorption of the sugars in white flour, plus they activate the enzymes required to break down the phytic acid. Even commercial sourdoughs contain less sugar than most other breads.

1 tablespoon coconut oil, olive oil, butter or ghee

1 large onion, finely chopped

3 cloves garlic, crushed

2 pounds ground beef

2 tablespoons curry powder

2 tablespoons tamari

2 cups grated or finely chopped vegetables (cabbage and zucchini are best, but use whatever you have in the fridge—celery, beans, sweet potatos, carrots)

1 cup frozen peas

Heat the oil, butter or ghee in a large skillet over medium-high heat. Add the onion and garlic and sauté until the onion softens (about 5 minutes). Add the ground beef, breaking it up with a wooden spoon. Cook until browned (about 5 minutes). Stir in the curry powder and tamari and cook for 1 minute. Add the grated or chopped vegetables and peas, stirring until cooked through. Serve as is or with toast or a fried or poached egg.

This dish keeps in the fridge for a week and is a great base for creating Leftover Mishmashes (pages 246–65).

1 SERVING VEG + FRUIT PER SERVING

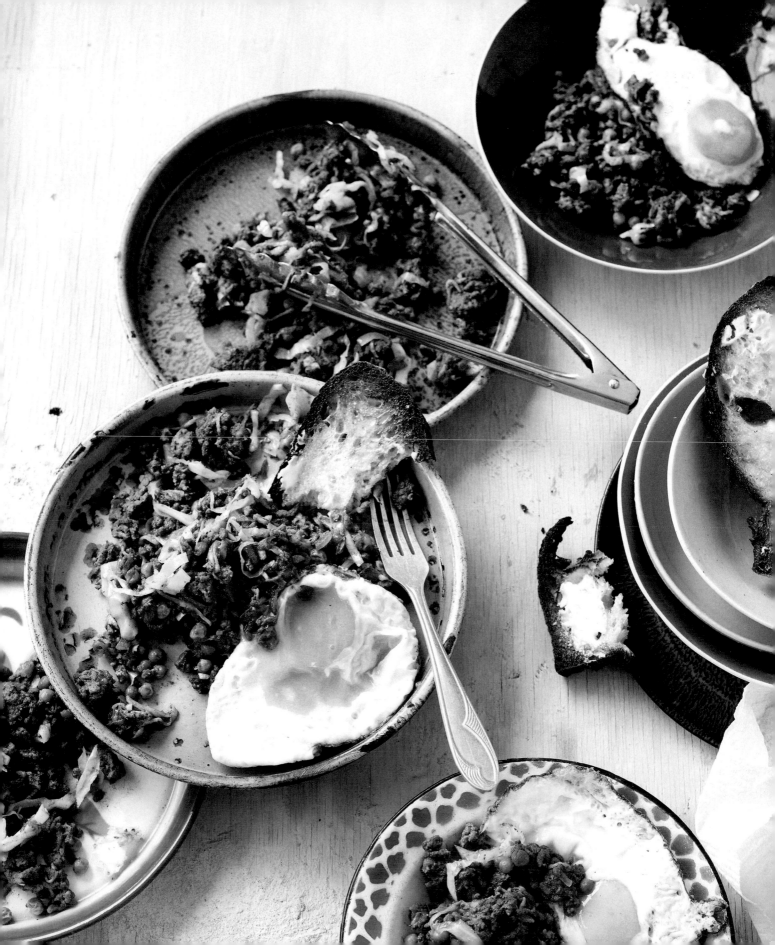

FOUR-INGREDIENT (or less) TOASTIES : *If you're going to eat toast, you should really make it count*

Layer up your ingredients between two slices of bread (see pages 113–14 for my homemade bread recipes), scrape with a bit of butter, and toast in a sandwich press, under a grill or in a skillet.

PUMPKIN SPICE BUTTER, WALNUT AND SAUERKRAUT

- Pumpkin Spice Butter (page 80)
- chopped walnuts
- Simplicious Sauerkraut (page 337), drained

even better with a smear of tahini

PINK BEET AND GOAT'S CHEESE

- Cooked 'n' Frozen Beets (page 23), thawed and sliced
- crumbled goat's cheese or sliced brie
- watercress, basil or spinach

🍴 1 SERVING VEG + FRUIT PER SERVING

which bread is best?

KIMCHEESE

- "But the Kitchen Sink" Kimchi (page 337) or Simplicious Sauerkraut (page 337), drained
- sliced Gruyère or Swiss cheese
- thinly sliced apple or pear

🍴 ½ SERVING VEG + FRUIT PER SERVING

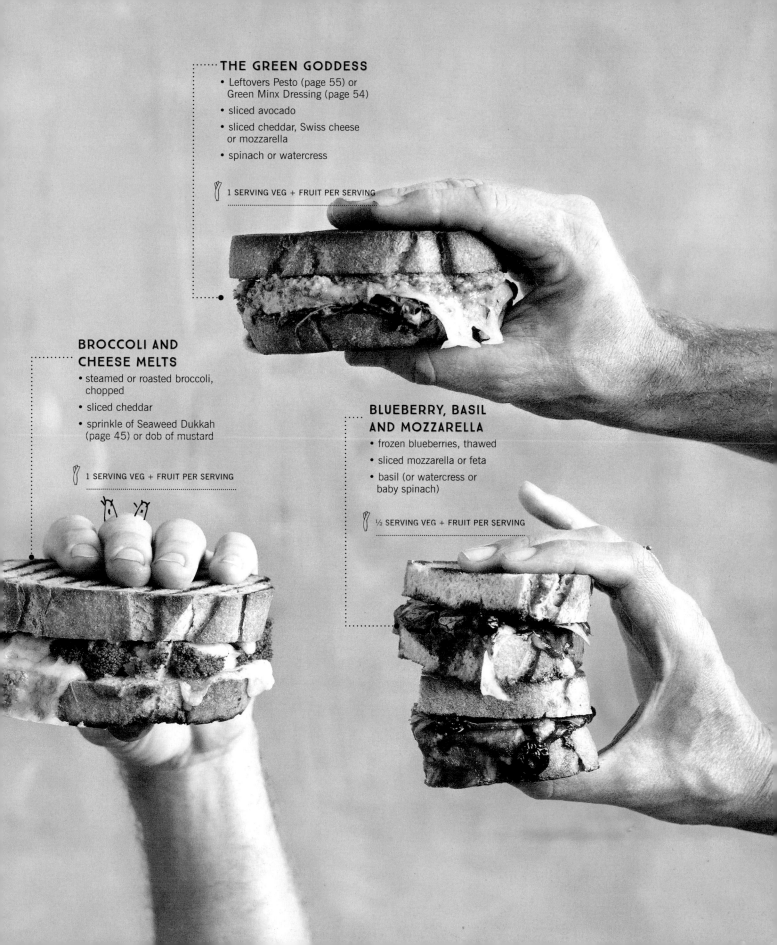

THE GREEN GODDESS
- Leftovers Pesto (page 55) or Green Minx Dressing (page 54)
- sliced avocado
- sliced cheddar, Swiss cheese or mozzarella
- spinach or watercress

1 SERVING VEG + FRUIT PER SERVING

BROCCOLI AND CHEESE MELTS
- steamed or roasted broccoli, chopped
- sliced cheddar
- sprinkle of Seaweed Dukkah (page 45) or dob of mustard

1 SERVING VEG + FRUIT PER SERVING

BLUEBERRY, BASIL AND MOZZARELLA
- frozen blueberries, thawed
- sliced mozzarella or feta
- basil (or watercress or baby spinach)

½ SERVING VEG + FRUIT PER SERVING

THE NEW GREEN "ZMOOTHIE"

Green smoothies are the new Starbucks-coffee-cup-as-accessory (worn with yoga mat slung over shoulder). Yawnful Instagram clichés aside, I tend to have a few issues with them: they can be mighty expensive, not particularly sustainable (um, carting coconuts across the globe?) and too complex and cold. Worry not. I've applied a few simplicious fixes to the formula, starting with my favorite vegetable, the zucchini, used in place of the less nutrient-dense cucumber, the more expensive avocado and the too-sweet banana. Blend on . . .

The zucchini is creamier and 200–300% denser in nutrients than the cucumber.

Smoothies vs. juices
Liquefying your breakfast or lunch has some health benefits—it can jam in a bunch of greenery while giving your digestion a bit of a break. But puréeing instead of juicing fruit and veggies is a far better way to go. It not only retains the fiber and extra nutrients from the skin but also helps you metabolize any sugar content. Oh, and it involves no waste.

CHOCOLATE CHERRY BLITZ

SERVES 2

½ cup frozen pitted cherries
(or any frozen berries)

1 cup grated or chopped fresh or frozen zucchini

2 handfuls of baby spinach leaves
(or just add extra zucchini)

¼ cup raw cacao powder

2 tablespoons vanilla protein powder
or 1 tablespoon chia seeds and a pinch
of powdered stevia (optional)

1 cup milk (any kind)

Place all the ingredients in a blender with ½ cup of water and blend until smooth. Add a little more water or milk if you need to.

 1½ SERVINGS VEG + FRUIT PER SERVING

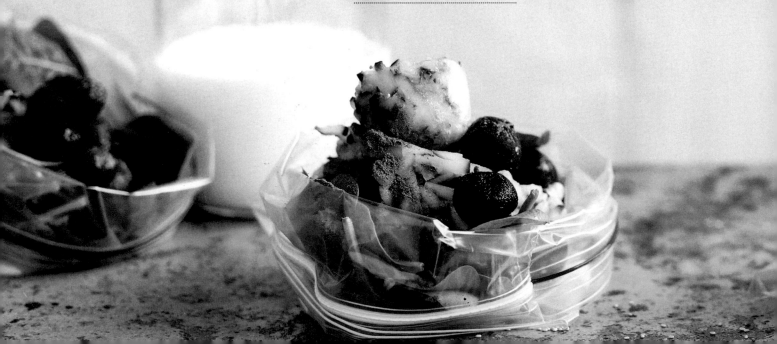

ZUCCHINI BREAD THICKIE

SERVES 2

Meet the thickie: a smoothie made over into a full meal. This thickie will keep you going 'til late lunch.

2 cups grated or chopped fresh or frozen zucchini

½ frozen banana (or add extra zucchini and a big pinch of powdered stevia)

1 cup milk (any kind)

½ cup Cooked Quinoa (page 26) or whole rolled oats (raw, soaked or cooked)

2 tablespoons nut butter (pecan or almond is best)

1 tablespoon chia seeds

1 teaspoon Pumpkin Spice Mix (page 45) or ¾ teaspoon ground cinnamon and ¼ teaspoon ground nutmeg

Place all the ingredients in a blender with ½ cup of water and blend until smooth. Add a little more water if you need to.

🥄 2 SERVINGS VEG + FRUIT PER SERVING

MY GUT-HEALING BREW

SERVES 2

When I pitched the idea of a smoothie made with bone broth/stock to the I Quit Sugar office, they thought I was mad. But then they tasted it. Makes a great lunch or light dinner, too.

1–2 cups grated or chopped fresh or frozen zucchini

½ cup frozen peas

½ avocado

2 cups Homemade Stock (page 42; beef or chicken is best)

juice of 1 lemon

1 clove Good for Your Guts Garlic (page 340), minced

sea salt and freshly ground black pepper

1 teaspoon Fermented Turmeric Paste (page 340)

2 cups watercress leaves (optional)

full-fat organic plain yogurt (optional)

Place all the ingredients in a blender and process until smooth. Add extra stock or water to achieve your desired consistency. Try not to serve this *too* cold as warm foods are more settling. In fact, feel free to heat it a little. Serve with a little yogurt if you like.

🥄 3 SERVINGS VEG + FRUIT PER SERVING

Smoothie bags: Freeze ingredients together in zip-lock bags and have them ready to place in your blender.

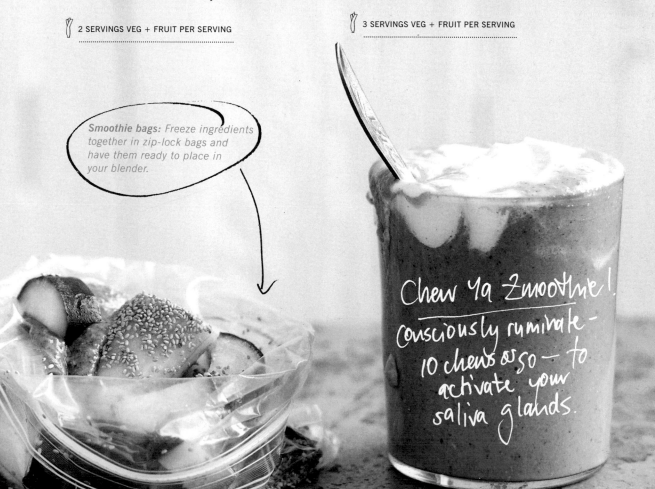

Chew ya smoothie! consciously ruminate - 10 chews or so - to activate your saliva glands.

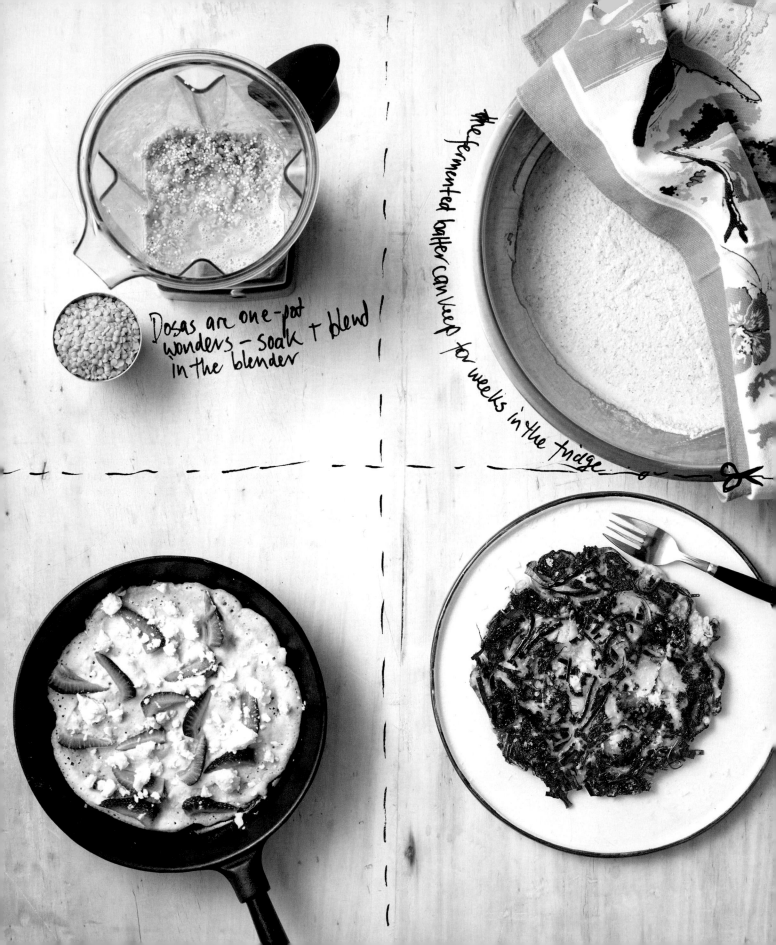

Dosas are one-pot wonders — soak + blend in the blender

the fermented batter can keep for weeks in the fridge

FERMENTED DOSAS

MAKES 10–16 PANCAKES

Does a dosa do things for you like it does for me? Not tried one? Well, let's get you dosed up. These traditional Indian pancakes tick a buncha boxes for me.

Dosas are:

* **Fermented.** Flick back to page 26 to read why fermenting grains is a win-win-win and kind of non-negotiable.

* **Low-toxin.** Especially mine. Traditional dosas are made with lentils and rice. I make mine with red lentils—the least toxic legume on the planet—and quinoa, which is gluten-free.

* **Brimful of protein.** Especially mine. Quinoa has both more and better protein than any other grain and one serving deals up 28% of your daily protein intake. But wait! Lentils contain double the amount of protein in quinoa. A protein punch right there.

1 cup quinoa

1 cup red lentils

1 tablespoon ground fenugreek

1 teaspoon sea salt

olive oil, coconut oil or ghee, for frying

Place all the ingredients in a blender. Add 2 cups of water and let sit for 4–6 hours or overnight. The next day, blend until smooth. Pour the batter into a large bowl and leave it to sit for 1–2 days, covering the bowl with a dishtowel to prevent bugs taking their fill. Bubbles will form and the batter will puff up a lot, so ensure the bowl is big enough for this. If it's cold or wintry, add 2 teaspoons of apple cider vinegar, lemon juice or whey (see page 46) to oomph the fermenting process.

When ready to cook, heat a skillet with 1 teaspoon oil or ghee. Stir the batter a little (adding extra water if necessary to ensure a pouring consistency) and pour in ¼ cup or so. Swirl or use a spatula to spread the mixture to the pan's edge. Feel free to make a thicker pancake (called an igli), covering with a lid when you cook it.

Once the batter has big bubbles on top, flip it over and cook for another minute or two. Make as many as you need, then put the rest of the batter in the fridge. Before using again, stir it (and add a little water if necessary) each time.

MAKE IT AN ONION CURRY DOSA:
Add a sprinkle of ground turmeric or cumin to the batter before cooking. Slice half a red onion and sauté in the hot pan before adding the batter. Serve with Watercress Sauce (page 176) or Green Minx Dressing (page 54) and a dollop of yogurt.

I keep a batch in the office fridge and the team dips in when they need a quick snack or lunch accompaniment.

SNACKALICIOUS

Weird lunch things and couch-side treats that work to a totally savory vibe.

BROC BITES

These are like lovely little scones and are delicious served warm or cold. Make up a big batch and freeze them—they make great health-bombs for the lunchbox.

coconut oil, olive oil, butter or ghee, for greasing

2–3 cups Parcooked 'n' Frozen broccoli (page 22), thawed and chopped

1½ cups grated cheese (cheddar, Parmesan or whatever you have)

3 eggs

1 cup flour (plain, gluten-free or almond)

1 teaspoon dried oregano or 1 tablespoon chopped oregano

sea salt

Preheat the oven to 375°F. Line two baking sheets with parchment paper and lightly grease the paper.

Combine all the ingredients in a large bowl and mix well. Roll the mixture into bite-sized balls and place on the prepared sheets. Bake for 25 minutes or until golden. Store in an airtight container in the fridge for 4–5 days, or freeze for up to 1 month.

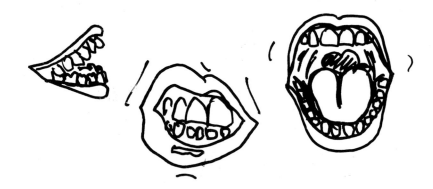

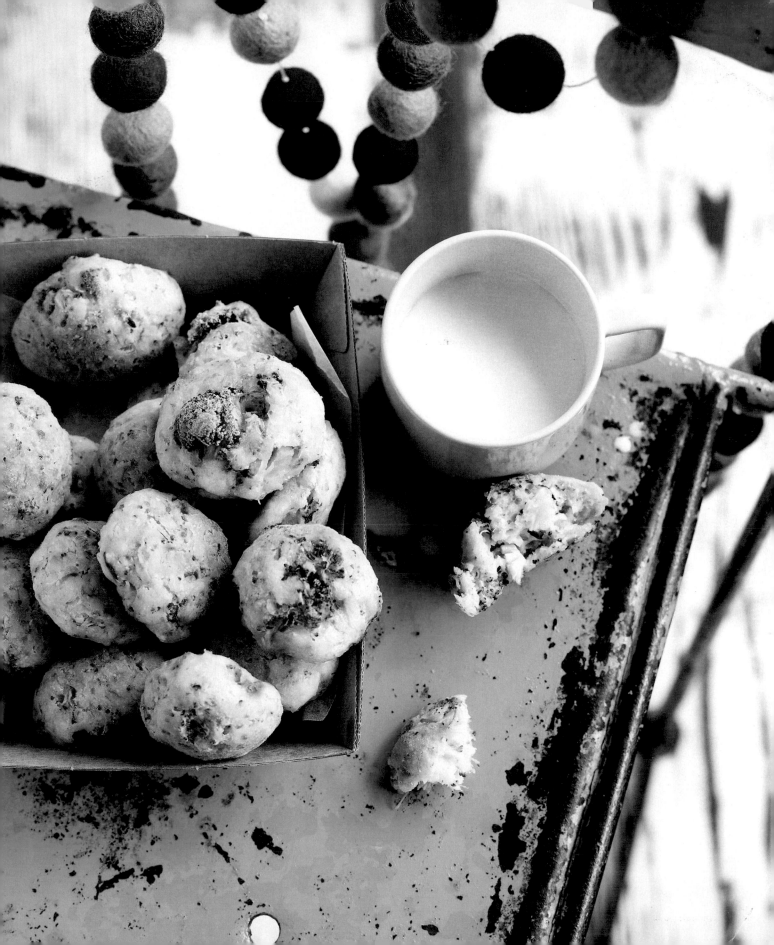

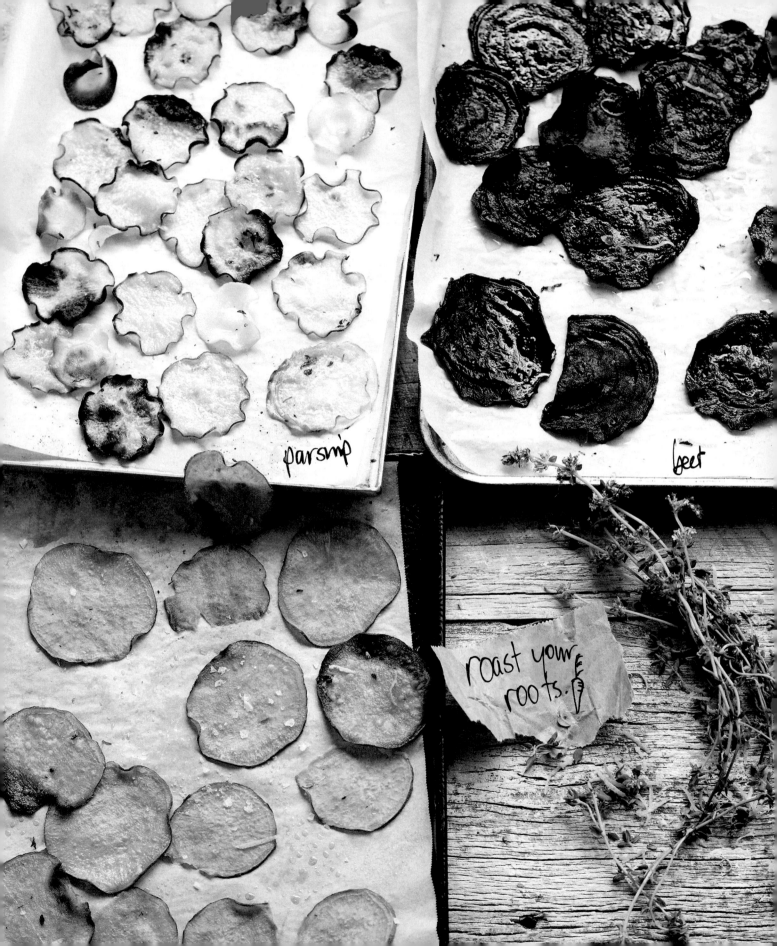

parsnip

beet

roast your roots.

ORANGE AND THYME RAINBOW CHIPS

SERVES 12

Make these when you do your Sunday cook-up. Try to buy even-sized roots for this recipe, so your chips match nicely.

1 parsnip

1 turnip, peeled

1 beet, peeled

1 sweet potato

1/3 cup coconut oil, butter or ghee, melted

zest of 1 orange

1/2 cup orange juice

1 tablespoon finely chopped fresh thyme

1 teaspoon sea salt

Preheat the oven to 400°F and line two baking sheets with parchment paper.

Using a sharp knife or a mandoline, slice all of the vegetables into even, very thin rounds. Mix the oil, butter or ghee, orange zest and juice, thyme and salt in a large bowl. Add the parsnip and turnip and toss to coat. Transfer the rounds to the first baking sheet in a single layer (no overlapping). Repeat the process with the beet and sweet potato, placing them on the other sheet.

Bake the parsnip and turnip chips for around 15 minutes and the beet and sweet potato chips for 25 minutes, or until golden. Remove from the oven and transfer to wire racks to cool. You can store them in an airtight container for 2–3 days, though they'll lose a bit of their crunch.

1/2 SERVING VEG + FRUIT PER SERVING

SLICE 'N' BAKE MISO BUTTER BISCUITS

MAKES ABOUT 48

The beauty of these is twofold: four ingredients only, and you can portion out what you need to bake a fresh batch.

1¼ cups buckwheat flour

2 tablespoons sesame seeds, plus extra for sprinkling

⅓ cup red miso paste

1 stick butter, cubed

2 tablespoons ice water

coconut oil, butter or ghee, for greasing

You can use black, white or a combo.

Place the flour, sesame seeds and miso in a food processor and blend for a few seconds until combined and crumbly. Add the butter cubes and ice water and process, turning the processor off and on frequently, until the mixture starts to ball around the blade.

Turn the dough out onto a floured surface and knead very lightly. Halve the dough and place each portion on a piece of plastic wrap. Roll each half, with the help of the wrap, into a log 1½ inches in diameter. Wrap the log up completely and place in the fridge to chill for 30 minutes. You can keep these in the fridge for up to a week before baking, or in the freezer for 2 months before thawing and baking.

When ready to bake, preheat the oven to 400°F and lightly grease two baking sheets. Cut the dough into ¼-inch slices and arrange on the prepared sheets. Sprinkle each with a pinch of extra sesame seeds. Bake for 12–15 minutes, or until light golden and crisp. Transfer to a wire rack to cool. These biscuits are best eaten fresh, though you can store them in an airtight container for 3–4 days.

Cut + bake what you need as you need

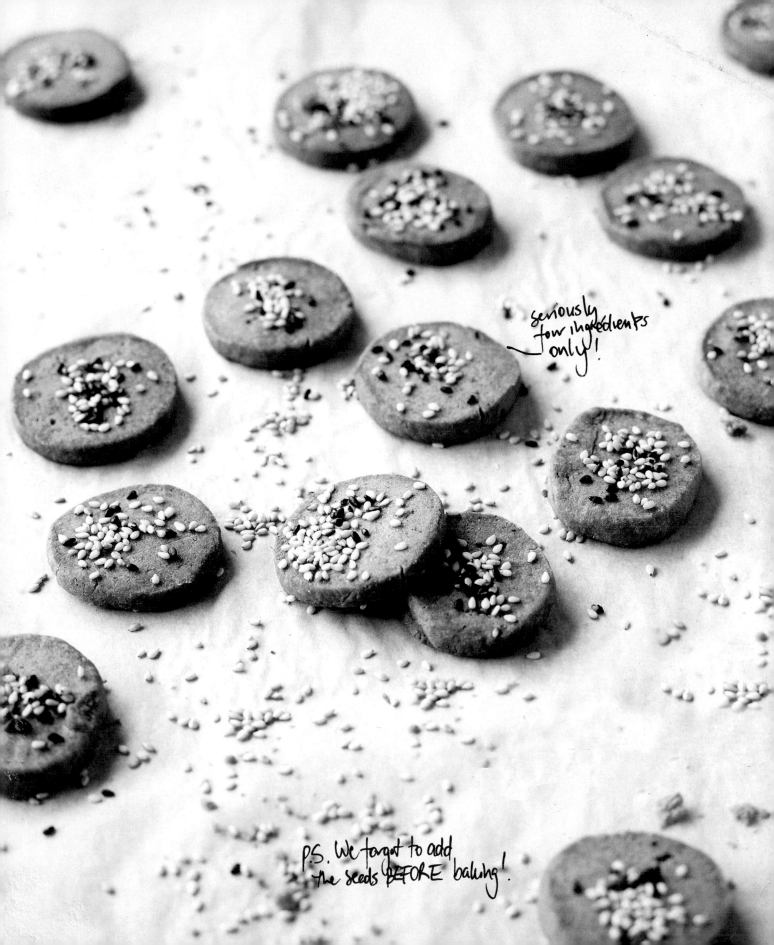

seriously four ingredients only!

P.S. We forgot to add the seeds BEFORE baking!

ROAST CHICKEN "MEFFINS"

Meffins are meat muffins. Eat two for lunch. Meffins that make a meal out of a deconstructed roast dinner are the money.

2 teaspoons coconut oil, olive oil, butter or ghee, plus extra for greasing

1 small onion, chopped

1 pound ground chicken

2 eggs

1½ cups Sweet Potato Purée (page 23)

¾ cup frozen peas, thawed

3 sprigs thyme, leaves chopped

1 sprig rosemary, leaves chopped

juice of ½ lemon

1 clove garlic, minced

sea salt and freshly ground black pepper

Preheat the oven to 350°F and grease an 8-cup muffin pan.

Heat the oil, butter or ghee in a skillet over medium heat. Add the onion and sauté until soft (about 3 minutes). Transfer the onion to a bowl and toss in the ground chicken, eggs, ½ cup of the Sweet Potato Purée, ½ cup of the peas, half the thyme, the rosemary, lemon juice and garlic, then season with a good pinch each of salt and pepper. Using your hands, mix the ingredients together until well combined. Divide the mixture into eight portions and press firmly into the prepared muffin pan. Bake for 25 minutes, or until the meat is cooked through and the tops are lightly browned. Remove from the oven and cool before serving.

To serve, place 1 tablespoon of Sweet Potato Purée on each of the meffins and sprinkle with the remaining peas and thyme. These will keep in the fridge for 2–3 days. Or you can freeze them (without the purée or peas) for 2–3 months.

½ SERVING VEG + FRUIT PER SERVING

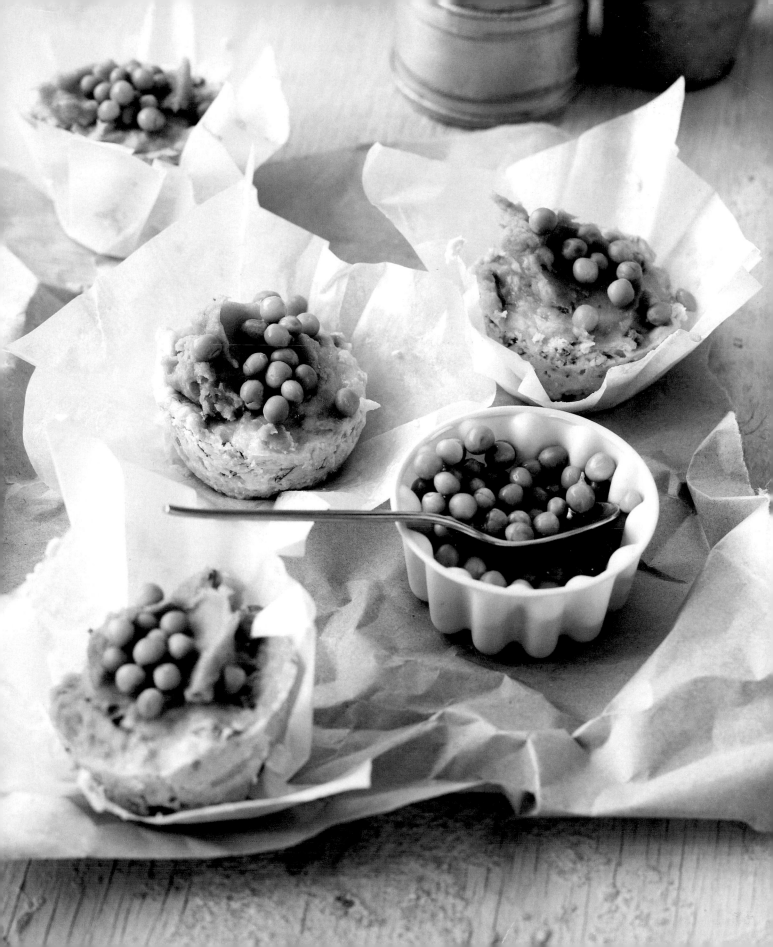

CAULI POPCORN

¼ cup coconut oil, melted

½ teaspoon paprika (smoked or sweet) or ground turmeric

¼ teaspoon ground cinnamon

1 teaspoon sea salt

1 large head cauliflower, cut into bite-sized florets

Preheat the oven to 400°F. Place the oil, spices and salt in a large bowl. Toss in the cauliflower and coat well. Transfer the cauli to a baking sheet and bake, tossing once, for 30 minutes or until golden brown and popcorny.

MAKE IT CHEESY CAULI POPCORN:
Add 2 tablespoons of nutritional yeast powder or grated Parmesan and omit the cinnamon.

1 SERVING VEG + FRUIT PER SERVING

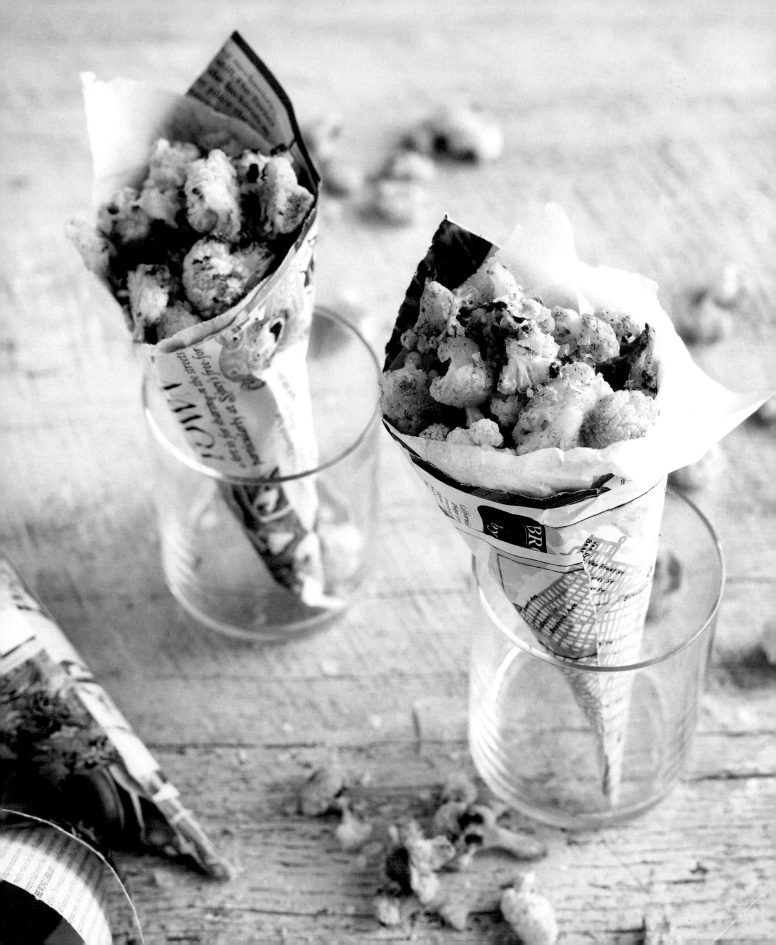

CHEESEBURGER WONTONS
Yep, seriously!

So much potential wrongness, right? But I tell you,
this is close to my favorite recipe in this book.

2 teaspoons coconut oil, olive oil,
butter or ghee

1 small onion, finely diced

½ pound ground beef

¼ cup buckwheat flour
or all-purpose flour

½ cup grated beet

8 small pickles (preferably no sugar added),
finely diced (or 1 tablespoon capers, finely
chopped)

2½ ounces cheddar, grated

sea salt and freshly ground black pepper

15 rice paper sheets (8½ inches diameter)

Nomato Sauce (page 51), to serve

Preheat the oven to 350°F and line a large baking sheet with parchment paper.

Heat the oil, butter or ghee in a skillet over medium heat. Add the onion and
cook until translucent (about 3 minutes). Transfer to a mixing bowl along with the
ground beef, flour, beets, pickles or capers, and cheese. Season to taste with salt
and pepper and use your hands to combine.

Fill a shallow dish (large enough to fit a rice paper sheet) with warm water.
Submerge a sheet in the water for 15 seconds, or until soft. Transfer to a clean
chopping board and use a sharp knife to slice it in half.

Place 1 tablespoon of the ground beef mixture in the center of each half, fold
to form a parcel and place on the prepared tray. Repeat with the remaining rice
paper sheets and mixture. Bake for 10–15 minutes, or until the meat has cooked
through. Serve with Nomato Sauce.

These were done with whole pickles. It's much easier to chop & mix it with the beef.

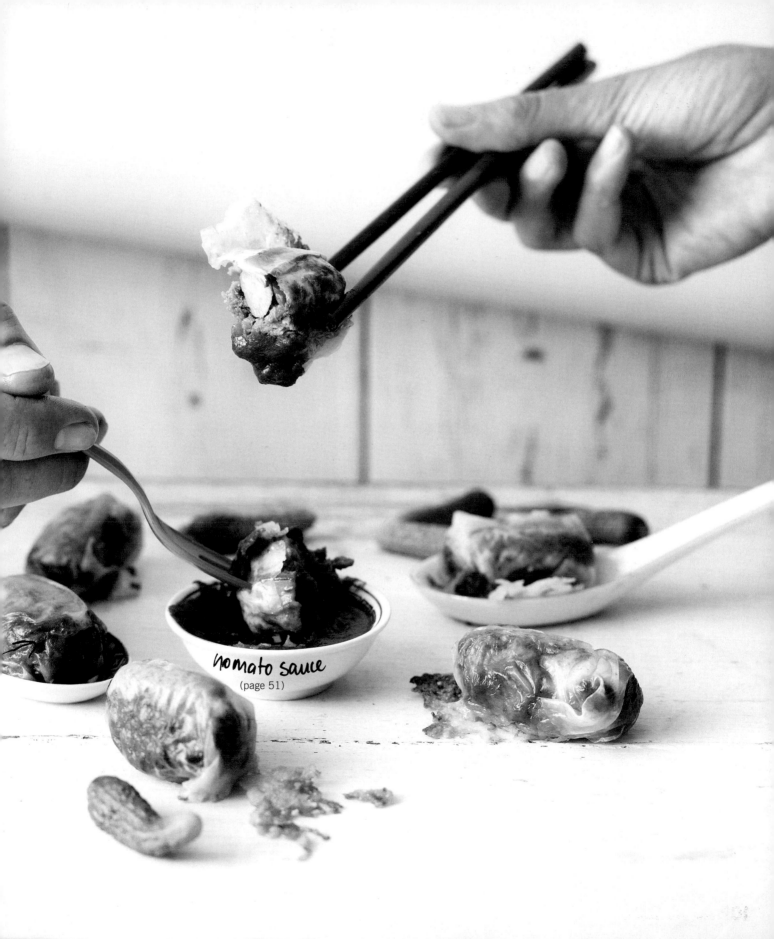

tomato sauce
(page 51)

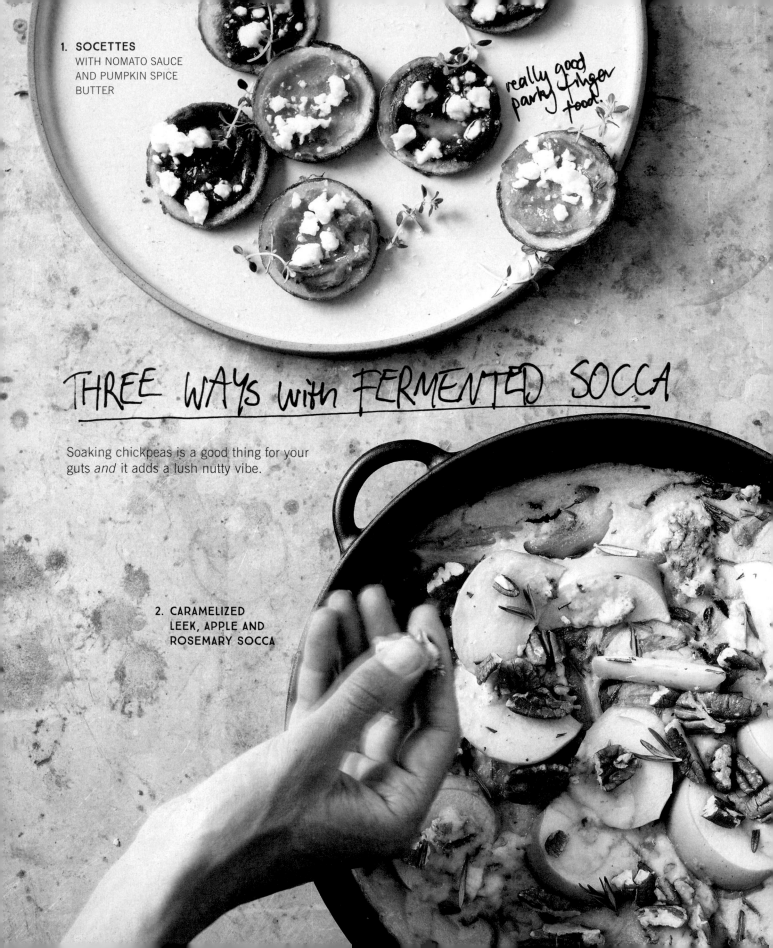

1. **SOCETTES**
WITH NOMATO SAUCE
AND PUMPKIN SPICE
BUTTER

really good party finger food!

THREE WAYS with FERMENTED SOCCA

Soaking chickpeas is a good thing for your guts *and* it adds a lush nutty vibe.

2. **CARAMELIZED
LEEK, APPLE AND
ROSEMARY SOCCA**

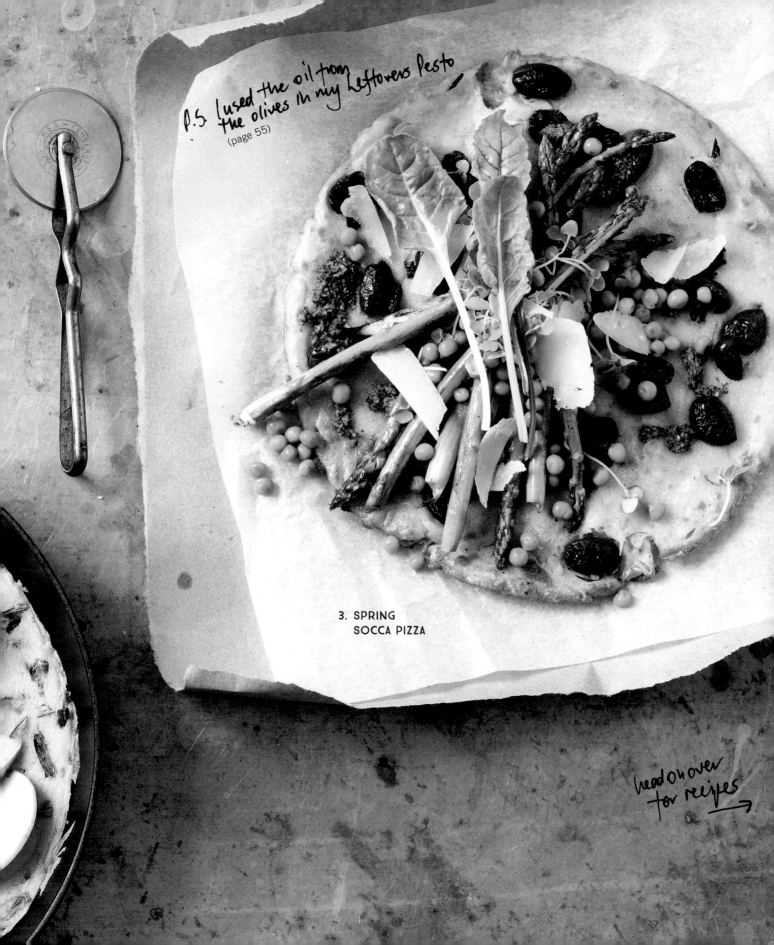

P.S. I used the oil from the olives in my Leftovers Pesto
(page 55)

3. SPRING
   SOCCA PIZZA

head on over for recipes →

First make your...

BASIC SOCCA

SERVES 6 AS A SIDE

1 cup chickpea flour

1 teaspoon apple cider vinegar, Homemade Whey (page 46) or lemon juice

1½ tablespoons coconut oil, butter or ghee, plus extra for greasing

½ teaspoon sea salt

Place the flour and vinegar, whey or lemon juice in a bowl with 1¼ cups of water. Whisk until combined. Cover with a dishtowel and allow to rest at room temperature overnight (24 hours is even better). The batter should bubble slightly and become lighter and airier. Whisk in the oil, butter or ghee and the salt until the mixture forms a thin, smooth batter.

Preheat the broiler to high and place the rack about 6 inches below the element. Place a dob of oil, butter or ghee in a cast-iron skillet and heat under the broiler for a few minutes, until hot. Pour half to one-third of the batter into the skillet, swirling to create a thin layer. Broil for 5–10 minutes, or until the edges crisp. Remove from the pan and repeat with the remaining batter. Cut into wedges and serve with soups, dips, stews, etc. Freeze any unused wedges to reheat and serve.

MAKE IT ON YOUR STOVETOP:
Heat a little oil, butter or ghee in a non-stick skillet over medium-high heat. Pour in the batter and swirl to evenly coat the pan. Cook, flipping once the batter comes away from the side (about 2–3 minutes). Cook for an extra 2 minutes on the other side.

then mix things up

1. SOCETTES

MAKES 24

Generously grease two 12-cup muffin pans with coconut oil and heat them in a 350°F oven for 2–3 minutes. Spoon 1 heaped tablespoon of Basic Socca batter into each muffin cup and return the pan to the oven for 8 minutes— the batter will pull away from the sides of the cups a little. Remove the socettes gently (using a butter knife or spatula) and cool on a wire rack. Turn the oven up to 400°F. Top each socette with Pumpkin Spice Butter (page 80), Nomato Sauce (page 51) or Zucchini Butter (page 189); a crumble of feta or Homemade Cream Cheese (page 46) and a sprinkle of thyme. Return to the oven for a few minutes or until the cheese melts.

2. CARAMELIZED LEEK, APPLE AND ROSEMARY SOCCA

SERVES 2 AS A LIGHT LUNCH

Preheat the broiler to high and place the rack about 6 inches below the element. Caramelize a sliced leek in butter or oil in a cast-iron skillet for a good 10 minutes, adding 1 tablespoon of chopped fresh rosemary after 5 minutes. Add ⅓ cup of Basic Socca batter to the leek and place under the broiler for 5–10 minutes or until the edge crisps. (Or you can do all of this on the stovetop as per the Basic Socca variation above.) Once cooked, layer with sliced apple, crumbled blue cheese and smashed pecans and place back under the broiler to melt the cheese a little (about 3 minutes).

3. SPRING SOCCA PIZZA

SERVES 2

Make as per the main recipe, but toss in ½ cup of pitted kalamata olives, halved, once you've poured the batter into the hot pan, and cook as above. While the broiler is on (and if there is enough room), cook a bunch of asparagus spears cut into shards and coated in a little oil. Once everything is cooked, smear your pizza with Leftovers Pesto (page 55) and layer with the asparagus as well as some mint, peas, watercress . . . whatever takes your fancy. Sprinkle with Parmesan gratings and a drizzle of lemon juice.

PEACH AND PEANUT BUTTER FROZEN YOGURT

SERVES 2

2 tablespoons natural peanut butter or other nut butter, softened

1 teaspoon brown rice syrup (optional)

½ cup full-fat organic plain yogurt (Greek-style is best)

pinch of sea salt

pinch of ground cinnamon (optional)

2 peaches, roughly chopped

Basic Raw Chocolate (page 56), to serve

crushed peanuts, to serve (optional)

In a bowl (or your immersion blender beaker), combine the peanut or nut butter and the brown rice syrup if using (you might need to heat them in the microwave for a few seconds so they combine properly). Add the yogurt, salt and cinnamon (if using) and stir. Place in the freezer for 45 minutes. Transfer to a blender with the peaches. Pulse a few times to mix but not purée. Return to the freezer for 1–2 hours. To serve, melt the chocolate in a cup in the microwave (do it gradually on low). Divide the frozen yogurt between two bowls and top with a swirl of melted chocolate and a sprinkle of crushed peanuts (if using).

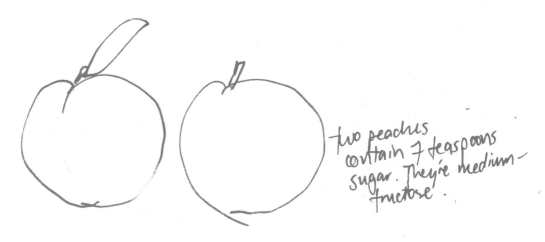

two peaches contain 7 teaspoons sugar. They're medium-fructose.

 ½ TEASPOON ADDED SUGAR PER SERVING

 1½ SERVINGS VEG + FRUIT PER SERVING

BACON GRANOLA

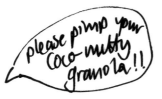

I was asked by precisely 23 of you to pimp my original granola recipe (the one featured in my first book, *I Quit Sugar*). However, I think this bacon version is the tastiest and most versatile of the cousins. Use as a soup topper, on savory yogurt or as a trail mix ("scroggin" for my Kiwi mates).

10 slices streaky bacon, rind removed (keep all the fat on)

3 cups coconut flakes

2 cups mixed nuts or seeds (use whatever you have—almonds, cashews, pecans, walnuts, pepitas), activated if possible (see page 28) and roughly chopped

2 tablespoons chia seeds

2 tablespoons Pumpkin Spice Mix (page 45) or 1½ tablespoons ground cinnamon and 2 teaspoons ground nutmeg

¼ cup brown rice syrup (optional)

I don't sweeten mine at all.

Preheat the oven to 150°F and line a baking sheet with parchment paper.

Place the bacon in a large, heavy-bottomed saucepan and add just enough water to completely coat the bottom of the pan. Cook over medium-high heat until the water has evaporated. Reduce the heat to medium and cook until the bacon is crisp (about 10 minutes—no need to turn). Remove the bacon and place in a strainer over the pan to drain all the fat. When cool, break the bacon into bits and retain the fat.

Combine the remaining ingredients in a big bowl. Add the bacon bits and stir in ¼ cup of the bacon fat (if you don't have enough, top it up with coconut oil). Spread the mixture over the tray and bake for 20–25 minutes, until golden, stirring after 10 minutes.

Store any leftover bacon fat in a sealed glass jar in the fridge and use it instead of cooking oil. It will keep for up to 1 month.

MAKE IT FASTER:
Use ¼ cup of coconut oil instead of the bacon fat and add ⅓ cup of frozen Bacon Bits (page 44) in the last 5 minutes of baking.

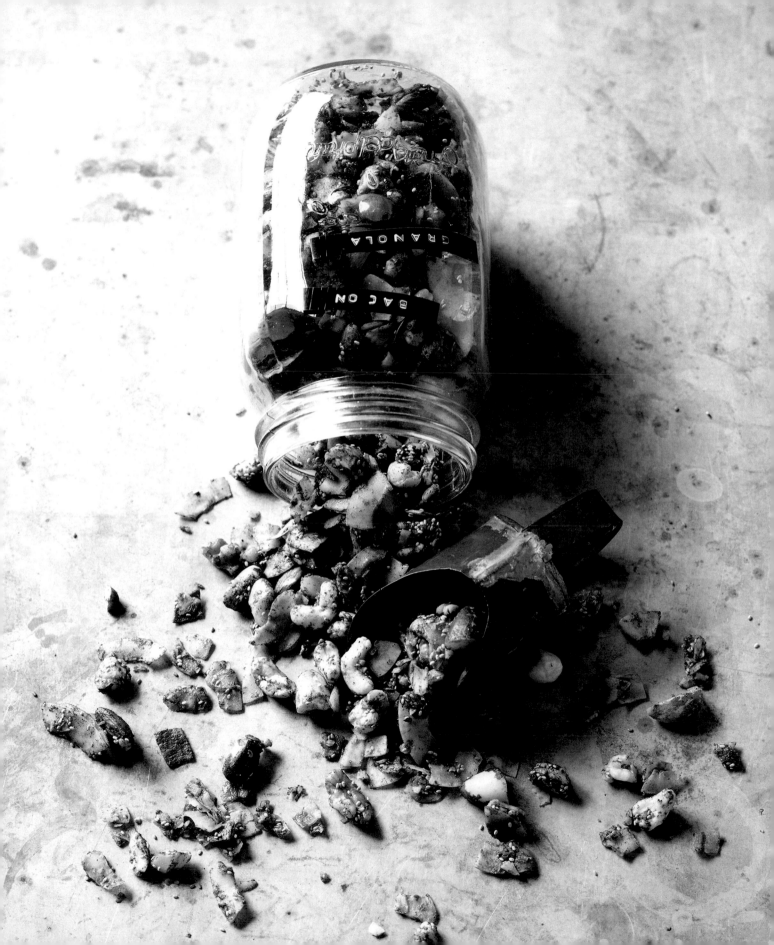

SPICED PANEER 'N' PEAS

IN WHICH I "PIMP" ANOTHER OF MY CLASSICS

SERVES 2 ——————————————————————————————

I was also asked by you guys to overhaul the "Salted Caramel" Haloumi and Apple recipe from my first book, which all of us got a bit obsessed about. Rather than go another sweet route I thought I'd just share my latest cultured cheese obsession.

1 teaspoon ghee or coconut oil

½ cup Homemade Paneer (page 48), cubed

¼ red onion, finely diced

½ teaspoon garam masala or Ras el Hanout Mix (page 45)

½ teaspoon ground cinnamon

1 bay leaf (optional)

½ cup frozen peas, thawed

Powerhouse Dressing (page 53), to serve

Heat the ghee or coconut oil in a skillet over medium heat. Add the paneer and cook for 1–2 minutes. Add the onion, spices and bay leaf, if using. Cook until the paneer is golden and the onion is soft. Add the peas and a dash of water and cook briefly to combine and reduce the liquid.

Serve with a drizzle of Powerhouse Dressing.

½ SERVING VEG + FRUIT PER SERVING

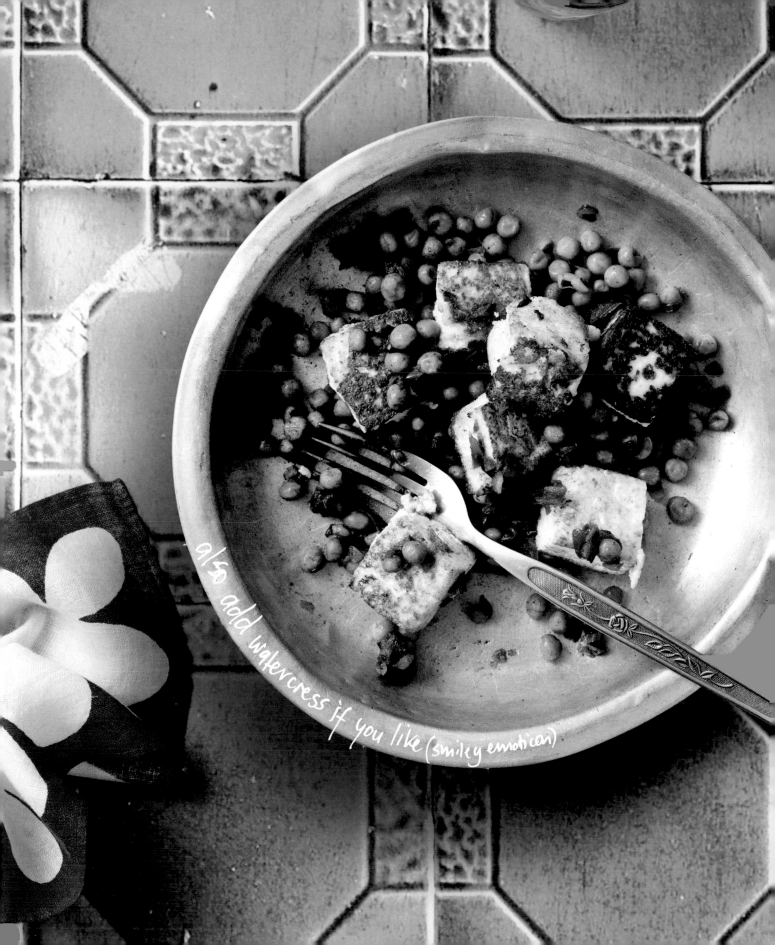

also add watercress if you like (smiley emoticon)

100% Allergy-free bread!

Inside-out Kitchen loaf.

baked stuffing loaf

(page 305)

MY ALLERGY-FREE BREAD

This stuff suits most paleo peeps, vegans, lactose intolerants, nut sensitives, gluten-frees and anyone in between or beyond.

2 cups buckwheat groats

¼ cup chia seeds

1½ teaspoons gluten-free baking powder

1 cup grated sweet potato

¼ cup coconut oil

1 onion, chopped

1 teaspoon sea salt

¼ cup sunflower seeds

Rinse the buckwheat well. Place in a large bowl or jar and cover amply with water. Allow to soak for at least 4 hours (preferably overnight).

Preheat the oven to 325°F and line a 9 × 5-inch loaf pan with parchment paper.

Place the chia seeds in a glass jar with 1 cup of water. Seal with the lid and shake every few minutes until a chia gel forms (about 10 minutes).

Drain the buckwheat using a sieve—it might be slimy, so make sure you rinse it well. Allow all the water to drain out.

Place the drained buckwheat, chia gel, baking powder, sweet potato, coconut oil, onion and salt in a food processor or high-powered blender and process until a thick paste forms. Spoon into the prepared loaf pan and sprinkle the sunflower seeds on top.

Place the bread on the middle rack of the oven and cook for 1 hour. When cooled, remove from the loaf pan and allow to cool completely before cutting into ⅜-inch slices. Serve as is, or toasted and spread with coconut oil (or butter or olive oil, depending on your dietary needs).

This bread will last 4–5 days in the fridge. To freeze, cut into slightly thicker (½-inch) slices and layer between parchment paper. The slices can be thawed and toasted very successfully.

INSIDE-OUT SPROUTED KITCHERI LOAF

MAKES 1 LOAF

This bread is great on your guts and wonderfully balanced to keep your doshas calibrated (see page 362). I've also sprouted the beans to reduce the phytic acid and make it even gentler on the guts—not a big deal if you don't have time, but it creates a more textured bread, so consider doing so. Why is it "inside-out"? Well, I've taken my standard kitcheri recipe and put the toppers (the egg and coriander) and the sweet potato variation all on the inside of the bread to bring you a meal in one loaf.

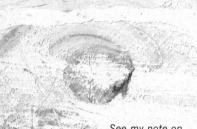

See my note on page 23 about the benefits of eating resistant starch in this way. →

1 tablespoon ghee or coconut oil, plus extra to serve (optional)

1 small red onion, finely chopped

1 teaspoon each of black mustard seeds, cumin seeds and fennel seeds

1 teaspoon each ground coriander seeds and ground turmeric

1 tablespoon grated ginger

1½ cups sprouted mung beans or brown lentils (see page 352)

1 cup cooked basmati rice

1 cup grated sweet potato

1 cup arrowroot

1 teaspoon baking powder

1 teaspoon sea salt

3 eggs

¼ cup ground chia seeds

shredded coconut, to garnish

Homemade Cream Cheese (page 46), to serve

Preheat the oven to 350°F. Grease and line a 9 × 5-inch loaf pan with parchment paper.

Melt the ghee or coconut oil in a small skillet over medium-high heat. Add the onion and sauté for 1–2 minutes. Add the mustard, cumin and fennel seeds, spices and ginger, and sauté for 1–2 minutes, until the mustard seeds start to pop and the onion is translucent. Set aside to cool.

Transfer the onion to a food processor with the sprouts, rice, sweet potato, arrowroot, baking powder, salt, eggs and chia seeds and process until combined. Pour into the prepared pan and smooth the top of the batter. Sprinkle with shredded coconut. Bake for 1 hour, or until a skewer inserted in the middle comes out clean. Leave to sit for 5 minutes before transferring to a wire rack. Once the loaf is completely cool, cut into thick slices and store in a container (or wrapped in foil) in the fridge. It will keep for up to 5 days. Alternatively, slice and freeze for up to 1 month.

Serve the kitcheri loaf warm, spread with cream cheese, coconut oil or butter.

½ SERVING VEG + FRUIT PER SERVING

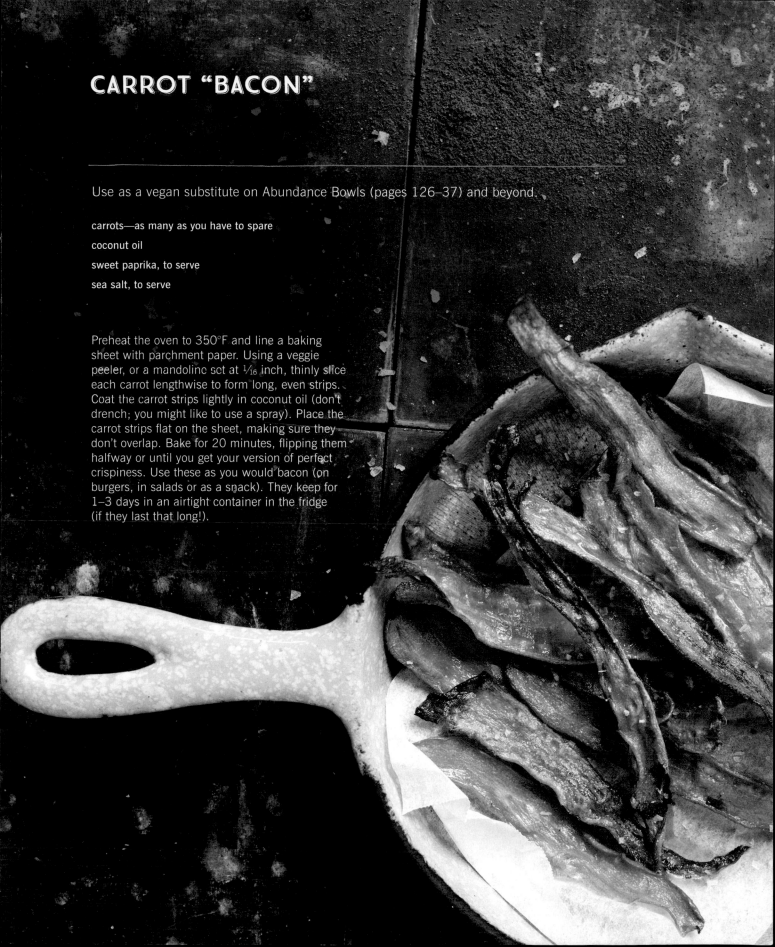

CARROT "BACON"

Use as a vegan substitute on Abundance Bowls (pages 126–37) and beyond.

carrots—as many as you have to spare

coconut oil

sweet paprika, to serve

sea salt, to serve

Preheat the oven to 350°F and line a baking sheet with parchment paper. Using a veggie peeler, or a mandoline set at $\frac{1}{16}$ inch, thinly slice each carrot lengthwise to form long, even strips. Coat the carrot strips lightly in coconut oil (don't drench; you might like to use a spray). Place the carrot strips flat on the sheet, making sure they don't overlap. Bake for 20 minutes, flipping them halfway or until you get your version of perfect crispiness. Use these as you would bacon (on burgers, in salads or as a snack). They keep for 1–3 days in an airtight container in the fridge (if they last that long!).

TWO-MINUTE DESK LUNCH NOODLES

SERVES 1

Pack this up in a big jar in layers, take it to work, add hot water and stir with a chopstick (or your pen). Done.

The frozen veggies keep things cool 'til lunch.

What shrimp should you buy?
Look for Marine Stewardship Council–certified shrimp (they certify shrimp in 15 countries around the world).

Not too many.
All shrimp have sustainability issues in part because the bycatch is shocking. Depending on where they are trawled, for every shrimp caught, up to 27 other species are trapped in the bycatch and tossed away. *Please, pause on this.*

Go farmed rather than trawled, due to bycatch issues. Or go local estuary or river shrimp, which aren't trawled.

1–2 teaspoons red curry paste

1 teaspoon red miso paste

dash of fish sauce

small handful of rice noodles

¼ cup coconut milk or cream (or use 3 cubes frozen coconut milk or cream; see page 25)

small handful of frozen peas (or thinly sliced snow peas)

½ cup Parcooked 'n' Frozen broccoli (page 22)

5 cooked jumbo shrimp, peeled and deveined, or a small handful of Shredded Chicken (page 214)

3–4 green onions, thinly sliced on the diagonal

cilantro leaves and lime wedges, to serve

Pop them in a separate zip-lock bag.

Place all the ingredients, except the cilantro and lime, in a large jar in the order given above. Throw in the fridge when you get to work. At lunchtime, pour over enough boiling water to just cover everything, pressing the ingredients down. Cover and leave for 2 minutes, stirring once or twice. Top with the cilantro and a squeeze of lime juice. Eat.

MAKE IT KIMCHI INSTANT NOODLES:
Use ½ cup of "But the Kitchen Sink" Kimchi (page 337) instead of the pastes and sauce, and replace the jumbo shrimp with Pulled Beef (page 223), Some Beefin' Good Jerky (page 209) or cubed tofu. Add some chili sauce if you like.

MAKE IT ITALIAN "PASTA" NOODLES:
Add, in this order: ⅓ cup of Cooked Quinoa (page 26); 1 zucchini, sliced into thin strips; ⅓ cup of Nomato Sauce (page 51); a small handful of Shredded Chicken (page 214) and the broccoli and peas (as per the recipe above). Serve with fresh basil leaves or Leftovers Pesto (page 55).

2 SERVINGS VEG + FRUIT PER SERVING

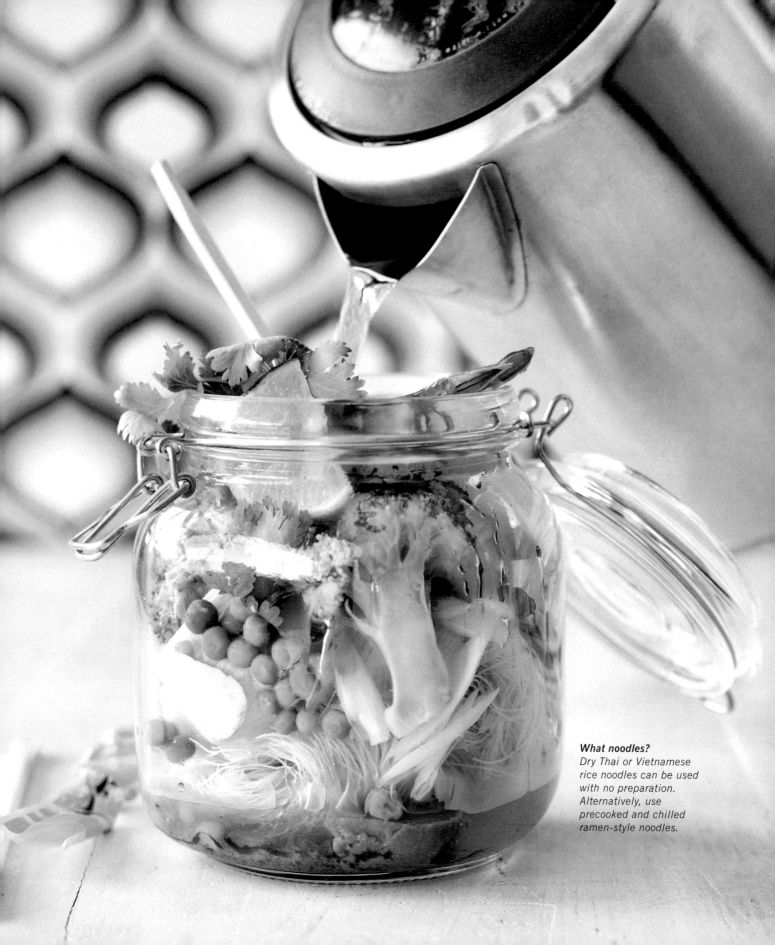

What noodles?
Dry Thai or Vietnamese rice noodles can be used with no preparation. Alternatively, use precooked and chilled ramen-style noodles.

A SUPER-GREENS COUCH FONDUE

You can use any leftover leafy greens for this cheesy dipper dinner—beet greens work well! Eat on the couch with a DVD.

Referencing outdated technologies = sure sign one is getting old.

coconut oil, olive oil, butter or ghee, for greasing

1 bunch chard, stalks removed, leaves very finely chopped

1 onion, roughly chopped

2 cloves garlic, minced

1½ cups sour cream

2 cups grated vintage cheddar (or your favorite hard cheese)

sea salt and freshly ground black pepper

Preheat the oven to 350°F and grease an ovenproof dish with oil, butter or ghee.

Combine the chard, onion and garlic in a food processor and process until finely chopped (not puréed). Add the sour cream and half the cheese, and season to taste with salt and pepper. Process briefly to combine, then transfer to the prepared dish. Sprinkle with the remaining cheese and bake for 15–20 minutes, or until the cheese is melted and golden.

Serve with fun dipping things: scrubbed baby carrots, sliced baby cucumbers, sliced radish, endive "cups," fennel sticks, purple carrot sticks, sliced raw turnip, Socca wedges (see page 106), seed crackers . . .

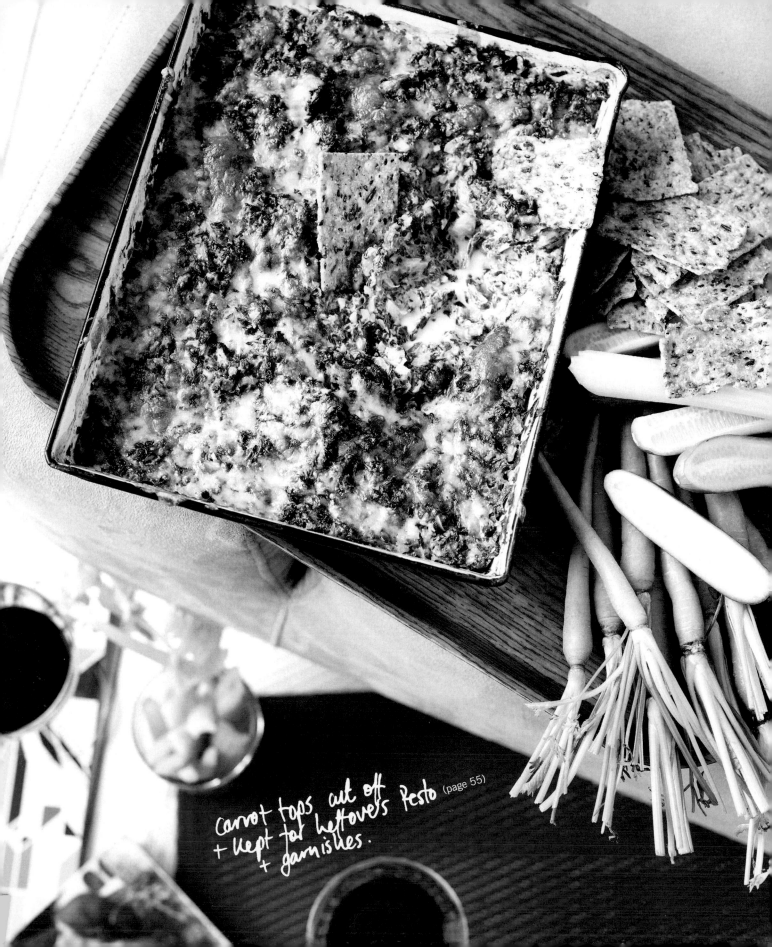

carrot tops cut off
+ kept for leftover's Pesto (page 55)
+ garnishes.

Just a Page of THREE-INGREDIENT Snacks

Things I tend to eat for breakfast or for weekend "lunch-lites."

These are the three-ingredients-or-less things I "snack" on, often as part of my breakfast or a light weekend lunch.

Why I don't *really* snack

The concept of snacking was developed by nutritionists in the 1990s to help treat the huge numbers of people who had developed diabetes (and everyone else on the planet riding a blood-sugar roller coaster and needing to fuel themselves every couple of hours). But we are not designed to eat in this way—it is inefficient and taxing on our bodies. Once you're off sugar for a few months, you'll find you don't need to snack anyway—you'll be used to eating full meals that are nutritionally dense.

So, if I snack, it's directly at the end of a meal if I find myself still hungry. Or in lieu of a meal if I'm not that hungry.

1. **CHOC-NUT SPOON POPS**
   Mix 1 tablespoon coconut oil with 1 heaping teaspoon raw cacao powder and a big sprinkle of rock salt in a small cup (you can add a tablespoon of nut butter as well and a drizzle of brown rice syrup if you like). Pile onto a dessert spoon and freeze for 15 minutes.

2. **APPLE AND PEANUT BUTTER WITH PUMPKIN SPICE BUTTER**
   Spread a slice of apple with natural peanut butter and a dob of Pumpkin Spice Butter (page 80).

3. **UNCANNED SARDINES (PAGE 156) WRAPPED IN A LEAF**

4. **TURNIP CHEESEBURGERS**
   Place slices of mature cheddar between thinly sliced raw turnip.

5. **SOME BEEFIN' GOOD JERKY (PAGE 209) WRAPPED IN A MUSTARD LEAF**

6. **MISOMITE IN A CUP**
   Place a dollop of Misomite (page 54) in an endive cup or lettuce leaf.

7. **BRUSSELS SPROUT, HALOUMI AND SAUERKRAUT SLIDERS**
   MAKES 16

2 tablespoons coconut oil	16 large brussels sprouts, trimmed and halved
1 tablespoon tamari	8½ ounces haloumi
½ teaspoon ground cumin	Simplicious Sauerkraut (page 337), to serve
¼ teaspoon cayenne pepper	

   Preheat the oven to 400°F and line a large baking sheet with parchment paper.

   In a large bowl, combine 1 tablespoon of the coconut oil with the tamari and spices. Toss through the sprouts until well coated. Place them cut side down on the baking sheet and bake for 5 minutes.

   Meanwhile, cut the haloumi in half lengthwise and then into ¼-inch-thick slices, giving you about 16 squares of haloumi roughly the size of your sprout halves.

   Place on the baking sheet with the sprouts and cook for another 10–15 minutes, turning halfway, or until everything is golden.

   Assemble the sliders by layering a slab of haloumi and some sauerkraut between two brussels sprout halves and securing with a toothpick.

Ever tasted raw turnip? Oh, it's so good and sweet and creamy-crunchy.

I also like using radicchio leaves.

MICHAEL POLLAN

These are great at
cocktail dos, too.

1.

endive

3.

6.

a collard leaf

7.

4.

5.

2.

A WEEK of LUNCHBOXES:

Five days of interesting food combos that look cute in a box.

I appreciate that kids want more interesting lunches. But I also don't think parents should be spending all evening assembling them. Here are some quick fixes. In my experience, the best way to get your kids to eat the stuff in their lunchboxes is to have them make/assemble it with you.

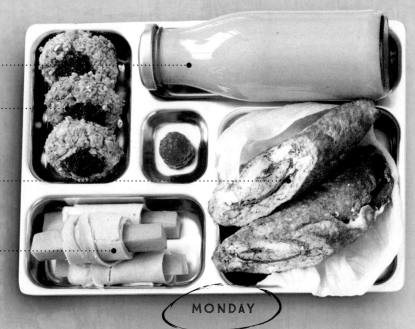

KERMIT SLUSHIE ⋯⋯⋯⋯⋯
(page 125)

SUNFLOWER STRAWBERRY THUMBLES ⋯⋯⋯⋯
(page 298)

MONSTER-MASH ROLL-UPS ⋯⋯⋯⋯
(page 124)

HAM-WRAPPED CARROT STICKS ⋯⋯⋯⋯

MONDAY

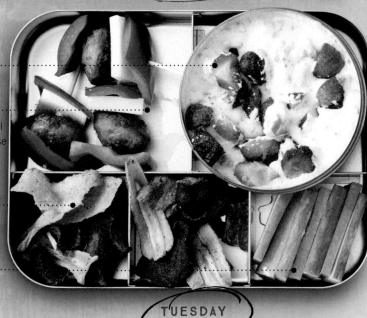

STRAWBERRY FROZEN YOGURT ⋯⋯⋯⋯
(page 125)

CHEESEBURGERS ⋯⋯⋯⋯
Thread a leftover cooked meatball (page 144) and a chunk of cheese between two chunks of red bell pepper on a toothpick.

ORANGE AND THYME RAINBOW CHIPS ⋯⋯⋯⋯
(page 95)

CARROT AND CUCUMBER STICKS ⋯⋯⋯⋯

TUESDAY

CUCUMBER AND CARROT FLOWERS
You can make these with your kids; buy a bento cutter online or from an Asian supermarket. Use the leftover bits in your own smoothie or salad.

STRAWBERRY FROZEN YOGURT
(page 125)

ROAST CHICKEN "MEFFINS"
(page 98)

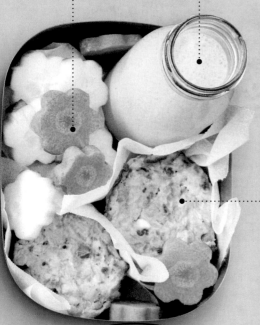

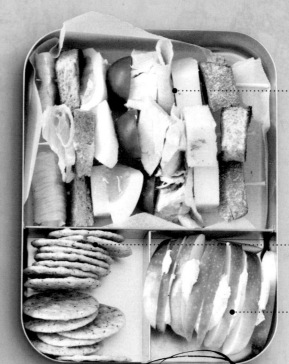

CHICKEN CAESAR ON A STICK
(page 125)

RICE CRACKERS OR SLICE 'N' BAKE MISO BUTTER BISCUITS
(page 96)

APPLE WEDGES AND CREAM CHEESE

WEDNESDAY

THURSDAY

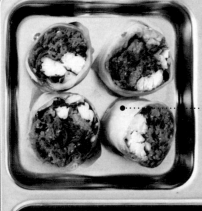

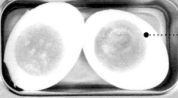

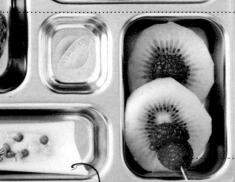

HARD-BOILED EGGS

check out my favorite egg-peeling trick (page 44)

RAINBOW ROLLS
(page 124)

KIWI AND RASPBERRY KEBABS

FRIDAY

raisin-free + nut-free ants on a log

What should a healthy lunchbox contain?

This list is based on international dietary guidelines and works to the idea that a lunchbox contains about one-third to half of your kids' nutrition for the day.

2–3 servings VEGGIES
(1 serving = 1 cup leafy greens or ½ cup other veggies)

1 serving FRUIT (1 serving = 1 peach or 2 kiwi fruit or ½ cup berries)

1 serving PROTEIN
(1 serving = 2 eggs or 1 kid-sized handful of meat or 1 cup cooked legumes or 2 tablespoons nuts/seeds)

1 serving DAIRY (1 serving = 1 cup milk or 2 slices cheese or ¾ cup yogurt)

Most guidelines also advise 2½ servings of grains. Which I don't feel needs to be factored in consciously. We get enough grains without trying.

MONSTER-MASH ROLL-UPS

SERVES 1–2

2 eggs

1 tablespoon chia seeds

1 tablespoon full-fat milk

1 tablespoon chopped fresh herbs (try dill or basil) or ½ teaspoon dried herbs

1 teaspoon coconut oil

handful of baby spinach leaves

1 tablespoon crumbled feta

Whisk the eggs, chia seeds, milk and herbs together and leave to sit for 5 minutes. Heat the oil in a skillet over medium-high heat. Pour in the egg mixture. Sprinkle with the spinach and feta. Reduce the heat to medium-low and cover with a lid (or a large plate or another pan). Cook for 2–3 minutes until the egg is set.

Lay a piece of parchment paper on a flat surface. Slide the omelette onto the paper. Use the parchment paper to tightly roll the omelette. Cut in half to serve.

MAKE IT EXTRA-NUTRITIOUS:
Add 1 teaspoon Fermented Turmeric Paste (page 340) to the eggs before whisking and lay a sheet of nori on top of the omelette before rolling.

1 SERVING VEG + FRUIT PER SERVING

RAINBOW ROLLS

MAKES 4

If you're organized, you can make this mixture the night before with the kids, and the next morning get them to help make the rolls.

1 beet, trimmed, scrubbed and grated

1 large carrot, grated

2 tablespoons chia seeds

⅓ cup Green Minx Dressing (page 54) or Whey-Good Mayo (page 50)

4 rice paper sheets (8½-inch diameter)

½ cup snow pea sprouts or green leaves (mint, spinach, watercress)

½ cup Shredded Chicken (page 214)

Toss the beet, carrot, chia seeds and dressing or mayo in a bowl and let the chia work its soaking-up-the-sogginess magic for 5 minutes.

Set up a work area with a chopping board, a plate and a large pan filled with warm water. Submerge a sheet of rice paper in the water for 30 seconds, or until soft. Place on the chopping board and spread over ¼ cup of the beet mixture. Top with some sprouts or green leaves and some chicken. Fold one side in and then roll to form a log. Plonk one or two in each lunchbox.

1 SERVING VEG + FRUIT PER SERVING

what should a healthy lunchbox contain?

2-3 servings Veggie + 1 serving fruit + 1 serving Protein + 1 serving dairy

CHICKEN CAESAR ON A STICK

MAKES 4 SKEWERS

2 hard-boiled eggs, halved

2 cherry tomatoes, halved

big wedge of iceberg lettuce, cut into cubes

1 slice bread, toasted and cut into cubes

1 cucumber, sliced

4 pieces Shredded Chicken (page 214) and/or cheddar

Thread the ingredients onto 4 skewers.

 ½ SERVING VEG + FRUIT PER SERVING

STRAWBERRY FROZEN YOGURT

SERVES 4

1 cup full-fat organic plain yogurt

1 cup frozen strawberries (or any other berries)

1 cup coconut flakes

Place the ingredients in a blender and blend until smooth (or just mash with a fork). Transfer to containers with wide necks and firmly fitting lids, and freeze.

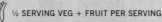 ½ SERVING VEG + FRUIT PER SERVING

KERMIT SLUSHIE

SERVES 4

1 frozen banana

2 cups greens (baby spinach, romaine, zucchini, mint)

1½ cups coconut water (or water)

3 cubes frozen coconut cream (see page 25)

 This little thing will keep lunch cool and thaw to become a slushie.

Place all the ingredients in a blender and blend until smooth. Place in a lunchbox brick or resealable plastic bag and freeze.

 ½ SERVING VEG + FRUIT PER SERVING

Peanuts vs. seeds
"Peanuts, tree nuts and nut products" are the focus for anaphylaxis policies in schools and are often banned. Seeds, however, are often suggested as good alternatives and are allowed in most schools. Which is why I use tahini and seeds instead of nut butter and peanuts when creating my healthy lunchboxes.

ABUNDANCE
BOWLS

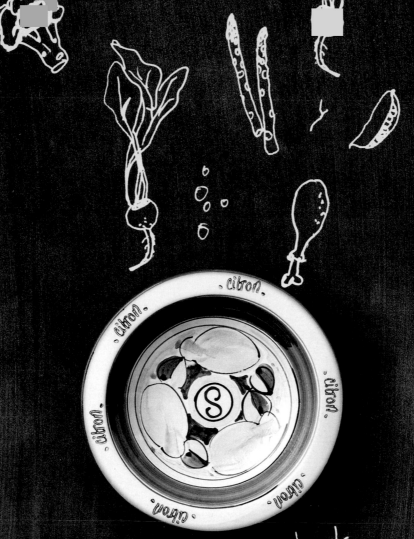

All the **MISH MASH** bowls
of <u>nutrient - dense</u> goodness I bore you
with on social media @_sarahwilson_ #sarahwilsoneats

HERE'S HOW I SHAPE MY BOWLS

These one-pan, two-minute mélanges are my standard lunch (or breakfast, or dinner) fare. I feel weird putting them into recipe format because I mostly make them on a whim, using what I've got (and a few too many lax cooking techniques). But I've been asked by my publisher to do so. So . . . here's how I shape my bowls:

1 serving → 1 cup leafy greens → ½ cup all other veg

Raw bowls vs. cooked bowls
Both have benefits.

The raw bowl argument:
Cooking reduces a food's enzymes, and the fewer enzymes in a food, the more our own body's enzymes must be drawn upon to break down a meal. The more of our own enzymes we use, the quicker we age.

The cooked bowl argument:
Many of the vitamins and minerals in vegetables are embedded in the plant's cellulose cell walls, which require cooking to break them down. So many of the valuable nutrients in raw vegetables end up not being absorbed by the body.

In conclusion: I advocate a mix across a meal/your day of 70% cooked, 30% raw (varying a little from winter to summer). The best way to get your raw fix is via ferments (where the fermentation breaks down the tough cellulose walls) and eating vegetables that are meant to be eaten raw—e.g., lettuce and cucumber.

Step 1: Start with 3 servings of veggies
Sauté in oil or sweat in 2 frozen stock cubes (page 25) or ferment brine (page 334).

Step 2: Add 1 serving of protein
Deglaze, if required, with a big splash of ferment brine or apple cider vinegar, or a squeeze of lemon juice.

2 eggs, a palm-sized portion of meat, or 1 cup properly prepared legumes (page 28).

Step 3: Stir through 1–3 tablespoons of fat
As you all know, you need saturated fat to absorb essential vitamins A, E, K and D, and to digest meat protein. You're wasting your time without it.

Step 4: Add an enzyme kick
1–2 tablespoons fermented veggies (see page 334) or enzyme-rich foods like sprouts (see page 352) or bitter vegetables.

Dressing, oil, cheese or avocado.

Step 5: Flavor-bomb
Soup Toppers (page 245), Seaweed Dukkah (page 45), Kale Flakes (page 179), Celery Leaf Salt (page 265), capers, dulse flakes, fresh herbs, etc.

CLEAN BITTERS BOWL

2 handfuls of chopped radicchio, red endive and/or red cabbage

½ cup thinly sliced fennel or radish

1 celery stalk and leaves, thinly sliced

small handful of mint or cilantro leaves, torn

¼ avocado, chopped

2 tablespoons Powerhouse Dressing (page 53)

½ cup cooked Puy or brown lentils (page 28)

smashed activated almonds (see page 28), to serve

Toss together the radicchio, red endive and/or red cabbage with the fennel or radish, celery and mint or cilantro. Add the avocado, dressing and lentils, and top with the almonds.

ADD KICK: 2–3 tablespoons Pink Sauerkraut (page 337).

Big fennel vs. baby fennel
Large fennel bulbs are best for baking and soups; small ones are best for salads. But don't worry too much if you have the wrong one for the job. Both work.

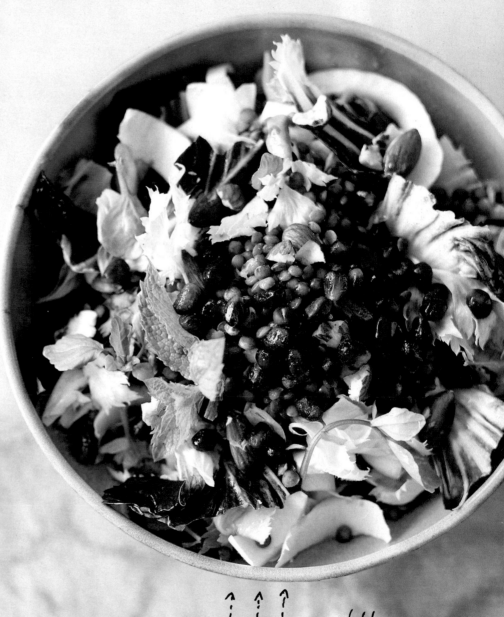

? ? ?
Add prettiness: a tablespoon of pomegranate seeds, half an APPLE or 4 strawberries

4½ SERVINGS VEG + FRUIT PER SERVING

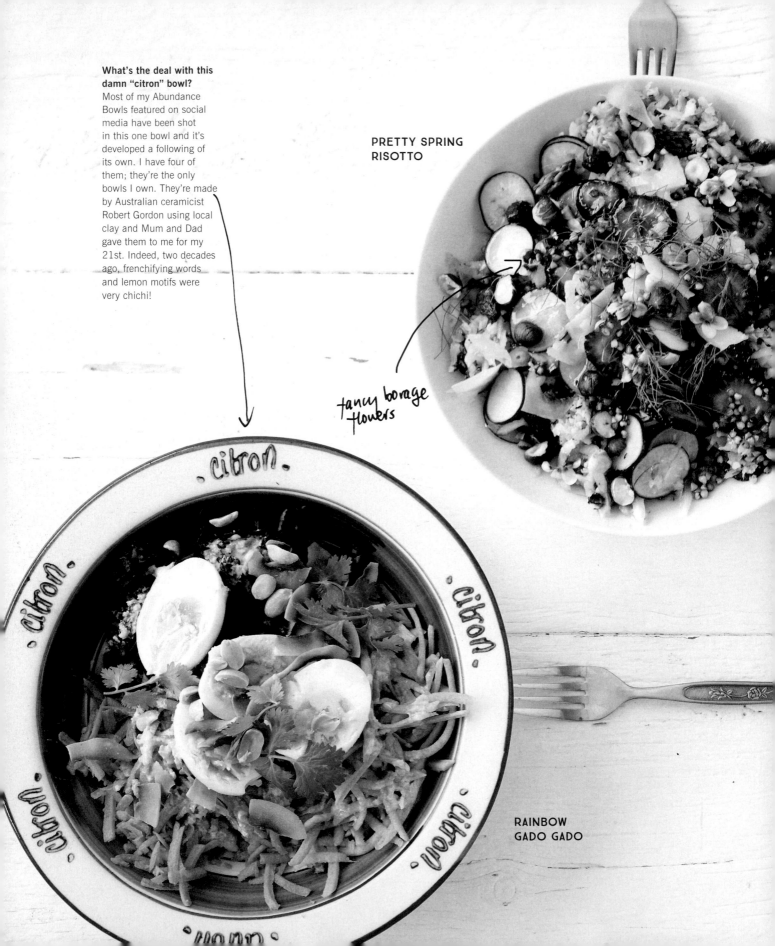

What's the deal with this damn "citron" bowl?
Most of my Abundance Bowls featured on social media have been shot in this one bowl and it's developed a following of its own. I have four of them; they're the only bowls I own. They're made by Australian ceramicist Robert Gordon using local clay and Mum and Dad gave them to me for my 21st. Indeed, two decades ago, frenchifying words and lemon motifs were very chichi!

PRETTY SPRING RISOTTO

fancy borage flowers

RAINBOW GADO GADO

· citron ·

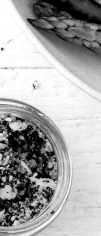

TMT Dressing

NORI ROLL
IN A BOWL

Seaweed dukkah

All recipes on the next page ⟶

PRETTY SPRING
RISOTTO

1 teaspoon olive oil, butter or ghee

3 cups grated spring veggies (asparagus, zucchini, broccoli, fennel bulb and stalks)

1 frozen stock cube (see page 25) or 1 tablespoon water

3 strawberries and/or radishes, sliced

shaved Parmesan and chopped hazelnuts (preferably activated; see page 28), to serve

Powerhouse Dressing (page 53), to serve

Heat the oil, butter or ghee in a skillet or small saucepan over medium heat. Sauté the grated vegetable "rice" for 1 minute, then deglaze with the stock or water. Serve with the sliced strawberries and/or radishes, a smattering of Parmesan flakes and chopped hazelnuts and a good dollop of dressing.

ADD BULK: Sprinkle over ½ cup of Activated Groaties (page 27).

RAINBOW
GADO GADO

1 cup grated beet (or red cabbage)

1 cup grated butternut squash

1 cup grated carrot

2 boiled eggs, halved

¼ cup TMT Dressing (page 53) or 1 tablespoon each natural peanut butter, miso paste and coconut milk, whisked together

toasted peanuts and cilantro leaves, to serve

Arrange the grated veggies in a bowl, top with the eggs and dressing and scatter with the toasted peanuts and cilantro.

ADD KICK: 1–2 tablespoons of "But the Kitchen Sink" Kimchi (page 337) or Sprouts in a Jar (page 352), and a sprinkle of Seaweed Dukkah (page 45).

NORI ROLL
IN A BOWL

4 asparagus spears

½ cup Cooked Buckwheat (page 27), Cooked Quinoa (26) or Cauliflower Rice (page 22)

3½ ounces Simplicious Smoked Salmon (page 160) or 3-ounce can Italian canned tuna in olive oil

2 radishes, sliced

½ avocado, sliced

small handful of Sprouts in a Jar (page 352)

1 nori sheet, crumbled, or 2 teaspoons Seaweed Dukkah (page 45)

TMT Dressing (page 53), to serve

1 teaspoon black sesame seeds

Blanch the asparagus in boiling water for a few minutes (or zap in the microwave if you're at work). Place the buckwheat, quinoa or cauli rice in a bowl. Top with the fish, radish, avocado, sprouts, nori or dukkah and asparagus. Drizzle with the dressing and sprinkle with sesame seeds.

MAKE IT VEGETARIAN:
Replace the fish with 3½ ounces fried tempeh strips.

Why tempeh, not tofu?
I'm not a fan of soy, for a range of reasons, one of which is the phytic acid content. Tempeh, however, is fermented, which breaks down many of these problematic toxins.

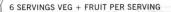 6 SERVINGS VEG + FRUIT PER SERVING

6 SERVINGS VEG + FRUIT PER SERVING

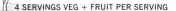 4 SERVINGS VEG + FRUIT PER SERVING

FOUR-INGREDIENT GREEN CHICKEN SHRED-UP

1 bunch broccolini, roughly chopped

1 frozen stock cube (see page 25) or 1 tablespoon water

½ cup Shredded Chicken (page 214)

1 tablespoon Leftovers Pesto (page 55)

½ avocado, chopped, or 2 tablespoons crumbled feta

In a skillet or small saucepan, sweat the broccolini in the stock or water for 1–2 minutes, adding a little more water if needed. Add the chicken. Mix the pesto with the avocado or feta and add to the pan, stirring to heat through.

ADD KICK: My Indian Kimchi (page 338) and Seaweed Dukkah (page 45).

ADD BULK: 1 portion Cooked Quinoa (page 26).

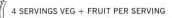 4 SERVINGS VEG + FRUIT PER SERVING

THE SIX-STAR WALDORF

1 cup Massaged Kale (page 23)

1 celery stalk and leaves, chopped

8 snow peas or sugar snap peas, sliced

½ peach, chopped

a dash of apple cider vinegar

2 tablespoons smashed pecans (preferably activated; see page 28)

1–2 tablespoons crumbled feta

Toss the kale, celery, peas and peach with the apple cider vinegar. Top with the pecans and feta.

2 SERVINGS VEG + FRUIT PER SERVING

VATA BALANCING BOWL

Sweet Potato Chips (below), to serve

1 cup Parcooked 'n' Frozen chard (page 22), thawed, or 2 cups sliced chard

½ cup Pulled Beef (page 223), Shredded Lamb (page 220) or Pulled Pork (page 222)

½ cup frozen peas, thawed

steamed zucchini rounds or yellow squash wedges, to serve

Make the sweet potato chips. *Dead simple and fast (due to secret tricks).* Remove from the pan and keep warm.

Deglaze the pan with a little water or ferment brine (page 334). Add the chard, meat and peas and cook for 2–3 minutes, or until heated through. Serve with steamed zucchini rounds or yellow squash wedges and sweet potato chips.

ADD KICK: A dollop of Pink Sauerkraut (page 337) and TMT Dressing (page 53).

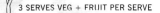 3 SERVES VEG + FRUIT PER SERVE

SWEET POTATO CHIPS

Slice ½ sweet potato into ¼ inch rounds. Heat a generous dollop of coconut oil in a skillet over medium-high heat. Add the sweet potato slices and sprinkle liberally with sea salt (this speeds up the cooking!). Cook both sides until dark golden (about 5 minutes).

1 SERVING VEG + FRUIT PER SERVING

PUTTANESCA FESTIVAL

small handful of watercress or radicchio leaves

1 zucchini, carrot or parsnip, cut lengthwise into thin ribbons with a veggie peeler or spiralizer

1 celery stalk and leaves, thinly sliced

4 cherry tomatoes, quartered

¼ red onion, thinly sliced

handful of pitted black olives

½ cup Uncanned Sardines (page 156) or 3-ounce can Italian canned sardines or tuna in olive oil

1 tablespoon Leftovers Pesto (page 55)

¼ cup Activated Groaties (page 27) or toasted sourdough cubes

Place all the veggies and the olives in your bowl and toss. Top with the fish and pesto and scatter with the groaties or sourdough cubes.

MAKE IT WARM:
If you have digestion or thyroid issues, you might like to sauté the vegetable ribbons (you can use the oil or brine from your fish), then add the other ingredients to heat through.

Zucchini in a salad
The great thing about using zucchini instead of cucumber or salad greens is that you can add the dressing in the morning and the whole thing marinates nicely—rather than going soggy—ready for lunch.

3 SERVINGS VEG + FRUIT PER SERVING

recipes back over this way!

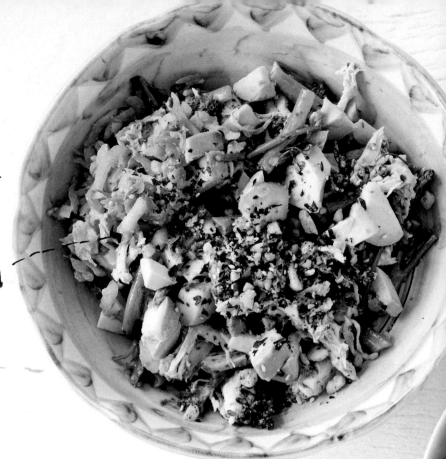

FOUR-INGREDIENT
GREEN CHICKEN
SHRED-UP

Indian KIMCHI

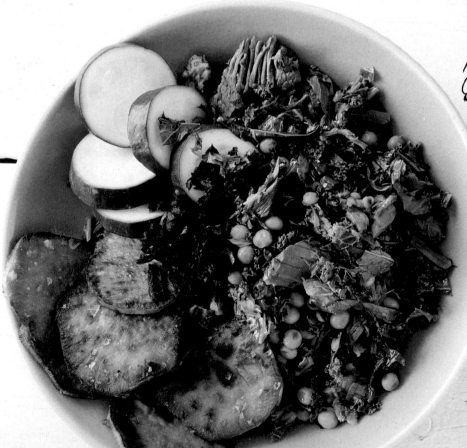

My "Anxiety Busting Bowl"
(great for AUTOIMMUNE-Y DAYS)

VATA BALANCING
BOWL
WITH PINK
SAUERKRAUT AND
SWEET POTATO CHIPS

**PUTTANESCA
FESTIVAL**
WITH SOME
ACTIVATED
GROATIES AS
THE "PASTA"
ELEMENT

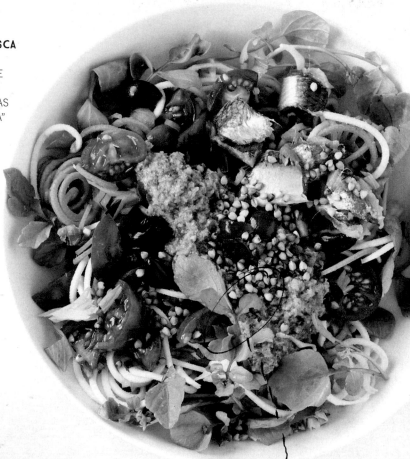

Activated
GROATIES

**THE SIX-STAR
WALDORF**

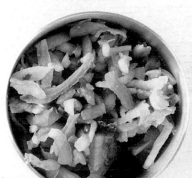

**MY INDIAN
KIMCHI**
(page 338)

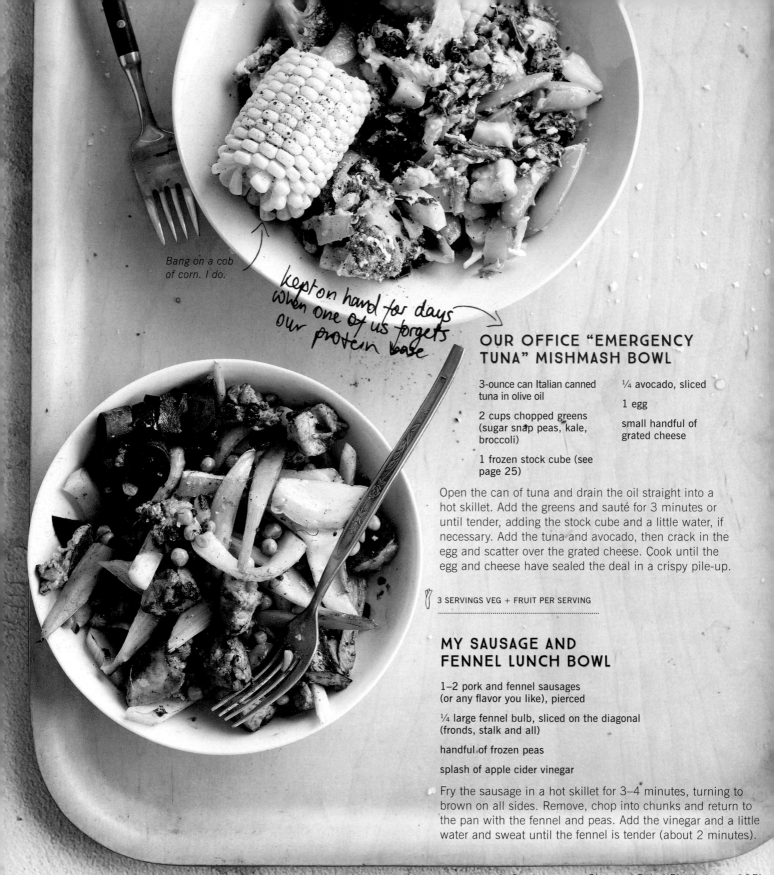

Bang on a cob of corn. I do.

Kept on hand for days when one of us forgets our protein base

OUR OFFICE "EMERGENCY TUNA" MISHMASH BOWL

3-ounce can Italian canned tuna in olive oil

2 cups chopped greens (sugar snap peas, kale, broccoli)

1 frozen stock cube (see page 25)

¼ avocado, sliced

1 egg

small handful of grated cheese

Open the can of tuna and drain the oil straight into a hot skillet. Add the greens and sauté for 3 minutes or until tender, adding the stock cube and a little water, if necessary. Add the tuna and avocado, then crack in the egg and scatter over the grated cheese. Cook until the egg and cheese have sealed the deal in a crispy pile-up.

3 SERVINGS VEG + FRUIT PER SERVING

MY SAUSAGE AND FENNEL LUNCH BOWL

1–2 pork and fennel sausages (or any flavor you like), pierced

¼ large fennel bulb, sliced on the diagonal (fronds, stalk and all)

handful of frozen peas

splash of apple cider vinegar

Fry the sausage in a hot skillet for 3–4 minutes, turning to brown on all sides. Remove, chop into chunks and return to the pan with the fennel and peas. Add the vinegar and a little water and sweat until the fennel is tender (about 2 minutes).

ADD KICK: 1–2 tablespoons Chopped Salad Pickle (page 335).

2 SERVINGS VEG + FRUIT PER SERVING

PRETTY IN PASTEL PINK PARSNIP PASTA

1 Cooked 'n' Frozen Beet (page 23), chopped into ½-inch cubes

½ cup full-fat organic plain yogurt

1 small clove garlic, crushed

big pinch of ground cumin

sea salt and freshly ground black pepper

½ teaspoon coconut oil or olive oil

2 parsnips, peeled and cut lengthwise into long strips with a veggie peeler or spiralizer

small handful of walnuts (preferably activated; see page 28), roughly chopped

small handful of flat-leaf parsley, roughly chopped

⅓ cup Green Minx Dressing (page 54), Watercress Sauce (page 176) or Leftovers Pesto (page 55) mushed with ½ avocado

Place a quarter of the beet in a food processor with the yogurt, garlic and cumin. Season to taste with salt and pepper, then blend until smooth.

Heat the oil in a skillet over a medium heat. Add the parsnip strips and fry for 1–2 minutes, or until just soft. Add the pink sauce and remaining beet cubes to the pan and heat through. Serve with the walnuts, parsley and dressing.

This one serves two for a light lunch

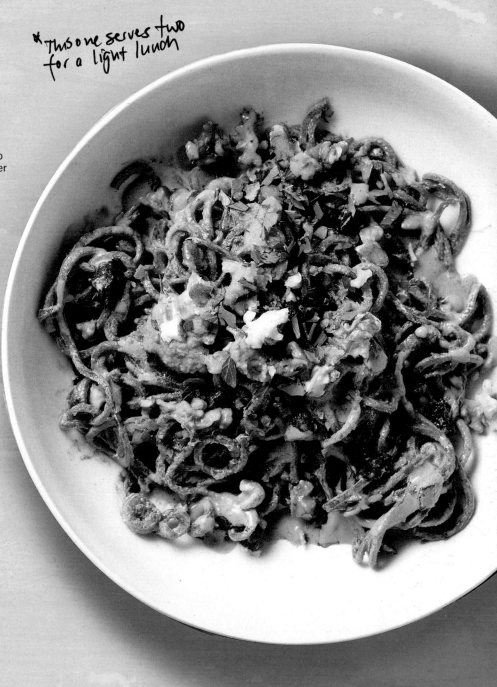

3 SERVINGS VEG + FRUIT PER SERVING

A CHAPTER DEDICATED TO

GROUND MEAT

It's cheap, easy to extend and
BOMB PROOF (culinarily speaking.)

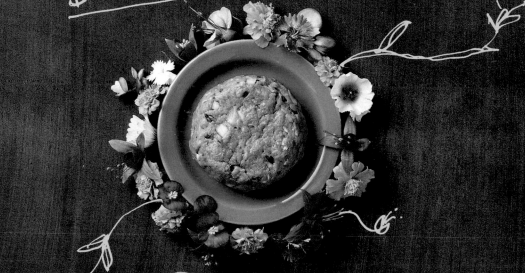

(P.S.) Most recipes in this chapter allow you
to use different ground meats interchangeably

SUPERFOODIE LASAGNA CAKE

SERVES 6

I don't subscribe to the notion of superfoods. Any meal laden with veggies and really low in toxins is super.

9 rice paper sheets
(8½-inch diameter)

2 cups spinach leaves
(or 1 cup Parcooked 'n' Frozen spinach
or beets [page 22], thawed and drained)

2 nori sheets, torn into large pieces
(or 1 tablespoon dulse flakes)

MEAT SAUCE

1 tablespoon coconut oil, olive oil,
butter or ghee

1 red onion, finely chopped

1 pound ground meat

2 cloves garlic, crushed

¼ teaspoon cayenne pepper,
or to taste

1 teaspoon Fermented Turmeric Paste
(page 340) or freshly grated turmeric
(or ¼ teaspoon ground turmeric)

1 cup Nomato Sauce (page 51)
or 1½ cups diced tomatoes and
1 teaspoon dried oregano

2 cups grated pumpkin
or 1 cup Squash or Sweet
Potato Purée (page 23)

sea salt and freshly ground
black pepper

CHEESY CAULIFLOWER SAUCE

1 head cauliflower, chopped

2 tablespoons butter

½ cup milk (any kind)

½ cup grated Parmesan,
plus extra for the topping

sea salt and freshly ground
black pepper

Preheat the oven to 350°F and grease a 9-inch springform cake pan.

To make the meat sauce, heat the oil, butter or ghee in a large skillet over medium-high heat. Add the onion and ground meat and cook for 3–4 minutes. Stir in the garlic, cayenne and turmeric, and cook for 1–2 minutes. Add the Nomato Sauce or tomatoes, then reduce the heat and cook for 15–20 minutes, or until the sauce has thickened.

Meanwhile, to make the cheesy cauliflower sauce, steam or boil the cauli in a saucepan of water until tender (about 8 minutes). Drain. Add the butter, milk, Parmesan, salt and pepper and purée with an immersion blender until smooth and creamy (or use a food processor).

To assemble the lasagna, spread one-third of the meat sauce over the base of the cake pan, cover with three rice paper sheets, then top with one-third of the cheesy cauliflower sauce. Repeat for the remaining two layers, placing a layer of spinach and nori after the second and third layers of cheese sauce. Top the lasagna with the extra Parmesan and a good grind of pepper. Cook for 40 minutes, or until the top is browned and the cheese is melted. Allow to sit for 10 minutes before serving.

3 SERVINGS VEG + FRUIT PER SERVING

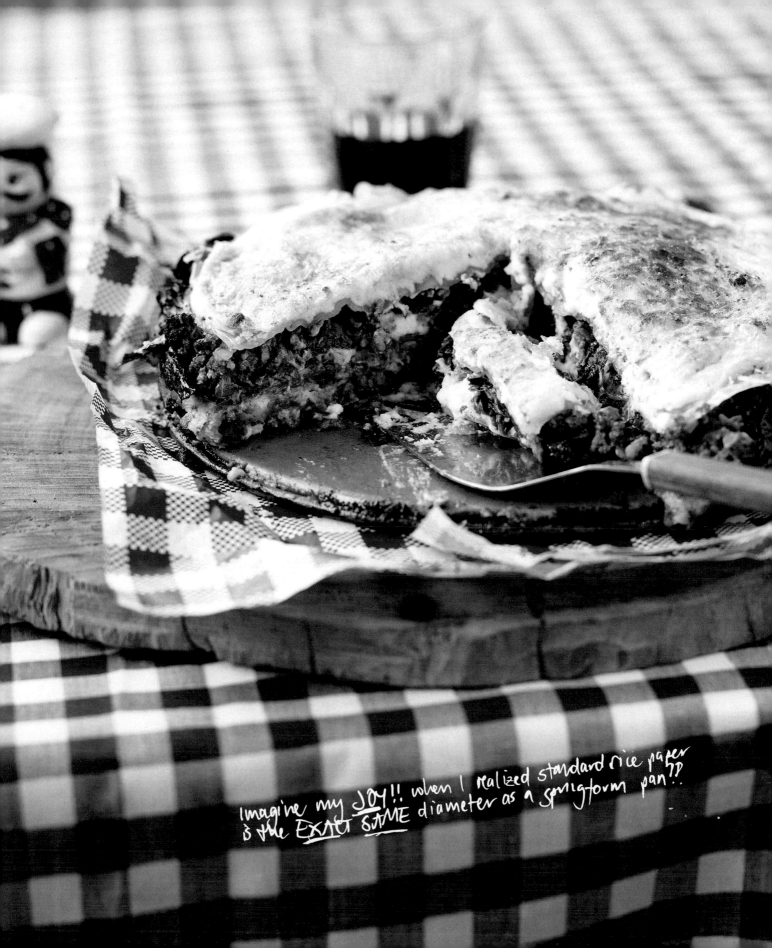

Imagine my JOY!! when I realized standard rice paper
is the EXACT SAME diameter as a springform pan!!

THREE WAYS with MEATBALLS:

Make in bulk, freeze raw + use in these recipes...

1. ONE-POT SPAGHETTI AND MEATBALLS

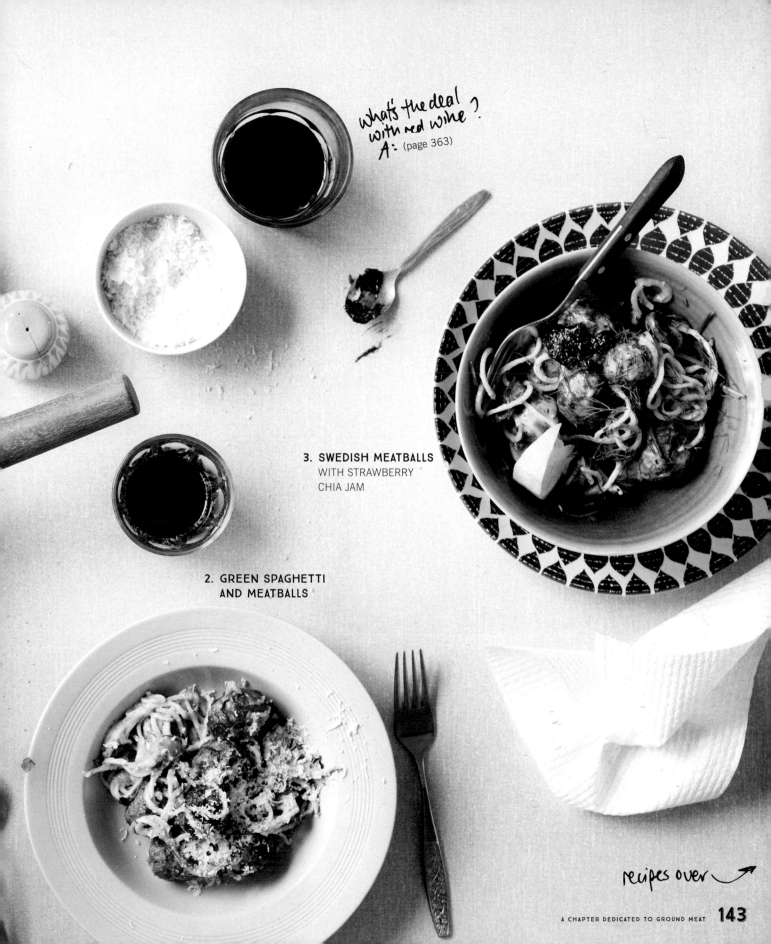

what's the deal with red wine? A: (page 363)

3. **SWEDISH MEATBALLS**
WITH STRAWBERRY
CHIA JAM

2. **GREEN SPAGHETTI
AND MEATBALLS**

recipes over →

BASIC MEATBALLS

first make your → *and then turn them into* →

MAKES ABOUT 80 SMALL BALLS
(16 SERVINGS)

2 pounds fresh
ground meat   *Use beef, chicken, lamb, turkey or pork.*

1 onion, finely chopped

½ bunch flat-leaf parsley
or basil, leaves finely chopped

1 teaspoon each sea salt and
freshly ground black pepper

olive oil, for frying

Place all the ingredients in a large bowl and, using your hands, mix until well combined. With wet hands, roll the mixture into walnut-sized balls.

To freeze: Line a baking sheet with parchment paper. Place the uncooked balls in a single layer on the sheet and freeze for 2 hours, or until frozen. Transfer to freezer-proof containers in meal-sized batches (5 per person) and return to the freezer.

To cook the meatballs now: Heat a little olive oil in a skillet over medium heat. Cook the meatballs on all sides (5–8 minutes in total). Remove from the heat, cover and allow to rest for a couple of minutes before serving.

MAKE IT YOUR OWN HOUSE MIX:
Add 1 teaspoon of cumin or fennel seeds (great with ground pork) or 1 teaspoon of oregano (great with lamb) to the recipe above.

A few tips

* Buy in bulk when you see it on sale, divide into meal-sized portions and freeze.

* Your ground meat is brown? Forget it—it's fine. It's just that it's not been exposed to oxygen. Leave it on the counter and it will go pink again.

* Freeze flattened out; thaw in the fridge and don't refreeze (unless you cook it first).

* Thinking of using a spatula to press down on that burger patty as it's cooking? Don't. You'll squeeze out all the juice and flavor. Ditto poking holes with a fork.

* RESPECT YOUR GROUND MEAT!

1. ONE-POT SPAGHETTI AND MEATBALLS

SERVES 2

This recipe breaks *all* the cooking rules. Everything is cooked in the same pot: no boiling the pasta separately, no defrosting the meat first. The spag starch is not drained out, so it makes for a slightly "canned spaghetti" kind of vibe, which kids especially love.

2½ cups Nomato Sauce (page 51)
or tomato purée   *If you use store-bought tomato purée, water it down (3:1) to reduce the sugar content.*

1 teaspoon dried parsley
(or 1 tablespoon chopped flat-leaf parsley)

1 teaspoon dried basil or oregano

¼ teaspoon fennel seeds

sea salt and freshly ground black pepper

10 frozen Basic Meatballs

3½ ounces spaghetti (gluten-free, if desired)

finely grated Parmesan, to serve (optional)

Place the Nomato Sauce or tomato purée in a large saucepan with 1 cup of water and bring to a boil over high heat. Stir in the parsley, basil or oregano, and fennel seeds and season to taste with salt and pepper. Add the frozen meatballs and reduce the heat to medium-high. (The meatballs should just be covered by the sauce.) Allow to simmer, uncovered, for 20 minutes.

Break the spaghetti in half and add it to the pan, stirring to coat. Cook for 12 minutes, uncovered, or until the pasta is tender. (Be sure to stir the spaghetti to prevent it from sticking to the base of the pan.) If the sauce becomes too dry, add up to 1 cup of boiling water. Serve topped with Parmesan, if you like, and a good grind of pepper.

MAKE IT MORE NUTRIENT-DENSE:
Toss in 1–2 cups of grated zucchini and a few cubes of frozen Squash Purée (page 23) in the final 5 minutes of cooking.

2½ SERVINGS VEG + FRUIT PER SERVING

2. GREEN SPAGHETTI AND MEATBALLS

SERVES 2

1 tablespoon coconut oil, olive oil, butter or ghee

10 Basic Meatballs, thawed

⅓ cup Leftovers Pesto (page 55) or Green Minx Dressing (page 54)

1 avocado

2–3 zucchini

sea salt and freshly ground black pepper

chili flakes, to serve (optional)

Parmesan shavings, to serve (optional)

Heat the oil, butter or ghee in a large skillet over medium-high heat. Cook the meatballs for 5–8 minutes, until browned and cooked through. Meanwhile, blend the pesto or dressing and avocado in a food processor (or use an immersion blender and beaker) until smooth.

Use a spiralizer, julienne peeler, mandoline or grater to make zucchini "spaghetti." Transfer to a saucepan and cover with boiling water for 1 minute (or leave raw if you like). Drain, then stir through the avocado sauce. Season with salt and pepper and a sprinkle of chili flakes and Parmesan, if desired.

MAKE IT MORE NUTRIENT-DENSE:
Toss in 1 cup of chopped baby spinach leaves or a few cubes of Parcooked 'n' Frozen spinach or kale (page 22).

3. SWEDISH MEATBALLS

SERVES 2

1 celeriac, peeled

2 tablespoons butter

10 Basic Meatballs, thawed

1½ teaspoons caraway seeds

½ teaspoon ground allspice

1½ cups milk (any kind)

1½ tablespoons cornstarch

¼ cup chopped dill, plus extra to serve

sea salt and freshly ground black pepper

1 cup baby spinach leaves

juice of ½ lemon, plus wedges to serve

Strawberry Chia Jam (page 57), to serve

steamed greens, to serve

Can't find celeriac? Use 2 or 3 parsnips instead.

When a recipe calls for a small amount of fresh dill, I generally use fennel fronds rather than buying a whole bunch of dill. Parsley will also do the job if you're stuck (or 3 teaspoons dried dill).

Cut the celeriac into several long chunks, then use a spiralizer, potato peeler or mandoline to make noodles. (Exposed celeriac turns brown quickly, so if you're not cooking it immediately, immerse the slices in water and lemon juice.)

Heat 1 tablespoon of the butter in a large skillet over medium-high heat. Add the meatballs and cook for 5–8 minutes until browned. Sprinkle with the caraway seeds and allspice, and cook for another minute until fragrant. Remove the meatballs from the pan.

Add the milk and cornstarch to the pan and stir well. Cook, scraping up any brown bits from the bottom, for 1–2 minutes, or until thickened. Add the dill, celeriac noodles and meatballs to the pan and cook, covered, for 2–3 minutes or until heated through. Season with salt and pepper, then stir through the spinach. Remove from the heat and stir in the lemon juice. Serve with the jam, lemon wedges, steamed greens and a sprinkle of extra dill.

Celeriac vs. celery root
They're the same thing, but bear in mind some folks like to call the bottom of a bunch of celery "celery root." Ignore them. Possibly the ugliest-looking veggie around, celeriac tastes a bit like celery (with a dash of parsley, to my mind), is bursting with fiber, and can be found in the root-veggie section in winter (they keep quite well, so can be found into spring, too). Always choose heavy ones (the light ones are fluffy and sad to eat).

3 SERVINGS VEG + FRUIT PER SERVING

2 SERVINGS VEG + FRUIT PER SERVING

GREEK SAN CHOI BAU

Or use 10 ounces ground pork or lamb meat

1 tablespoon coconut oil, olive oil, butter or ghee, melted

10 frozen Basic Meatballs (page 144)

1 small eggplant, chopped into ½-inch cubes

1 teaspoon dried oregano

½ teaspoon ground cumin

½ teaspoon sweet paprika

juice of ½ lemon, plus wedges to serve

sea salt and freshly ground black pepper

½ savoy cabbage (or regular white or purple cabbage)

½ cup full-fat organic plain yogurt

1 zucchini or Lebanese cucumber, grated

TO SERVE

cherry tomatoes, quartered

mint leaves and/or flat-leaf parsley leaves, chopped

pine nuts, toasted (optional)

Heat the oil, butter or ghee in a large skillet over medium-high heat. Add the frozen meatballs or ground meat and cook for 5 minutes, or until browned and the insides of the meatballs are slightly defrosted. (You can break them apart a little to aid cooking.) Add the eggplant, oregano and spices and cook for 2–3 minutes, until the eggplant is tender. Add the lemon juice and season to taste with salt and pepper.

Meanwhile, carefully separate the cabbage leaves, keeping them whole if you can, then steam for 5 minutes in your double steamer or in a bamboo steamer.

To make tzatziki, combine the yogurt and grated zucchini or cucumber in a small bowl. Season with salt and pepper.

Serve the meatballs in the cabbage leaves topped with the cherry tomatoes, tzatziki, herbs, toasted pine nuts (if using) and a squeeze of lemon juice.

USE THE LEFTOVER CABBAGE:
Cook 1 cup of finely chopped cabbage with the eggplant and meatballs if you like.

4 SERVINGS VEG + FRUIT PER SERVING

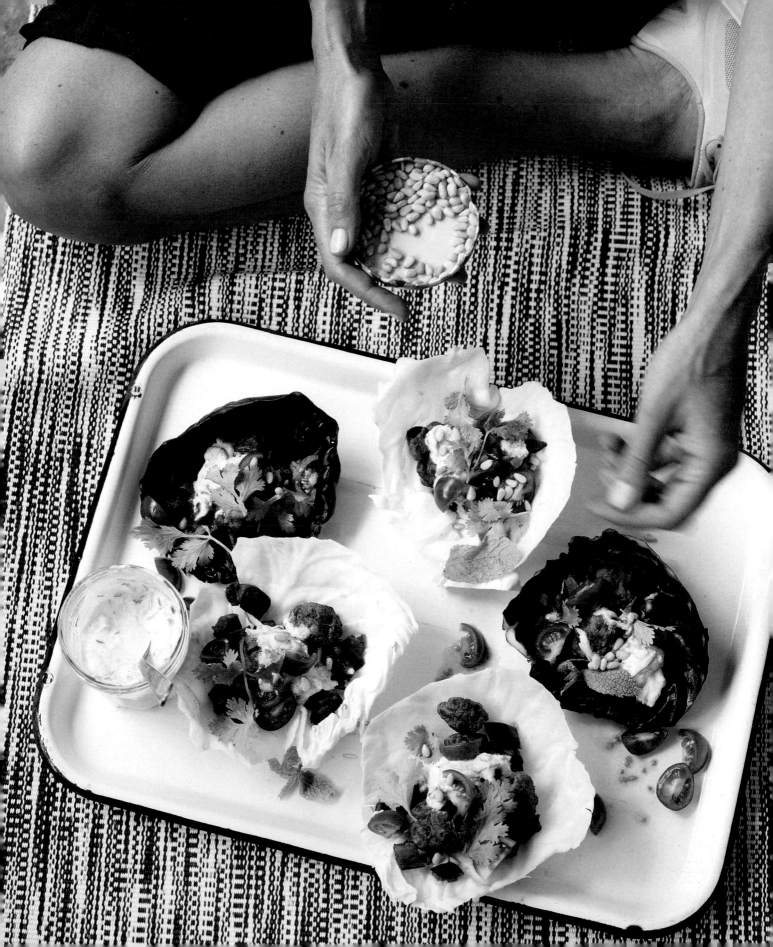

MIDDLE EASTERN
EGGPLANT

1 large eggplant

2 tablespoons coconut oil, melted

1 small onion, chopped

½ pound ground meat

Or 8 frozen Basic Meatballs

1 teaspoon ground allspice

2 teaspoons ground cinnamon

2 teaspoons ground cumin

Or use 1 tablespoon Ras el Hanout Mix (page 45).

sea salt and freshly ground black pepper

2 tablespoons finely chopped mint and/or flat-leaf parsley, plus extra leaves to serve

¼ cup full-fat organic plain yogurt (preferably Greek-style), plus extra to serve

¼ cup pine nuts, toasted

TO SERVE

1 cup baby spinach leaves

1 cup string beans, steamed

Preheat the oven to 400°F and line a baking sheet with parchment paper.

Pierce the eggplant several times with a fork then halve it lengthwise and lightly coat both sides with 1 tablespoon of the oil. Place the halves, cut side down, on the prepared sheet and bake for 20–30 minutes, or until tender. Leave to cool slightly. Using a spoon, scoop the flesh from the eggplant halves, leaving a ½-inch border. Finely chop the flesh.

Meanwhile, heat the remaining oil in a skillet over medium heat and brown the onion and meat (about 3–4 minutes). Add the allspice, cinnamon and cumin to the pan and cook for 1–2 minutes. Add the eggplant flesh and season with salt and pepper. Stir in the herbs, yogurt and pine nuts and remove from the heat.

Spoon the mixture into the eggplant shells and cover with foil. Bake for 10 minutes, then remove the foil and bake for a further 5 minutes to allow the meat to brown.

Serve with the spinach, beans, and the extra herbs and yogurt.

4 SERVINGS VEG + FRUIT PER SERVING

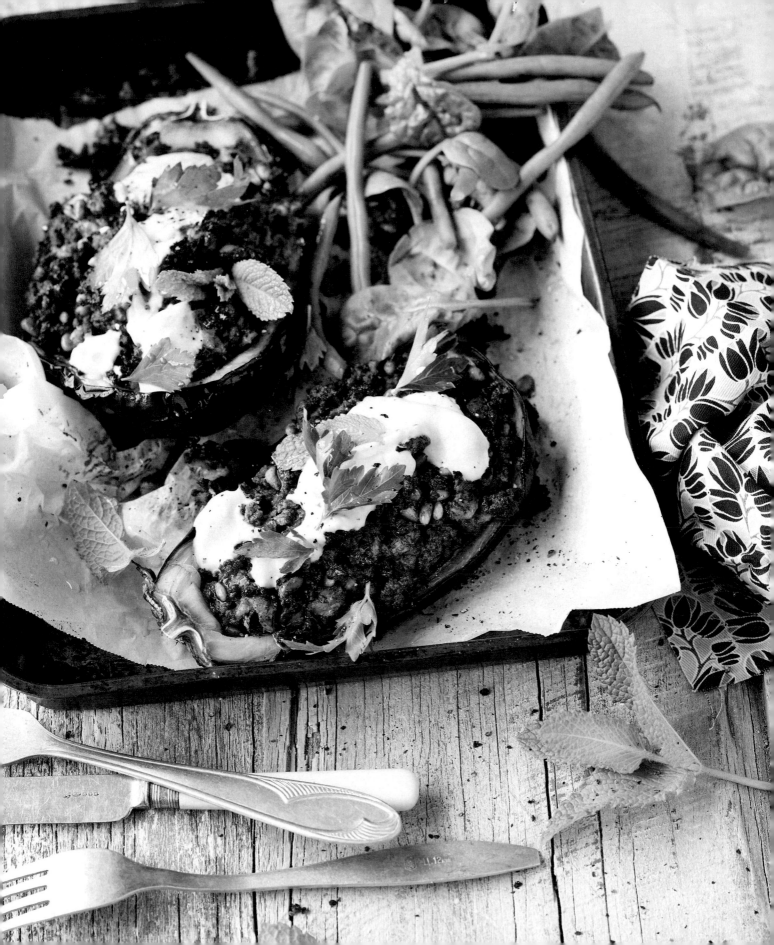

VIETNAMESE TURKEY PANCAKES

If you've got some dosa batter in the fridge (see page 89), use that instead.

RICE PANCAKES

½ cup rice flour

2 tablespoons chia seeds

½ teaspoon ground turmeric

⅔ cup milk (any kind; coconut milk works well)

½ cup ice water

2 teaspoons coconut oil, plus extra for frying

Ground pork or chicken is okay, too.

10 ounces ground turkey

2 green onions, thinly sliced

1 clove garlic, crushed

1 teaspoon finely grated ginger

1 long red chili, thinly sliced

1 tablespoon fish sauce

juice of 2 limes

1 cup cilantro and/or mint leaves

½ red bell pepper, thinly sliced

lime wedges, to serve

steamed Asian greens, to serve

To make the rice pancakes, mix all the ingredients together in a bowl and refrigerate while you prepare the meat mixture.

To make the meat mixture, heat the oil in a skillet over medium-high heat. Add the meat, green onions, garlic, ginger and chili. Cook for 5 minutes, breaking up any chunky bits with a wooden spoon, or until browned. Add the fish sauce and lime juice. Cook for a further 2 minutes. Remove from the heat.

To cook the pancakes, heat some oil in a skillet over medium-high heat. Stir the batter well. Add half the batter to the pan and swirl to cover the bottom. Cook for 3–4 minutes until golden, then flip and cook the other side for 2–3 minutes. Slide the pancake onto a plate. Repeat with the remaining batter.

Place half the meat mixture on each pancake. Top with half the herbs and bell pepper and fold to enclose. Serve with lime wedges and a side of steamed Asian greens.

MAKE IT FASTER:
Use lettuce cups instead of rice pancakes.

2½ SERVINGS VEG + FRUIT PER SERVING

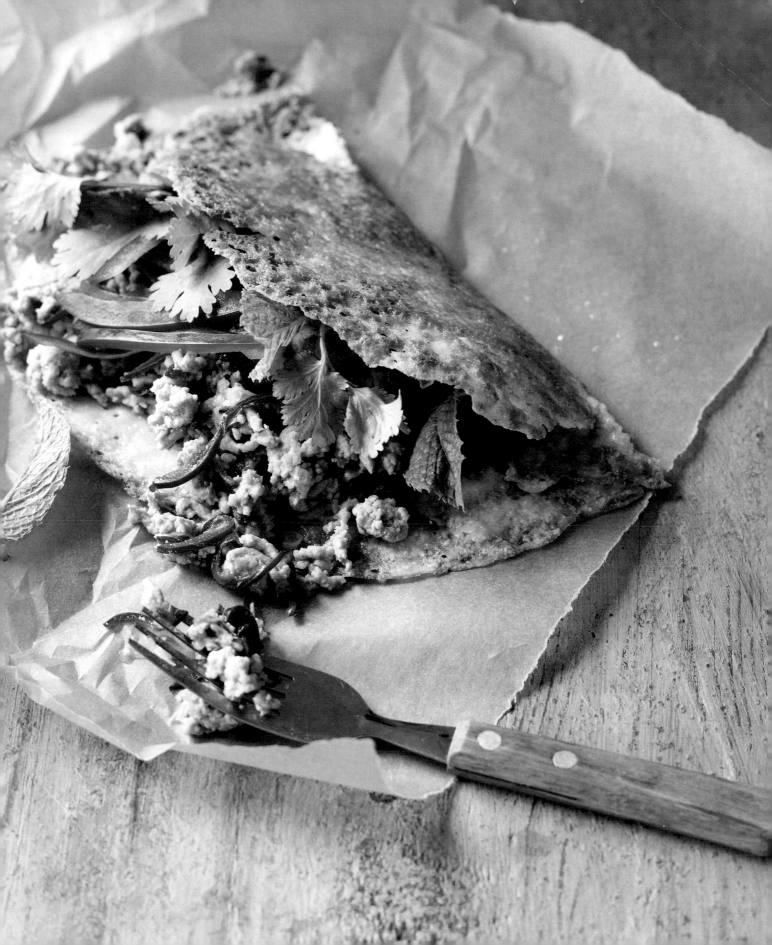

SUSTAINABLE FISH
IN A DISH

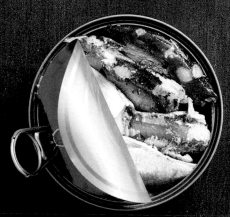

First choice   here's how as a few dot pointers:
1. small oily fish ps. 1 ♡ SARDINES
2. fish offcuts (ask your monger to keep them aside for you)
3. buy whole fish. And cook the carcass
4. white flesh fish
5. local and ethically sourced
6. check out The Kit for helpful apps + consumer guides.

(see page 5)

let's get started with:

THREE WAYS with an OILY FISH:

want to cut to the omega 3 + sustainable chase?
Just eat small, oil-ful fish - Sardines, anchovies + mackerel
(herring, too!)

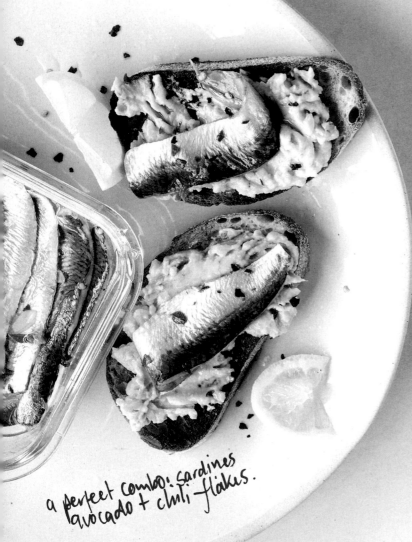

1. UNTINNED SARDINES ON AVOCADO TOAST WITH CHILI FLAKES

2. BAKED MEDITERRANEAN SUMMER SARDINES

a perfect combo: sardines
avocado + chili flakes.

I especially love eating the heads + tails of sardines. You don't? You should!

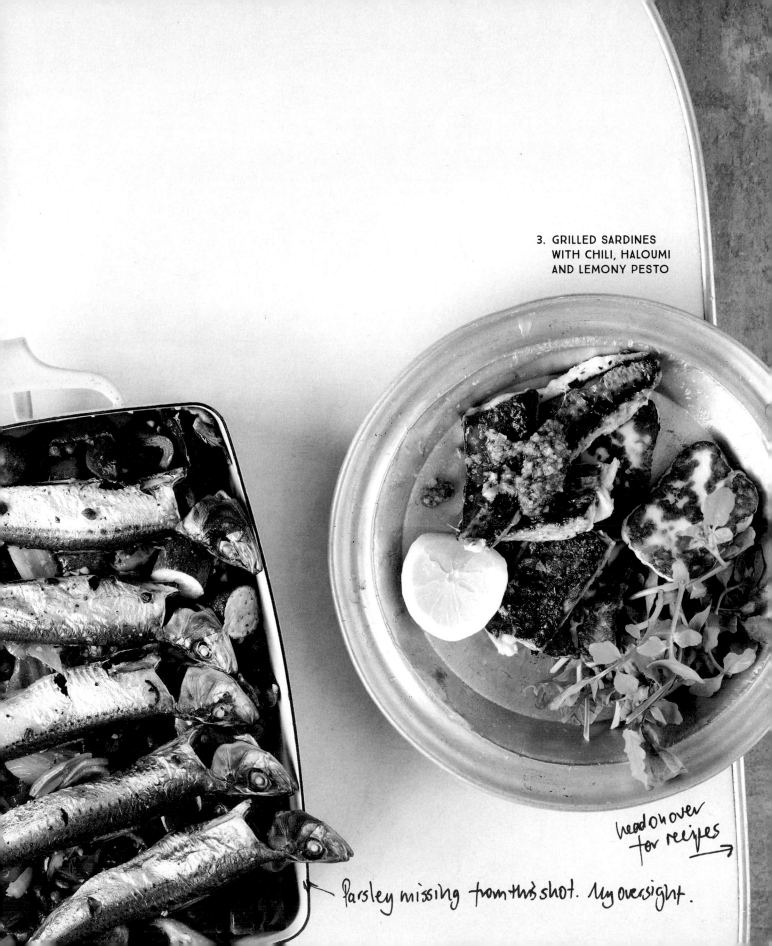

3. GRILLED SARDINES
WITH CHILI, HALOUMI
AND LEMONY PESTO

head on over
for recipes →

Parsley missing from this shot. My oversight.

1. UNCANNED SARDINES

SERVES 6

Why preserve your oily fish?
Oily fish can be hard to come by because they're seasonal and not wholly popular . . . yet (I'm working on it). So when you find them, it's worth buying a lot. But they oxidize quickly (see opposite). Kill two birds by preserving in bulk so you have them ready to fly whenever you get the briny incline.

I've played with various ways to preserve my oilies. Many fish fans work with vinegary cures or oil and/or salt, but these use a lot of ingredients that get tossed, which I'm not happy with. The recipe below is the most efficient, economical one and leaves you with condiments, too.

1 pound filleted sardines, anchovies, herring or mackerel (cut the bigger fish into smaller pieces)

½ red onion, thinly sliced

½ baby fennel, including stalks and fronds if you like, sliced

2 bay leaves

½ teaspoon chili flakes

2 tablespoons Homemade Whey (page 46) or apple cider vinegar

2 teaspoons sea salt

Don't worry if you're all out of big jars—a glass bowl or dish covered with plastic wrap will do just as well.

FIVE WAYS TO EAT SARDINES:

1. As a soup topper.

2. Spread on toast with avocado and chili flakes.

3. Stirred through an Abundance Bowl (hot or cold); see pages 126–37.

4. On a platter with radishes, Homemade Cream Cheese (page 46) and crackers.

5. Rolled up in a radicchio leaf or endive cup. (I do this. For breakfast.)

In a large jar (broad enough for each fillet to lie flat), arrange the fish in layers with the onion, fennel, bay leaves and chili. Add the whey or vinegar and salt along with 1 cup of water.

Fill a smaller clean jar with water, then seal and place inside the big jar (or bowl) as a weight to press the fish under the liquid (or use a plate). Drape a clean dishtowel or cloth over the top and put the jar or bowl in a dark place for 24 hours to ferment.

Remove the water-filled jar or plate, pop a lid on your main jar (or if using a bowl, cover with plastic wrap) and throw the jar or bowl in the fridge. It'll keep for 3–4 weeks.

MAKE IT "YOU'RE A BIT GREEK":
Use garlic instead of onion and fresh oregano instead of bay leaves.

2. BAKED MEDITERRANEAN SUMMER SARDINES

SERVES 6

1 large eggplant, cut into 1½-inch cubes

1 large red bell pepper, roughly chopped

2 zucchini, halved lengthwise and roughly sliced

8 ounces cherry tomatoes, halved

1 red onion, cut into wedges

2 cloves garlic, minced

2 tablespoons coconut oil, plus extra (melted) for drizzling

2 tablespoons apple cider vinegar or red wine vinegar

sea salt and freshly ground black pepper

12 fresh whole sardines (heads on), cleaned, scaled and gutted (or 1½ pounds other filleted oily fish)

2 tablespoons capers

lemon wedges, flat-leaf parsley and sourdough, to serve

Preheat the oven to 400°F and line a large baking sheet with parchment paper.

Place the eggplant, bell pepper, zucchini, tomatoes, onion and garlic on the prepared sheet and toss with the oil and vinegar. Season with salt and pepper. Bake for 15–20 minutes, until the vegetables are tender.

Meanwhile, prepare the fish by drizzling with oil and seasoning with salt and pepper. Remove the sheet from the oven, top with the fish fillets and capers, and continue cooking for another 20 minutes, or until lovely and crisp looking. Serve with lemon wedges, a sprinkling of parsley and some crusty sourdough.

3. GRILLED SARDINES WITH CHILI, HALOUMI AND LEMONY PESTO

SERVES 6 AS A STARTER

½ cup Leftovers Pesto (page 55) or Watercress Sauce (page 176)

zest and juice of 1 lemon

6 fresh whole sardines or 12 fresh whole anchovies (heads on), cleaned and gutted, or ¾ pound mackerel fillets, skin left on, cut into 6 pieces

2 teaspoons coconut oil, olive oil, butter or ghee, melted

½ teaspoon chili flakes

½ teaspoon sea salt

1¼ pounds haloumi, cut into ¼-inch-thick slices

watercress, to serve

lemon wedges, to serve (optional)

Make a lemony pesto by combining the Leftovers Pesto or Watercress Sauce with the lemon zest and juice. Set aside.

Preheat a broiler, grill pan or electric grill to medium-high. Rub the fish with the oil, butter or ghee and season with the chili flakes and salt. Place the haloumi and fish under the broiler, in the grill pan or on the electric grill and cook, turning once, for about 2–3 minutes each side, until lightly charred. Serve with watercress, lemony pesto and lemon wedges.

MAKE IT A MAIN COURSE:
Triple the fish and serve atop The Green Counterbalance Salad (page 309) or some Massaged Kale (page 23).

2 SERVINGS VEG + FRUIT PER SERVING

MY BROTHER PETE'S APP-AND-MAIN-IN-ONE KOKONDA

SERVES 6 PEEPS

Pete brought this cured fish recipe back from the Solomons, where he used to live, and made it for 15 of us at a family Christmas. I've kept to the instructions in his original wording, sent to me via e-mail, as much as I can.

When you go to the fish shop . . .

Bear in mind you use the whole fish for this two-part meal (appetizer = fish stock, main = kokonda). Ask your fishmonger to fillet and clean the fish, but ensure you get to take the carcass with you! Ask for an extra carcass or two while you're there to make a stronger stock.

Also, you're "cooking" (or denaturing) the fish in lemon so it's important to use fish that's super-fresh.

Pete catches his an hour before dinner and fillets it himself; for the rest of us he advises telling the fishmonger it's for marinating, not cooking, so they can ensure you're getting fresh stuff.

1¼ pounds whole fresh white non-oily fish, filleted (reserve the carcass for the stock) and cut into ¾-inch pieces

juice of 4–6 lemons (to cover the fish)

1 long red chili, sliced

6 green onions, thinly sliced

2 small yellow bell peppers, cubed

1 Lebanese cucumber, cubed

2 tomatoes, cubed

14-ounce can coconut cream

sea salt and freshly ground black pepper

cilantro leaves, to serve

The night or morning before: Place the fish in a glass or ceramic dish. Pour over the lemon juice, ensuring that the fish is completely covered by the juice. Cover and place in the fridge to marinate for at least 3 hours (preferably overnight). This method will "cook" the fish, leaving it firm and opaque.

Meanwhile, use the carcass to make fish stock (see page 42).

The next day or when ready to serve: Drain the fish (reserving the marinade; see below) and throw into a serving dish. Add the chili, green onions, bell pepper, cucumber and tomatoes and stir to combine. Pour the coconut cream over all and season to taste with salt and pepper.

Gently heat the stock and serve it first in mugs. ← *"No need to get fancy." —Pete*

Then serve the kokonda with cilantro leaves.

"Or with Usain Bolt's favorite, taro (unless you are paleo) to make it authentically South Pacific. And think yourself lucky." —Pete

USE THE LEFTOVER LEMON MARINADE:

Add it to the fish stock before you reheat it. Or use it to deglaze your next chicken or fish dish.

1½ SERVINGS VEG + FRUIT PER SERVING

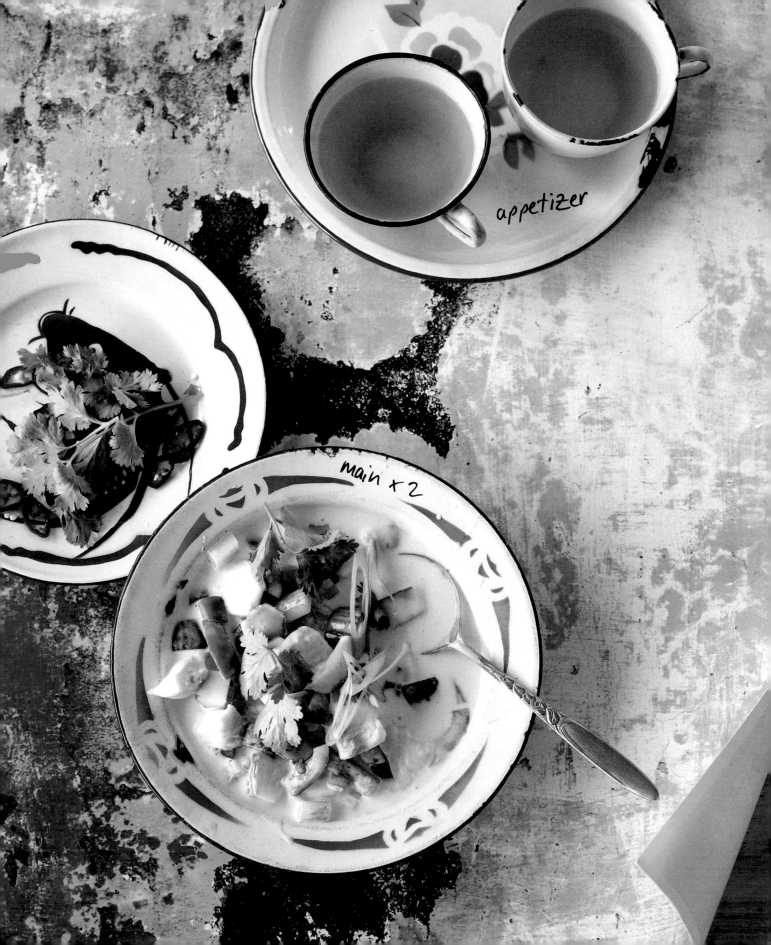

SIMPLICIOUS SMOKED SALMON

(WELL, KIND OF)

SERVES 12

I have a few issues with smoked salmon. It's expensive, it comes in a package and the smoking part means it can contain carcinogenic guff. Not conclusive, but enough to suspend question marks over it. And so all roads lead to making your own gravlox (also called gravlax). Most are cured in sugar. Mine isn't. Most take several palaver-y steps. I skip these.

Leaving the skin on makes it easier when you slice it later. And it wastes less.

If the salt is too fine the moisture will dissolve the crystals and the fish will absorb too much salt too quickly.

14 ounces salmon fillets, bones removed, skin left on

¼ cup coarse sea salt

zest of 2 lemons

2 teaspoons white peppercorns, ground using a mortar and pestle (or 2 teaspoons allspice)

1 small bunch dill, chopped

Which salmon is best?
Wild-caught salmon is best. Farmed salmon can be used as an occasional choice. Lots of small wild-caught fish are used to feed farmed salmon. So using wild-caught local fish is a better option.

Either way, my take is that if you're going to eat the stuff, then you should eat it in small amounts and savor it respectfully.

Dry the fish well, using paper towels. Combine the salt, lemon zest, pepper and dill and smother it over both sides of the fish (just use your hands, and make sure you cover it completely). Press the skinless sides of the fillets together and place in a large zip-lock bag, but don't completely seal it. You can also place it in a glass dish loosely covered with plastic wrap. Leave it on the counter for 2–6 hours.

Seal the bag properly (or tightly seal the plastic wrap) and put it in the fridge for 24–48 hours. Place a weight on top (such as a chopping board) to compress the fish.

Once done, the fish will be firm and sitting in a pool of liquid in the bag or bowl. Drain the fish and scrape off the excess salt mixture. If it's too salty, you can rinse it, but only JUST before you serve it (otherwise bacteria will grow). Slice it super-thinly and eat respectfully with eggs, on little rye squares with butter and radish disks.

It will keep in the fridge, covered, for 2–3 weeks.

MAKE IT WITH WHITE FISH:
Use 1 pound (you might need to use 3–4 fillets), skin left on.

My preferred option!

MAKE IT PINK:
Process 1 large peeled beet to a purée and spread this mixture between the salted fish fillets before placing them in the bag.

This is a really pretty option, especially served with Pink Devilish Googie Eggs (page 253).

ONE-PAN MOROCCAN FISH PILAF

SERVES 2 —————————————————————————————

This is the cleverest meal, truly. You cook your pilaf, vegetables and fish all in one hit.

1 cup Cooked Quinoa (page 26)

1 cup Homemade Fish Stock (page 42)

2 carrots, quartered lengthwise and sliced on the diagonal

½ cup frozen peas

2 tablespoons almonds or pistachios

2 tablespoons chopped fresh mint or cilantro, plus extra to serve

1 tablespoon olive oil

sea salt and freshly ground black pepper

2 sustainable white fish fillets

½ teaspoon Ras el Hanout Mix (page 45) or ¼ teaspoon each ground cumin and coriander

lemon wedges, to serve

Preheat the oven to 425°F. In a small baking dish or skillet, combine the quinoa, stock, carrots, peas, nuts, herbs and oil. Season with salt and pepper. Plonk the fish on top and sprinkle with the spice mix.

Cover (with lid or foil) and bake for 20 minutes. Serve with lemon wedges.

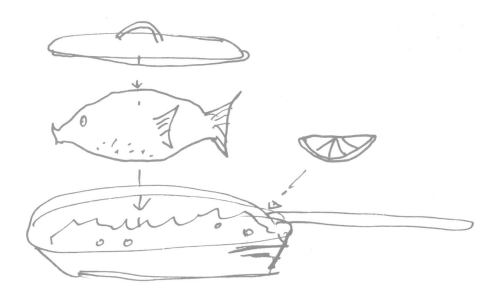

2 SERVINGS VEG + FRUIT PER SERVING

SKILLET FISH 'N' SUPERSLAW

This is my holier-than-thou version of fish 'n' chips and coleslaw.

1 bunch broccolini, chopped into bite-sized pieces

9 ounces bagged coleslaw mix (or 1 large carrot and ¼ cabbage, grated)

2 baby new potatoes, very thinly sliced (about 1/16 inch thick)

1 tablespoon chopped macadamias, almonds or cashews (preferably activated; see page 28)

1 teaspoon apple cider vinegar

2 teaspoons coconut oil

sea salt and freshly ground black pepper

10-ounce salmon fillet (see page 160), skin left on

1 teaspoon smoked paprika

juice of ½ lemon, to serve

Preheat the oven to 400°F and line a skillet or baking sheet with parchment paper.

In a large bowl, toss together the broccolini, coleslaw mix, potatoes, nuts, vinegar and oil, and season with salt and pepper.

Cut the salmon fillet in half lengthwise to create two even portions. Spread the coleslaw mix over half of the prepared tray and place the fillets skin-side down on the other. Sprinkle the salmon with the paprika. Bake for 12–15 minutes, uncovered. Serve the salmon on top of the superslaw with a squeeze of lemon.

MAKE IT SUMMERY:
Replace the potatoes with peach slices.

3 SERVINGS VEG + FRUIT PER SERVING

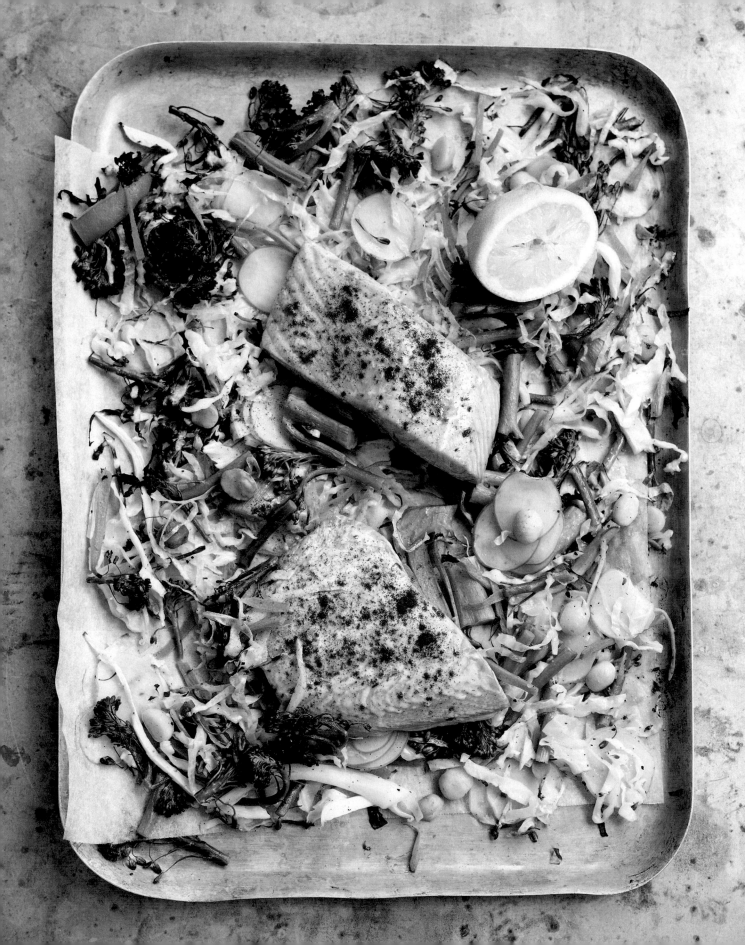

SUSTAINABLE SWEET
FISH CURRY

Too many people get scared if their fish has been sitting around in the fridge for more than a day or two. I don't. I make fish curry.

14-ounce can full-fat coconut milk, unshaken

¼ cup Thai red curry paste
(look for a brand that doesn't contain sugar—many do)

1 tablespoon minced lemongrass
(optional)

1 tablespoon grated fresh turmeric, Fermented Turmeric Paste (page 340) or ½ teaspoon ground turmeric

1 large onion, chopped

2 cups chopped sweet potato or squash (1½-inch chunks)

½ cup Homemade Chicken Stock
(page 42) or water

1¾ pounds sustainable firm white fish, cut into 1½-inch chunks
(offcuts are perfect)

3 cups chopped veggies (beans, zucchini and cauliflower are a good combo)

1 cup frozen peas

3 cloves garlic, minced (optional)

1 tablespoon fish sauce or lime juice

6 kaffir lime leaves, cut into fine strips *I buy these in bulk and keep them in the freezer.*

handful of mint, cilantro or basil leaves

1 long red chili, sliced (optional)

Heat a large skillet or wok over medium heat. Spoon the thick top layer of the coconut milk into the pan. Add the curry paste, lemongrass (if using) and turmeric and stir-fry for 2–3 minutes. Add the onion and sweet potato or squash and cook for 5 minutes. Pour in the remaining coconut milk and the stock. Add the fish, veggies, peas and garlic (if using).

Bring to a gentle boil. Simmer for 5 minutes, or until the fish is just cooked through. Stir in the fish sauce or lime juice, kaffir lime leaves, herbs and sliced chili (if using). Serve in bowls (it's quite soupy).

2 SERVINGS VEG + FRUIT PER SERVING

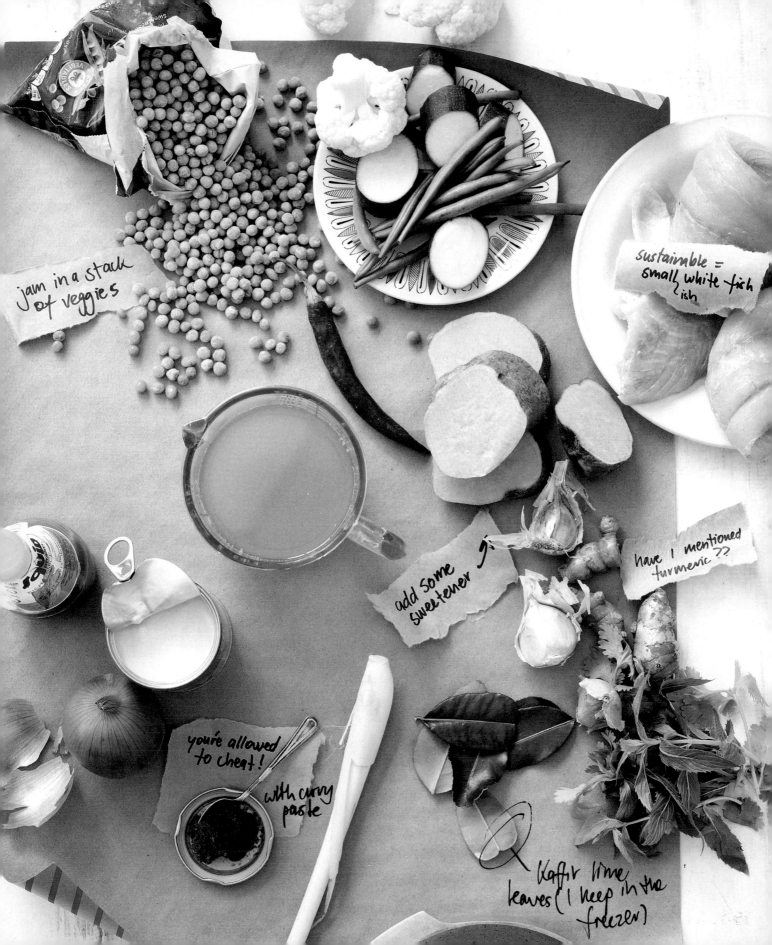

GIFT-WRAPPED MISO COD

SERVES 2 ——————————————————————————————

The original miso cod, invented by Nobu restaurant in Beverly Hills, is made with black cod, which is very sustainable in the United States. It's also glazed in a cacophony of Asian sugars, including mirin, rice wine and sweet miso. Here I cut out the mirin, which is full of sugar, but you'll never even miss it.

¼ cup red miso paste
(or ⅓ cup white miso paste)

1 teaspoon brown rice syrup

2 teaspoons grated ginger

2 teaspoons toasted sesame oil

2 black cod fillets

5 ounces string beans, thinly sliced on the diagonal

coconut oil, for drizzling

TO SERVE

2 green onions, thinly sliced on the diagonal

lemon wedges

1–2 teaspoons sesame seeds

In a glass (or other non-corrosive) bowl, combine the miso, brown rice syrup, ginger and sesame oil and stir until smooth. Add the fish fillets, douse and let sit for 5 minutes.

Preheat the oven to 400°F. Lay two sheets of parchment paper (each about 15 × 12 inches) side by side on your kitchen counter. Place half of the beans in the center of each sheet. Top each pile of beans with a fish fillet, spoon over the marinade and drizzle over some coconut oil. Wrap each into a parcel, gift-box style, making sure no juices can escape and no air can get in. This is super-important. Tie the parcels with baking twine for good measure.

Place the parcels on a baking sheet and bake for 9–11 minutes. Serve with the green onions, lemon wedges and a scattering of sesame seeds.

 ½ TEASPOON ADDED SUGAR PER SERVING

1½ SERVINGS VEG + FRUIT PER SERVING

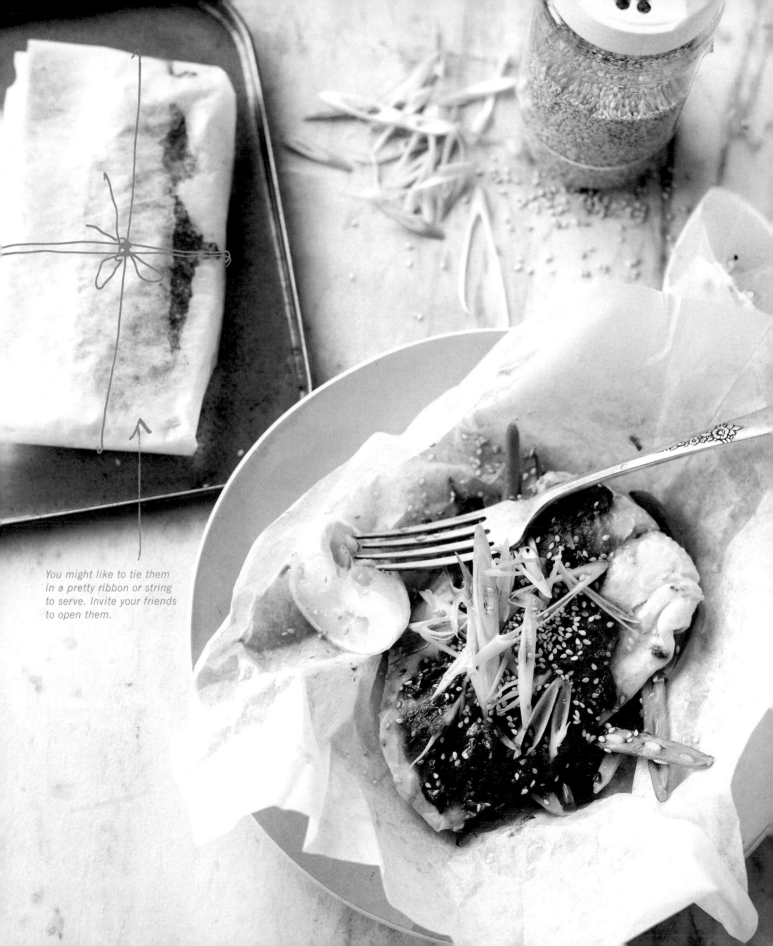

You might like to tie them in a pretty ribbon or string to serve. Invite your friends to open them.

SO I HAVE THIS STACK OF
VEGETABLES . . .

a chapter dedicated to using up that
STACK of BROCCOLI and that huge HEAD of CAULI
and making the most out of the fact that
ZUCCHINI IS ON SALE
right now + making
use of THAT
FROTHING of KALE
that's taking over my fridge.

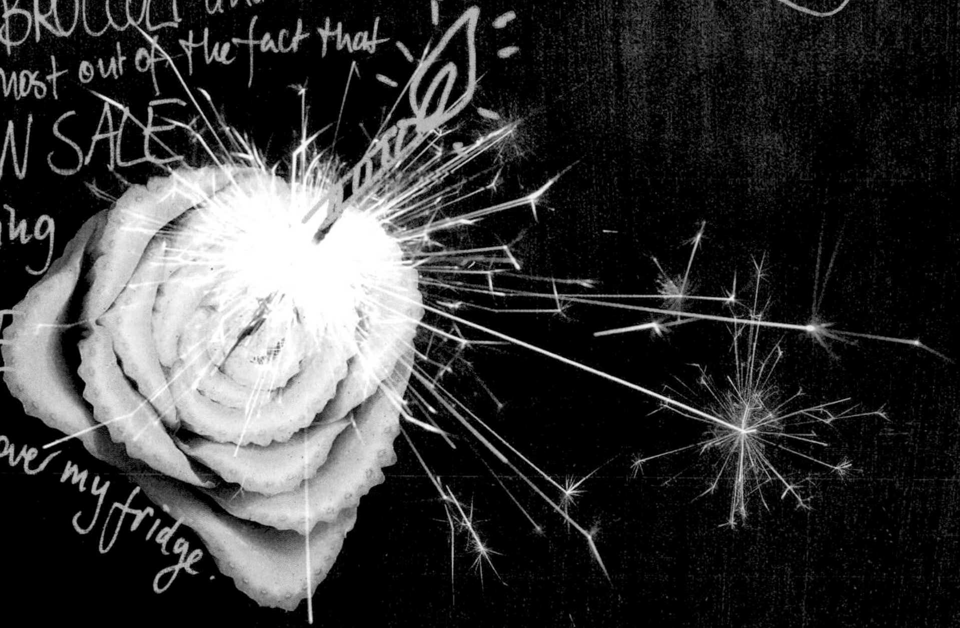

celebrating the
WHOLE VEGETABLE
since 2018

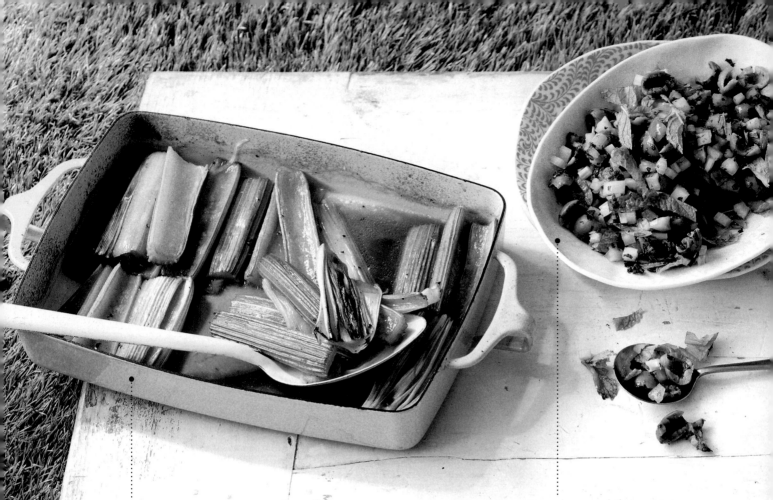

BRAISED CELERY AND LEEKS WITH VANILLA

SERVES 6 AS A SIDE

1 bunch celery, stalks cut into 4-inch lengths (slice the wider stalks in half lengthwise)

1 leek, halved lengthwise, then cut into 4-inch lengths

2 tablespoons butter

1 cup Homemade Stock (chicken or a veggie variation; page 42)

¼ teaspoon pure vanilla extract (or make your own; see page 45) or a pinch of pure vanilla powder

sea salt and freshly ground black pepper

Preheat the oven to 350°F. Arrange the celery and leek in a large baking dish. Dot with the butter. Combine the stock and vanilla and pour over the veggies. Season with salt and pepper. Cover with foil and braise for 30 minutes, then remove the foil and roast for another 30 minutes or until the liquid has reduced to a thick sauce. Serve.

1½ SERVINGS VEG + FRUIT PER SERVING

A SALAD OF CRUSHED OLIVES

SERVES 6 AS A SIDE

1½ cups green olives, pitted

½ bunch celery (including leaves), finely chopped

½ bunch mint, leaves finely chopped

½ cup Powerhouse Dressing (page 53)

Toss the olives with the rest of the ingredients in a serving bowl. Feel free to prepare in advance to slightly "pickle" things a bit.

To be honest, I rarely pit olives; I just warn guests to pit their own – the Italians do this, too. In this recipe, though, you need to.

Pitting olives hack
Place the olives on something flat and use a sturdy coffee mug to press and roll them firmly.

1 SERVING VEG + FRUIT PER SERVING

CELERY AND PINK GRAPEFRUIT GRANITA

SERVES 4–6

½ bunch celery, stalks only, roughly chopped

1 pink grapefruit, peeled, pith and pips removed, and segmented (finely sliced zest for garnish, if you like)

2 tablespoons brown rice syrup

Place the celery and grapefruit on a baking sheet in the freezer for 1 hour. Heat the syrup in a small saucepan with ¼ cup of water and boil for 3 minutes. Plonk the frozen celery and grapefruit in a blender with the syrup and blend until smooth. Pour into a freezer-proof container and freeze for 2 hours, removing every 30 minutes to rake with a fork. Serve as an appetizer or dessert in summer, garnished with zest, if you like. A drizzle of extra-virgin olive oil is nice, too.

USE THE LEFTOVER CELERY HEARTS:
Grow more celery (see page 33).

1 TEASPOON ADDED SUGAR PER SERVING

½ SERVING VEG + FRUIT PER SERVING

CELERY SODA

SERVES 6

I personally don't use a juicer for a number of reasons (see page 13 for some of them). But if I did, I'd make this. So fresh.

½ bunch celery, juiced (reserve a few of the paler, inner leaves)

2 cups coconut water

2 cups soda water

mint sprigs, to serve (optional)

Mix all the ingredients in a large jug. Serve cold with a sprig of inner celery leaf (or a sprig of mint if you prefer).

USE THE LEFTOVER CELERY LEAVES:
Make Leftovers Pesto (page 55) or Celery Leaf Salt (page 265).

½ SERVING VEG + FRUIT PER SERVING

BACK TO THE '70s LETTUCE SOUP

SERVES 6

Romaine lettuce is best in this soup. Or use two gem lettuces or an iceberg instead. A handful of arugula, if it's lying around, can be thrown in, too. I think what gives this the real "crockery and copper-goblet spin" is the frozen peas. Yes?

¼ cup butter

1 tablespoon flour (any kind)

1 leek or onion, chopped

2 cloves garlic, crushed

2 cups Homemade Stock (chicken or a veggie variation; see page 42)

1 nice and big romaine lettuce, chopped

2 cups frozen peas

½ cup mint leaves

juice of ½ lemon

½ teaspoon granulated stevia or 1–2 drops liquid stevia (optional)

sea salt and freshly ground black or white pepper

full-fat organic plain yogurt and your favorite Soup Topper (page 245), to serve

Lettuce is lovelier with white pepper.

Heat the butter in a large saucepan over medium-low heat. Stir in the flour. Add the leek or onion and the garlic and cook until soft (but not browned). Add the stock, 1 cup of water, lettuce and peas and bring to the boil. Plop on a lid, reduce the heat and simmer for about 5 minutes. Remove from the heat. Add the mint, lemon juice and stevia (if using). Purée in the pan using an immersion blender (or transfer to a blender) and season to taste with salt and pepper. Heat again to serve. Or cool, refrigerate and serve cold in summer! Serve with a blob of yogurt or some soup toppers.

USE THE LEFTOVERS FOR A WORK LUNCH:
Pour into jars, freeze and either microwave in the office or, in summer, drink cold like a smoothie.

2 SERVINGS VEG + FRUIT PER SERVING

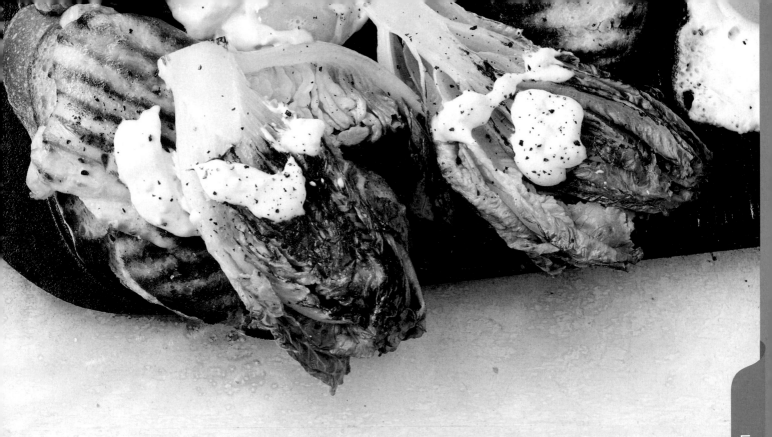

GRILLED CAESAR ON THE BARBIE

SERVES 4

Only trim the base of the lettuces so they don't fall apart when you cut them.

14 ounces chicken thigh fillets, cut into 8 pieces

sea salt and freshly ground black pepper

2 teaspoons olive oil

4 eggs

4 baby romaine lettuces, trimmed and halved lengthwise

4 slices leftover (stale) sourdough bread (optional)

CAESAR DRESSING

½ cup Whey-Good Mayo (page 50)

5 anchovies, finely chopped

1 clove Good for Your Guts Garlic (page 340), crushed

To make the dressing, combine the mayo, anchovies and garlic in a small bowl. Season with salt and pepper and mix well. Thin, if desired, with 1–2 teaspoons of water.

No barbie? Use a large skillet.

Season the chicken with salt and pepper. Preheat an electric grill on high heat. Reduce the heat to medium-high and grill the chicken for 3–4 minutes on each side, or until lightly charred and cooked through. While the chicken is cooking, add some oil to a skillet and fry the eggs for 2–3 minutes, or until set. Add the lettuce to the grill, cut side down, and the bread (if using), and grill for 1–2 minutes. Serve drizzled with the dressing.

2 SERVINGS VEG + FRUIT PER SERVING

HAVE SOME LETTUCE WITH YOUR DRESSING

SERVES 6 AS A SIDE

Bring your salad to the dressing party with this dead-simple concept.

1 iceberg lettuce, chopped into 12 thick wedges

1 cup Green Minx Dressing (page 54)

Arrange the wedges on a platter and pour the dressing over them.

½ SERVING VEG + FRUIT PER SERVING

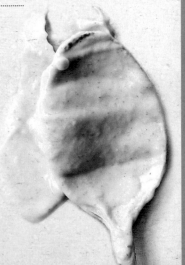

Know your LEAFY GREENS

Don't have kale? Most leafy greens can be used interchangeably. Mix it up!

Why bitter greens?
* They rank as the most nutrient-dense of all vegetables.
* They stimulate enzymes and bile, assisting digestion.
* They balance sugar cravings.

BEET LEAVES
Use as you would chard.

CAVOLO NERO
Also called Tuscan kale, black cabbage or lacinato.

SPINACH

WATERCRESS
The most nutrient-dense vegetable on the planet, according to researchers at William Paterson University.

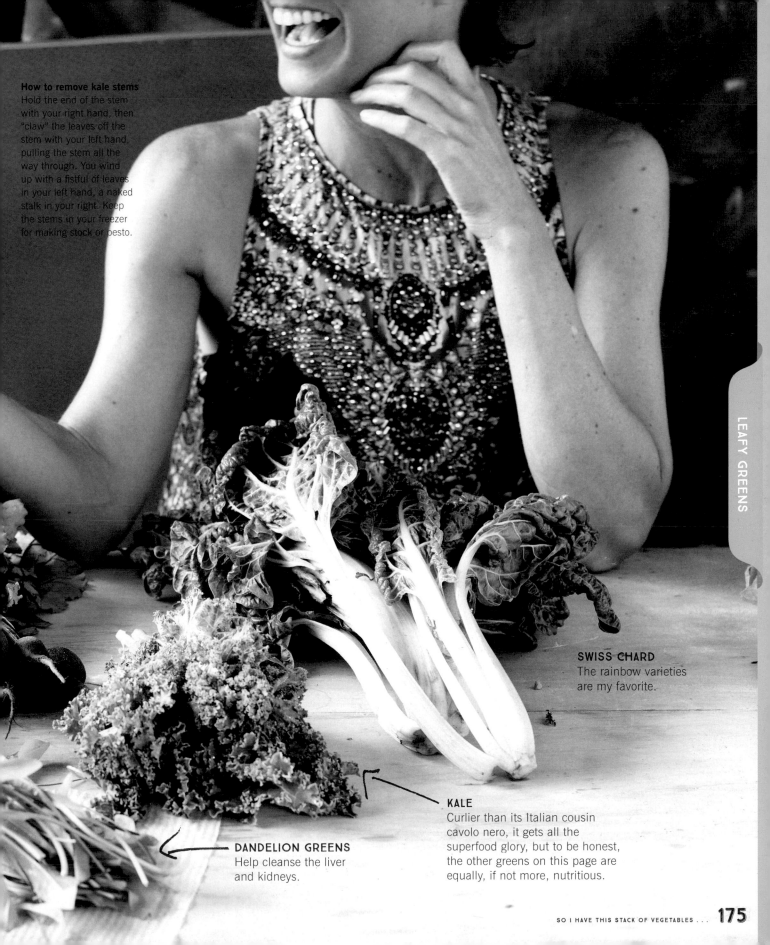

How to remove kale stems
Hold the end of the stem with your right hand, then "claw" the leaves off the stem with your left hand, pulling the stem all the way through. You wind up with a fistful of leaves in your left hand, a naked stalk in your right. Keep the stems in your freezer for making stock or pesto.

SWISS CHARD
The rainbow varieties are my favorite.

KALE
Curlier than its Italian cousin cavolo nero, it gets all the superfood glory, but to be honest, the other greens on this page are equally, if not more, nutritious.

DANDELION GREENS
Help cleanse the liver and kidneys.

SO I HAVE THIS STACK OF VEGETABLES . . . **175**

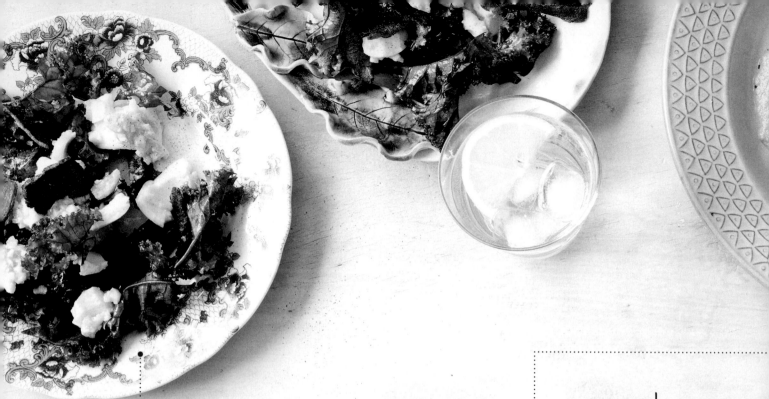

HIPSTER GRANDDADDY SALAD

SERVES 6 AS A SIDE, 2 AS A MEAL

A salad with bacon, egg and white pepper always reminds me of my granddad, who added white pepper and celery salt to everything. The massaged kale gives this old-school salad a modern edge.

1 batch of Massaged Kale (page 23)

4 hard-boiled eggs, roughly chopped

¾ cup Bacon Bits (page 44; optional)

1 teaspoon ground white pepper

Celery Leaf Salt (page 265) or sea salt, to taste

Toss your kale with the eggs, bacon, pepper and salt.

WATERCRESS SAUCE AND SOME EGGS

SERVES 2

⅓ cup extra-virgin olive oil

1 onion, thinly sliced

2 cloves garlic, minced

1 bunch watercress, washed, dried and chopped

sea salt

4 hard-boiled eggs, halved

Heat 1 tablespoon of the olive oil in a skillet over medium-low heat. Add the onion and sauté until translucent. Add the garlic and cook for a further 2 minutes or until fragrant. Add the watercress and allow to wilt until the stems are softened (about 5 minutes).

Transfer to a blender with the remaining oil and ⅓ cup of water. Blend until smooth. Season to taste with salt. To serve, place the eggs on a plate and drizzle with watercress sauce.

Reminder!

To dry watercress, place in a clean, sealable laundry bag in your washing machine and run on the last spin cycle for 30 seconds or so to remove water by centrifugal force.

2 SERVINGS VEG + FRUIT PER SERVING

2 SERVINGS VEG + FRUIT PER SERVING

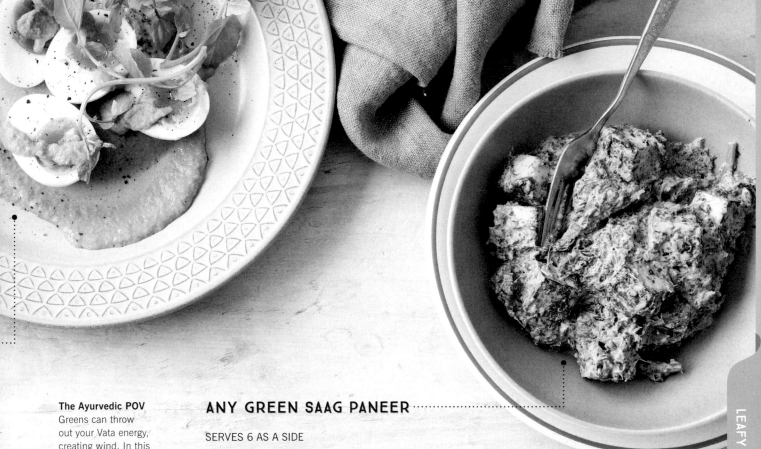

The Ayurvedic POV
Greens can throw out your Vata energy, creating wind. In this dish, paneer, a fresh cheese much like haloumi, comes to the rescue along with some good-quality fat and gently warming spices, reducing your Vata without aggravating your Pitta. Got it?

ANY GREEN SAAG PANEER

SERVES 6 AS A SIDE

2 tablespoons ghee (or coconut oil, though ghee is best)

9 ounces Homemade Paneer (page 48) or haloumi, cut into ¾-inch cubes

1 large onion, chopped

2 cloves garlic, minced

¾-inch knob of ginger, minced

2 teaspoons freshly minced turmeric or Fermented Turmeric Paste (page 340) or ½ teaspoon ground turmeric

3 teaspoons Ras el Hanout Mix (page 45) or 1 teaspoon each ground coriander, ground cumin and cayenne pepper

½ teaspoon freshly ground black pepper

18 ounces greens, rinsed and chopped

big pinch of sea salt

2–3 tablespoons full-fat organic plain yogurt (optional)

Green options: 2 small bunches of spinach (older, tougher spinach is best—baby leaves won't get the same result) or 1 small bunch of chard or 1 bunch of mustard leaves, dandelion greens, beet leaves, kale or watercress with ½ bunch of spinach.

Heat half the ghee or oil in a large saucepan over medium-high heat and cook the paneer or haloumi until golden. Set aside on a plate. Heat the remaining ghee or oil in the same pan and sauté the onion, garlic and ginger until soft. Add all the spices and sauté until very golden (about 5 minutes). If the spices start to stick, add a little water. Add the greens and salt, cover and cook for 5–10 minutes. (If your pan isn't big enough, add the greens gradually.) Once cooked, purée using an immersion blender or food processor. Stir in the yogurt only if you're after a creamier texture. Add the paneer or haloumi and heat for 5 minutes before serving.

MAKE IT VEGAN:
Use tofu instead of cheese.

 1 SERVING VEG + FRUIT PER SERVING

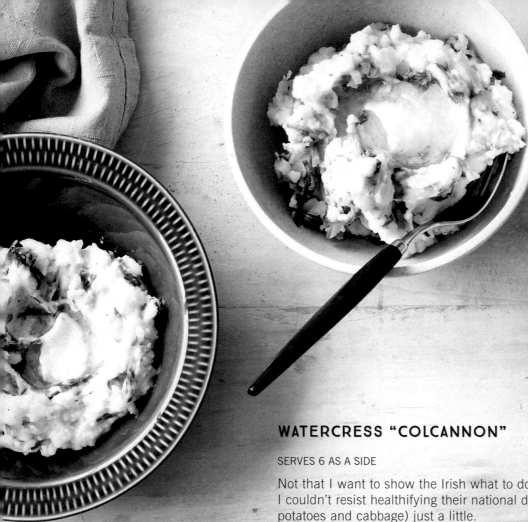

WATERCRESS "COLCANNON"

SERVES 6 AS A SIDE

Not that I want to show the Irish what to do with a spud, but I couldn't resist healthifying their national dish (usually made with potatoes and cabbage) just a little.

Just scrub the spuds; no need to peel. →

2 pounds "white" veggies (potatoes, cauliflower, parsnips, celeriac, turnip), chopped

⅓ cup butter, plus extra to serve

1 leek, chopped

1 bunch watercress, dandelion greens or chard, roughly chopped

1 cup milk

sea salt and freshly ground black pepper

MAKE IT ORANGE:
Replace half the white veggies with sweet potatoes and carrots.

MAKE IT MEATY:
Add 3 slices of bacon, chopped, when cooking the leek.

MAKE IT SUMMERY:
Mash in 1 cup of peas and ½ bunch of mint.

Place the white veggies in a stockpot or large saucepan with enough water to cover. Bring to the boil, covered, over a high heat. Reduce the heat and simmer for 15 minutes or until soft. Drain.

Meanwhile, melt the butter in a large stockpot over medium heat. Add the leek and cook for 3–5 minutes or until soft. Add the greens and cook for 5 minutes, or until the leaves are wilted and the stems are soft. Add the milk and heat until it bubbles. Add the cooked white veggies and season with salt and pepper. Mash with a potato masher or fork, leaving a few clumpy bits.

To serve, mound the mash into bowls. Use the back of a spoon to make an impression in the center and fill with a pat of softened butter. Once the butter melts, each forkful should be dipped into the well of butter before eating.

 3 SERVINGS VEG + FRUIT PER SERVING

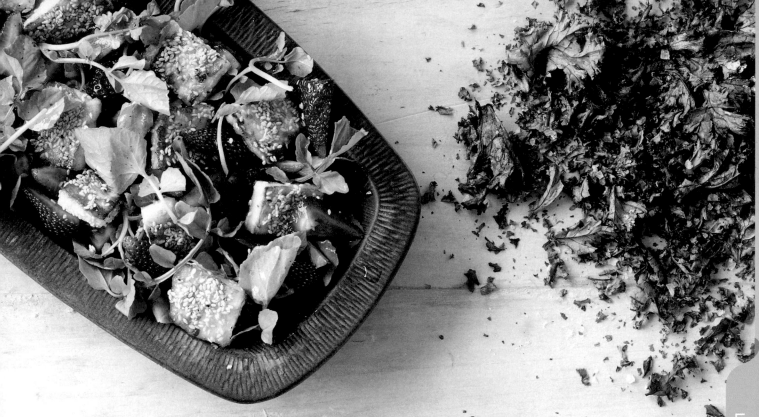

SESAME-CRUSTED HALOUMI AND STRAWBERRY SALAD

SERVES 6 AS A SIDE

¼ cup sesame seeds (white is best, but use what you've got)

sea salt and freshly ground black pepper

9 ounces haloumi (or Homemade Paneer; page 48), cut into 1¼-inch squares, ¼ inch thick

2 tablespoons coconut oil, melted

½ pound strawberries, hulled and quartered

1 bunch watercress, tough stems removed and leaves torn into bite-sized bits

½ cup Powerhouse Dressing (page 53)

Sprinkle the sesame seeds on a plate and season to taste with salt and pepper. Place the haloumi or paneer in a bowl with the coconut oil and toss gently to coat. Roll the cheese squares in the sesame seeds until evenly coated.

Cook the haloumi or paneer in a skillet over medium-high heat until lightly browned on both sides. Toss the remaining ingredients in a bowl and top with the cooked haloumi or paneer.

KALE FLAKES

MAKES ½–1 CUP

Use these salty green flakes as a salad, soup or stew topper or mix them with toasted sesame seeds and Activated Groaties (page 27) for a nutrient-dense snack.

1 bunch kale or cavolo nero, stems removed and leaves torn

1 teaspoon sea salt flakes

Preheat the oven to 400°F. Place the leaves on a baking sheet in a single layer (you may need two sheets) and sprinkle with salt. Bake for 10–15 minutes, until crispy and crunchy.

When cool, crumble in your hands into small flakes or process briefly in a food processor. Store in an airtight container for up to 1 week.

½ SERVING VEG + FRUIT PER SERVING

2 SERVINGS VEG + FRUIT PER SERVING

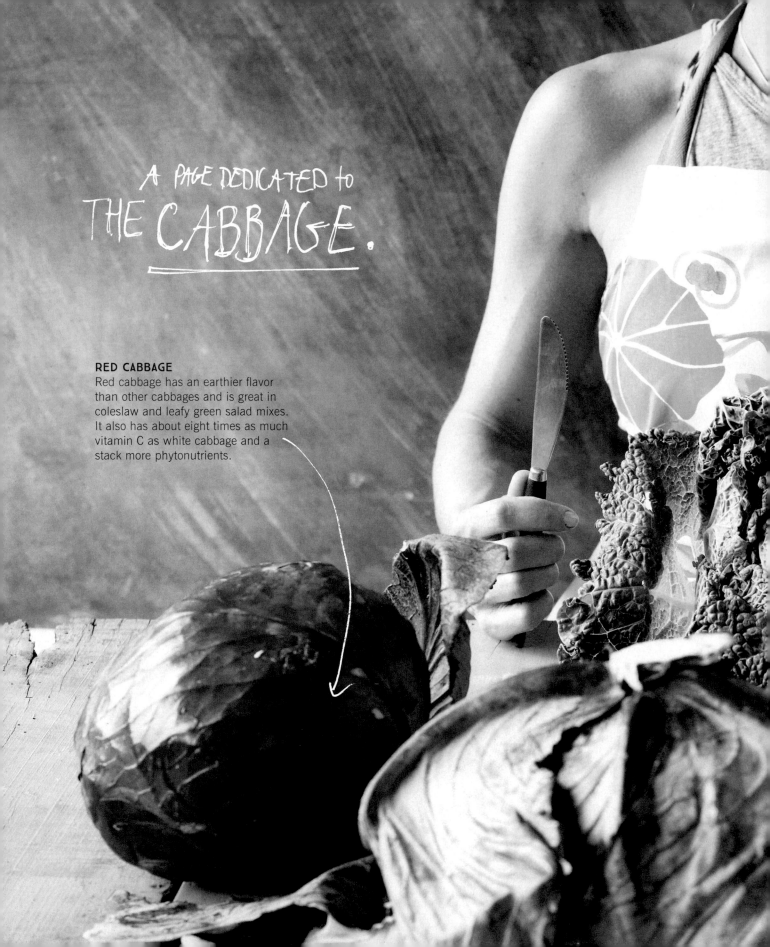

A PAGE DEDICATED to THE CABBAGE.

RED CABBAGE

Red cabbage has an earthier flavor than other cabbages and is great in coleslaw and leafy green salad mixes. It also has about eight times as much vitamin C as white cabbage and a stack more phytonutrients.

SAVOY
Leaves are tender, even when eaten raw. This makes them perfect for salads and wraps, and as a bed for other dishes. Savoy also lacks the sulfur-like pong when cooked, if that matters to you.

WHITE CABBAGE
Also known as patta gobi, it's held in high esteem as it works well in a multitude of dishes. Use it raw in salads or boiled or braised.

NAPA
Also called Chinese cabbage, it's widely used in East Asian cuisine. Great raw in salads and cooked in dumplings and spring rolls.

other cabbages not pictured: brussels sprouts, bok choy, choy sum

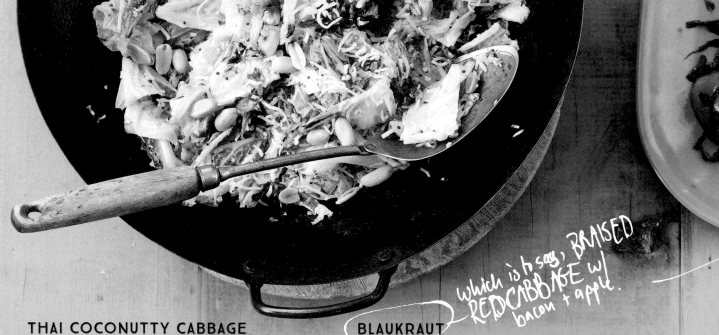

which is to say, BRAISED REDCABBAGE w/ bacon + apple.

THAI COCONUTTY CABBAGE

SERVES 2

2 tablespoons coconut oil

2 teaspoons mustard seeds

4 cloves garlic, minced

1–2 green chilies, sliced

1 teaspoon ground turmeric
or 2 tablespoons Fermented
Turmeric Paste (page 340)

1 teaspoon ground cumin

½ teaspoon freshly ground
black pepper

½ head cabbage (savoy or
napa), coarsely chopped

big pinch of sea salt

½ cup shredded coconut

chopped peanuts, to serve
(optional)

handful of cilantro leaves,
chopped, to serve (optional)

Heat the oil in a large wok or saucepan over medium-
high heat and cook the mustard seeds until they
start to pop. Add the garlic, chili, turmeric, cumin
and pepper and sauté for another minute. Add the
cabbage and salt and turn down the heat to very low.
Cook, covered, until the cabbage has softened (about
8 minutes). If the cabbage is still quite liquid-y, cook
for a few more minutes, uncovered. Remove from
the heat and add the coconut. Serve sprinkled with
chopped peanuts and cilantro, if desired.

MAKE IT A MEAL:

Add 1 cup of basmati rice and 2½ cups
of Homemade Stock (page 42) and cook for an
additional 15 minutes. Or toss through some
Shredded Chicken (page 214).

BLAUKRAUT

SERVES 6 AS A SIDE

6 slices bacon, cubed

1 onion, halved and
thinly sliced

2 apples, green or red,
cored and cut into
¾-inch wedges

1 red cabbage, cored,
quartered and thinly sliced

sea salt and freshly ground
black pepper

1 tablespoon caraway or
fennel seeds, lightly crushed
using a mortar and pestle

1 tablespoon apple
cider vinegar

1–2 tablespoons brown
rice syrup or ½–1 teaspoon
granulated stevia

½ cup Homemade Chicken
Stock (page 42) or water

¼ cup red wine (or
additional stock or water)

chopped hazelnuts
(preferably activated; see
page 28), to serve

Cook the bacon in a stockpot or large saucepan
over medium heat, stirring occasionally, until the fat
renders and the bacon is crisp (about 8 minutes). Add
the onion and apple and cook, stirring, until the onion
softens (4–6 minutes). Stir in the cabbage and season
with salt and pepper. Add the caraway or fennel seeds
and deglaze with the apple cider vinegar. Add the rest
of the ingredients and bring to a boil. Reduce the heat,
cover, and simmer until the cabbage is tender (20–25
minutes). Serve sprinkled with the hazelnuts.

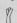 ½ TEASPOON ADDED SUGAR PER SERVING

1 SERVING VEG + FRUIT PER SERVING

1½ SERVINGS VEG + FRUIT PER SERVING

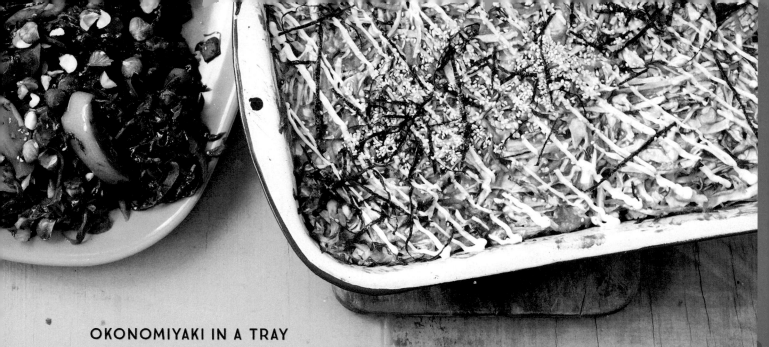

OKONOMIYAKI IN A TRAY

SERVES 6 AS A LIGHT MEAL

Okonomiyaki, usually served as a pancake for one, has always struck me as a fiddly dish crying out for a dumping of leftover veggies. So I bulked it up, packed in whatever I had in the fridge and threw it in a baking dish. Bam.

3 cups finely shredded cabbage and/or brussels sprouts

2 cups grated sweet potato or carrot (or another colorful veggie like leftover peas, corn, etc.)

½ bunch green onions, thinly sliced

6 eggs, whisked

2 tablespoons tamari

1 cup buckwheat flour (or any flour)

1 cup Whey-Good Mayo (page 50)

2 tablespoons sesame seeds

¼ cup "But the Kitchen Sink" Kimchi (page 337; optional)

1 nori sheet, cut into thin strips

Preheat the oven to 350°F and grease a large baking dish. Place the cabbage, grated veggies and green onions in a large bowl and toss. Stir through the eggs, tamari and flour until a batter forms. Dump the mixture into the baking dish. Bake for 30 minutes, or until the top starts to brown and the eggs have cooked through. Remove from the oven. Place the mayo in a zip-lock bag or small plastic bag and trim one corner (or use a piping bag) and squeeze out in even lines over the pancake. Sprinkle with the sesame seeds, kimchi (if using) and nori strips. Freeze the unused okonomiyaki in per-serve portions for up to 3 months.

2 SERVINGS VEG + FRUIT PER SERVING

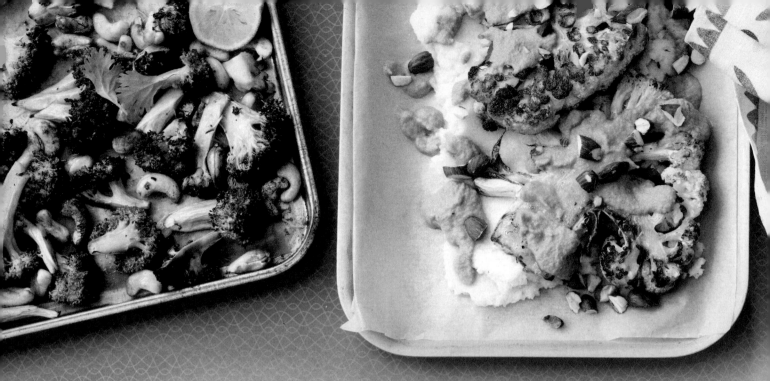

ASIAN CASHEW CRISP

SERVES 2

¼ cup coconut oil or ghee, plus extra for greasing

1 large head broccoli or cauliflower (or a combo of both), cut into small florets, including the stalk

½ teaspoon chili flakes

⅓ cup cashews (preferably activated; see page 28)

1 tablespoon fish sauce

lime wedges, to serve

cilantro leaves, to serve

Preheat the oven to 425°F. Line a baking sheet with parchment paper and brush (or spray) with oil. Toss all the ingredients together in a large bowl until well coated. Spread over the prepared sheet. Bake, turning once or twice, until the florets have crunchy blackened bits (about 20–30 minutes). Serve with lime wedges and fresh cilantro.

CAULIFLOWER TARTINES WITH GREEN GODDESS DRESSING AND HAZELNUTS

SERVES 2

1 head cauliflower

1 tablespoon coconut oil, plus extra for greasing

sea salt and freshly ground black pepper

a sprinkle of ground cumin

¼ cup chopped almonds or hazelnuts (preferably activated; see page 28)

1 tablespoon butter

2 tablespoons grated Parmesan

½ cup Leftovers Pesto (page 55) blended with ½ avocado or ½ cup Green Minx Dressing (page 54)

Preheat the oven to 425°F. Line a baking sheet with parchment paper and brush (or spray) with oil.

Remove any outer leaves from the cauliflower, but keep the stem intact. Place the cauli on a chopping board, stem side down. Cut two 1¼-inch-thick slices from the center of your cauli, ensuring they're nice and straight. Reserve the rest of the cauliflower for the purée, below.

Place the cauli steaks on the prepared sheet and rub with oil. Season generously with salt, pepper and cumin. Roast for 25–35 minutes, gently turning after 15 minutes, until the cauli is browned and the stems feel tender when pierced with a knife. In the final 10 minutes add the nuts to the sheet.

Meanwhile, steam (or microwave) the reserved cauliflower until soft. Place in a deep bowl with the butter and Parmesan. Using an immersion blender, purée until smooth.

Spoon the purée onto a platter and top with the steaks. Drizzle with the dressing and top with the toasted nuts.

You can also barbecue or pan-fry your cauli steaks—4–5 minutes for each side should do the job.

3 SERVINGS VEG + FRUIT PER SERVING

4 SERVINGS VEG + FRUIT PER SERVING

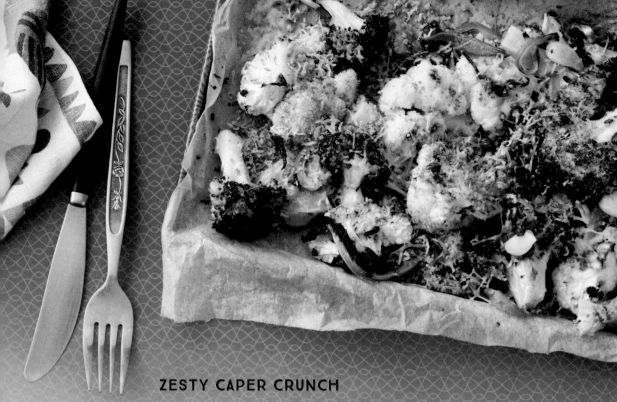

ZESTY CAPER CRUNCH

SERVES 2

¼ cup coconut oil or ghee,
plus extra for greasing

1 large head broccoli or cauliflower
(or a combo of both), cut into small
florets, including the stalk

1 red onion, halved and sliced into
thin wedges

5 cloves garlic, thinly sliced

¼ cup baby capers
(preferably in salt)

½ teaspoon chili flakes

½ teaspoon sea salt

½ cup Cooked Quinoa (page 26)
or Cooked Buckwheat (page 27)
or bread crumbs

¼ cup grated Parmesan

2 tablespoons lemon zest

*If you use a combo of
cauliflower and broccoli,
cut your cauli florets smaller
than your broccoli ones!*

Preheat the oven to 425°F. Line a large baking
sheet with parchment paper and brush (or spray)
with oil. In a large bowl, toss the broccoli and/or
cauli with the onion, garlic, capers, oil, chili and
salt, then spread over the prepared sheet. Bake,
turning once or twice, for 15 minutes. Sprinkle
with the quinoa, buckwheat or bread crumbs and
bake for a further 5–10 minutes, or until golden.
Serve sprinkled with Parmesan and lemon zest.

4 SERVINGS VEG + FRUIT PER SERVING

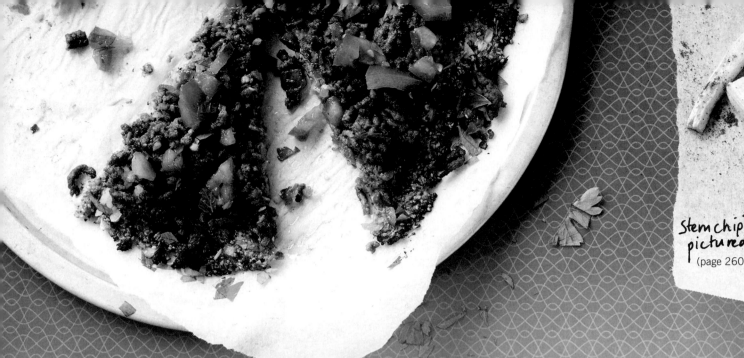

Stem chips pictured here (page 260)

LEBANESE ROLL PIZZA

SERVES 2

1 head broccoli, roughly chopped (including the stalk)

6 ounces cheddar (or any hard cheese)

¼ cup chia seeds

sea salt and freshly ground black pepper

2 tablespoons coconut oil, melted

½ red onion, chopped

1 clove garlic, chopped

9 ounces ground lamb or beef

1 teaspoon chili flakes

1 teaspoon ground coriander seeds

TO SERVE

½ cup roughly chopped flat-leaf parsley

1 large tomato, chopped

½ teaspoon finely chopped Good for Your Guts Garlic (page 340)

lemon wedges

Preheat the oven to 425°F and line a baking sheet with parchment paper.

Pulse the broc in a food processor to form small chunks, then transfer to a bowl. Place the cheese in the processor and pulse to form rough crumbs. Add the cheese to the broccoli, stir in the chia seeds and season with salt and pepper. Press the mixture onto the prepared sheet to make a thick "pizza" base. Drizzle with 1 tablespoon of the coconut oil and bake for 15 minutes.

Meanwhile, heat the remaining coconut oil in a large skillet over medium heat. Add the onion and sauté for a couple of minutes. Turn up the heat to medium-high, add the garlic and meat and cook for 2 minutes. Add the chili and coriander and cook for another 2 minutes or until most of the liquid has evaporated.

Remove the pizza base from the oven and scatter the meat and onion mixture over it. Return to the oven and bake for 5 minutes. To serve, scatter the parsley, tomato and garlic over it, and squeeze some lemon juice on top.

MAKE IT VEGAN:

Use Vegan "Ground Meat" (right) instead of the ground lamb or beef.

⸙ 4 SERVINGS VEG + FRUIT PER SERVING

VEGAN "GROUND MEAT"

MAKES 4 CUPS

Use in tacos, on pizza, or sprinkled over spaghetti. Just don't add it to a sauce as it will dissolve.

Yes, you read it right—this ain't no frankenfood, and the smoky, meaty taste is really rather remarkable!

1 head cauliflower, roughly chopped (including the stalk)

2 cups walnuts

2 tablespoons coconut oil

3 cloves garlic, minced

½ teaspoon smoked paprika

2 teaspoons ground cumin

1 teaspoon each sea salt and freshly ground black pepper

2 tablespoons tamari, soy sauce or coconut aminos

Preheat the oven to 350°F and line a baking sheet with parchment paper. Blend the cauli and nuts in a blender to a rice consistency (not a powder). Place in a large bowl and add the remaining ingredients, kneading with your hands to combine. Dump the mixture onto the baking sheet and spread out evenly. Bake for 45–75 minutes, tossing every 20 minutes or so to ensure the whole lot browns. Cool, then divide into ½-cup portions and freeze for up to 3 months.

⸙ 1 SERVING VEG + FRUIT PER SERVING

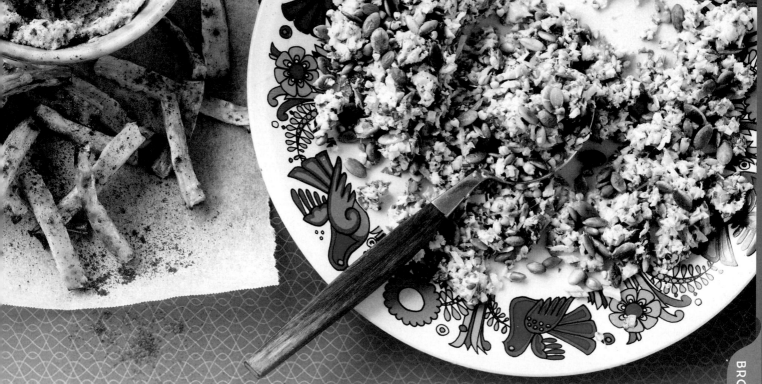

THE WHOLE BRASSICUS HUMMUS

MAKES 3 CUPS

This recipe ingeniously creates a hummin' hummus and some tasty stem chips to go with.

1 head broccoli or cauliflower (or a combo), chopped (reserve stems/stalks if you're making chips (see page 260), or just throw them in, too)

3 cloves garlic

¼ cup coconut oil, olive oil, butter or ghee, melted

½ cup TMT Dressing (page 53) or ¼ cup tahini mixed with the juice and zest of 1 lemon

½ teaspoon ground cumin

sea salt and freshly ground black pepper

Sweet Paprika Stem Chips (page 260), to serve (optional)

If you're not making the chips, feel free to steam the cauli and/or broc lightly instead of baking, and wring it out in a dishtowel to remove all the moisture. Saves turning on the oven!

Preheat the oven to 350°F. Place the broc and/or cauli and garlic on a baking sheet. Drizzle over 2 tablespoons of oil, butter or ghee and roast for 20 minutes, turning halfway. Transfer to a food processor or blender with the remaining oil and the dressing and cumin. Process until well combined. Add more oil if it's too dry, or some chia seeds if it's too moist. Season with salt and pepper. Store in a jar in the fridge for up to 1 week.

MAKE IT BULKIER:
Add 1 cup of cooked chickpeas, and some extra dressing.

1 SERVING VEG + FRUIT PER SERVING

CRUNCHY BROCCOLI BUCKWHEAT TABOULI

SERVES 6 AS A SIDE

1 large head broccoli, roughly chopped (including the stalk)

¼ cup pepitas (preferably activated; page 28)

½ cup Activated Groaties (page 27)

1 cup finely chopped flat-leaf parsley

1 cup finely chopped mint

½ red onion, finely chopped

½ cup Whey-Good Mayo (page 50) whisked with the juice and zest of 1 lemon

small handful of something small, red and lovely: pomegranate seeds, edible flowers, red currants, goji berries (very optional)

Process the broccoli in a food processor to a rice consistency. Transfer to a large heatproof bowl and pour over enough boiling water to cover. Set aside for 3–4 minutes. Drain, allow to cool and return to the bowl. Dry-roast the pepitas in a small skillet over medium heat and add to the broccoli, along with the remaining ingredients.

MAKE IT A MEAL:
Add hard-boiled eggs, halved, or Shredded Chicken (page 214).

1½ SERVINGS VEG + FRUIT PER SERVING

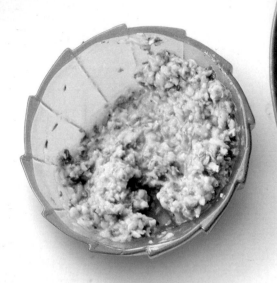

QUICK ZUCCHINI TZATZIKI

MAKES ABOUT 2 CUPS

1 cup grated fresh or frozen zucchini

1 cup full-fat organic plain yogurt

2 cloves Good for Your Guts Garlic (page 340) or 2 teaspoons minced garlic or other ferment

1 tablespoon brine (see page 334) or lemon juice

Combine all of the ingredients in a glass jar and store in the fridge for 2–3 days.

ZUCCHINI NO-CARBONARA

SERVES 2

1 pound zucchini (3–4 medium ones)

sea salt

1 egg, plus 1 egg yolk

¼ cup finely grated Parmesan, plus extra to serve

freshly ground black pepper

1½ tablespoons butter

½ cup Bacon Bits (page 44) or 3–4 strips bacon, rind removed, diced

Using a spiralizer or julienne peeler, slice the zucchini into noodles and place in a colander. Sprinkle with a little salt and leave for 10 minutes to drain. Blot gently with a dishtowel to remove excess moisture if required.

In a small bowl whisk together the egg, egg yolk and Parmesan until well combined. Season with freshly ground black pepper (the more the better!). Heat the butter in a large skillet over medium-high heat. Cook the Bacon Bits for 1–2 minutes or until hot; if using fresh bacon, cook for longer. Add the zucchini and cook for 1 minute. Add the egg mixture, tossing briefly to coat. Serve immediately, sprinkled with the extra Parmesan.

USE THE LEFTOVER EGG WHITE:
Make an omelette. You can freeze the egg white in the meantime by popping it in an ice-cube tray and then transferring the cube to a zip-lock bag. Or simply use 2 whole eggs and deal with a runnier sauce!

Pasta-making tip
The strips made from the center part of the zucchini tend to break more easily. If you want perfect-looking pasta, don't use the center parts (freeze them to make Zucchini Butter, right).

 ½ SERVING VEG + FRUIT PER SERVING

 1½ SERVINGS VEG + FRUIT PER SERVING

Make some zucchini booster
Grate a heap, freeze them in 1-cup servings and use them to bulk out nutrients. They dissolve and disguise themselves very easily, fooling most kids. Add to stews, pasta sauces, salads, smoothies (true story), muffins, cakes . . . You get the drift.

Note, however, that they will increase the liquid content of baked goods. So be sure to strain after grating (wring them robustly with your hands or in a clean dishtowel).

ZUCCHINI BUTTER

MAKES 2¼ CUPS

¼ cup butter

2–3 shallots (or 1 small onion), finely chopped

2 tablespoons thyme leaves

2 pounds zucchini (4–5 big ones), coarsely grated and squeezed to remove the juices

sea salt and freshly ground black pepper

Heat the butter in a large skillet over medium-high heat. Sauté the shallots or onion for 15 minutes until caramelized. Add the thyme and zucchini and season with salt and pepper. Cook, stirring a little, for 20 minutes, or until the zucchini has reduced by more than half. This will keep in the fridge for up to 1 month.

FIVE WAYS TO EAT ZUCCHINI BUTTER:

1. On a wedge of Socca (page 106).
2. Spread on toast.
3. As a soup topper.
4. Dolloped on pasta.
5. Added to a Salad of the Scoundrel (pages 252–53).

½ SERVING VEG + FRUIT PER SERVING

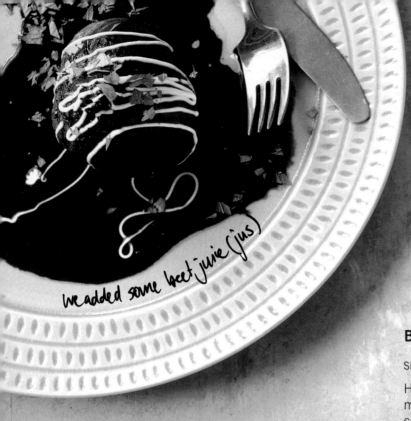

we added some beet juice (jus)

A REALLY FAT BEET
PLACED PRETTILY ON A PLATE

SERVES 6

6 large beets

coconut oil, melted, for drizzling

sea salt and freshly ground black pepper

chopped basil, to garnish

Preheat the oven to 350°F. Wash and dry the beets and place them in a baking dish. Drizzle with coconut oil and season with salt and pepper. Roast for 30–40 minutes. You can check if they're done after 30 minutes by sticking a knife in the center of the largest beet; if it slides in easily, they're done. Let them cool. Trim the stalks and peel the beets if you like—the skins will slip right off. Pour the beet juice into a small saucepan and heat over medium-high heat until reduced. Serve with the beets.

MAKE IT PRETTIER:
Drizzle with Whey-Good Mayo (page 50) or Homemade Cream Cheese (page 46)—use a piping bag or an old zip-lock bag with one corner snipped—and scatter with edible flowers.

. I eat the skins, or put into a sandwich

🍴 2 SERVINGS VEG + FRUIT PER SERVING

BEET HALWA

SERVES 6

Halwa is an Indian dessert mostly made with sweetened condensed milk. I provide, forthwith, a far more nutritionally grounding version.

⅓ cup ghee or butter

3 large beets, trimmed, scrubbed and grated (about 4½ cups)

2½ cups milk (any milk, but full-fat dairy is best)

¼ cup brown rice syrup

1 teaspoon ground cardamom

1 cup pistachios or cashews, activated (page 28) or toasted and chopped

Melt the ghee or butter in a heavy-bottomed saucepan over low heat. Add the beets and sauté gently for 5 minutes. Add the milk and bring to a boil. Reduce the heat and simmer for about 20 minutes (it might take longer, depending on how much liquid's in your beets), stirring occasionally, until the mixture thickens and begins to look glossy.

Add the brown rice syrup and stir for a few minutes. Keep stirring throughout to prevent sticking. Add the ground cardamom and continue to simmer, stirring constantly, until all of the liquid has evaporated and the mixture is thick and glossy and starts to pull away from the side of the pan. Pour into serving bowls, sprinkle with nuts and serve warm or chilled.

🍴 1½ TEASPOON ADDED SUGAR PER SERVING

🍴 1 SERVING VEG + FRUIT PER SERVING

feel free to reduce the amount of brown rice syrup, or use 1 tsp stevia instead.

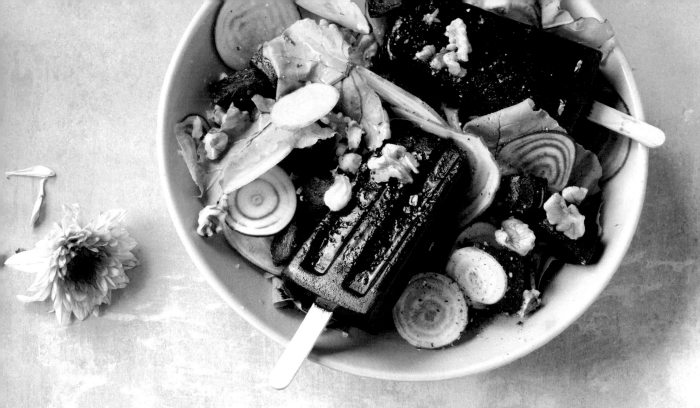

BEET THAT POPSTICK SALAD

SERVES 6

I made this at my 40th birthday, based on a dish I'd seen done by notoriously recalcitrant chef Colin Fassnidge at his sustainably minded restaurant 4Fourteen. As he told me via Twitter, he uses my first cookbook as a doorstop. I took it as a compliment.

USE THE LEFTOVER BIGGER, COARSER BEET GREENS:
Make Massaged Beet Greens (page 23)—my favorite—or Leftovers Pesto (page 55).

3 red beets, trimmed, peeled and chopped into ¾-inch chunks

¾ cup frozen raspberries

2 tablespoons lemon juice

2 yellow or other colored beets (if you can't find any, use 2 large carrots)

3 handfuls of baby beet leaves or arugula leaves

¼ cup walnuts (preferably activated; see page 28), roughly chopped

1 tablespoon apple cider vinegar

1 tablespoon extra-virgin olive oil

pinch of sea salt

If you'd like your beets a little crispier, pan-fry quickly in a little coconut oil.

Place the red beets in a saucepan with enough water to cover. Bring to a boil (with the lid on) and cook for 20 minutes, or until cooked through, but not mushy. Strain, reserving the precious bright-red beet water. Place 1½ cups of the beet water in a blender with the raspberries and lemon juice and blend until smooth. Pour into six ice pop molds, add the sticks, and place in the freezer to set for 6 hours.

Slice the yellow beets into super-thin rounds (with a mandoline if you have one) or peel the carrot into long ribbons with a vegetable peeler (or mandoline). Place in a serving bowl with the cooled red beet chunks, leaves and walnuts. Toss gently with the vinegar, olive oil and salt.

To serve, remove the beet popsticks from the molds by running them under hot water and place them on top of the salad.

 2 SERVINGS VEG + FRUIT PER SERVING

JUST LIKE

GRANDMA

USED TO MAKE

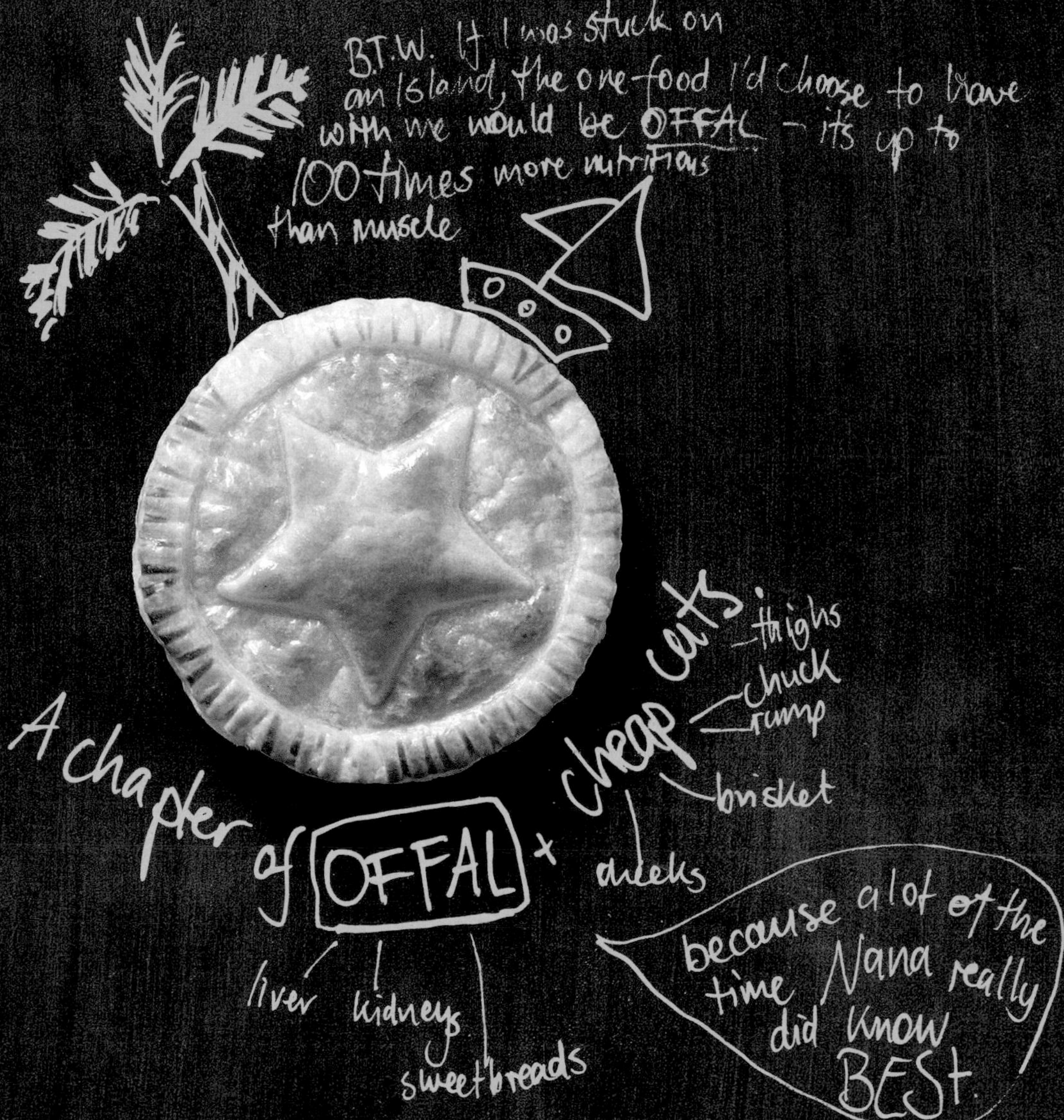

B.T.W. If I was stuck on
an island, the one food I'd choose to leave
with me would be OFFAL — it's up to
100 times more nutritious
than muscle

A chapter of OFFAL + cheap cuts :

— thighs
— chuck
— rump
— brisket
cheeks

liver kidneys
sweetbreads

because a lot of the
time Nana really
did know
BEST.

MUM'S STEAK AND KIDNEY STEW WITH HERBY DUMPLINGS

SERVES 6

Mum's original recipe comes from a little cookbook that her local butcher gave her when she got married at 21. It espoused using cheap cuts, and eating a little meat at each meal, including breakfast (with carbs and sugar limited). These principles were very much pivotal in my early eating.

I've tweaked her recipe a little, tossing in some mushrooms, which can help to "disguise" the kidneys if you're not used to them, and adding dumplings for an extra granny effect.

Why Mum made us eat kidneys

* They're high in iron: One kidney (about 3 ounces) = RDI of iron for women = 5 bags of baby spinach.
* They are one of the richest sources of selenium, an antioxidant that aids thyroid function and helps prevent tissue damage.
* They're stupidly cheap.

Buy your kidneys already skinned from your butcher.

1 onion, sliced

1½ cups cubed mushrooms (any variety is fine)

2 cloves garlic, sliced

2 pounds stewing beef (chuck is best, or blade or rump), cubed

2–4 sheep's kidneys (or 1 ox kidney), cored (remove the gristle on the inside with a small knife) and cubed

2 tablespoons plain flour (gluten-free if desired)

¼ teaspoon sea salt

½ teaspoon freshly ground black pepper

½ teaspoon dried mixed herbs or dried rosemary

¾ cup Homemade Beef Stock (page 42) or water

6 cups steamed greens (beans, zucchini, broccoli or frozen peas), to serve

HERBY DUMPLINGS

1½ tablespoons butter

2½ cups self-raising flour (gluten-free if desired) mixed with ½ teaspoon sea salt

3 teaspoons chopped thyme

3 teaspoons chopped flat-leaf parsley

1 tablespoon full-fat milk

Place the onion, mushrooms, garlic, beef and kidneys in a slow-cooker insert. Add the flour, salt, pepper and herbs and stir to coat the meat and kidneys. Pour over the stock or water, cover and cook on low for 8–10 hours or on high for 4–5 hours.

To make the herby dumplings, rub the butter into the flour and salt with your fingertips until the mixture resembles fine bread crumbs. Add the herbs and milk and mix to a soft dough. Roll into small balls.

Half an hour before serving, remove the slow-cooker lid and place the dumplings on top of the hot stew. Lay parchment paper over the top and replace the lid. Cook on high for 30 minutes until the dumplings are cooked. Serve with steamed greens.

1½ SERVINGS VEG + FRUIT PER SERVING

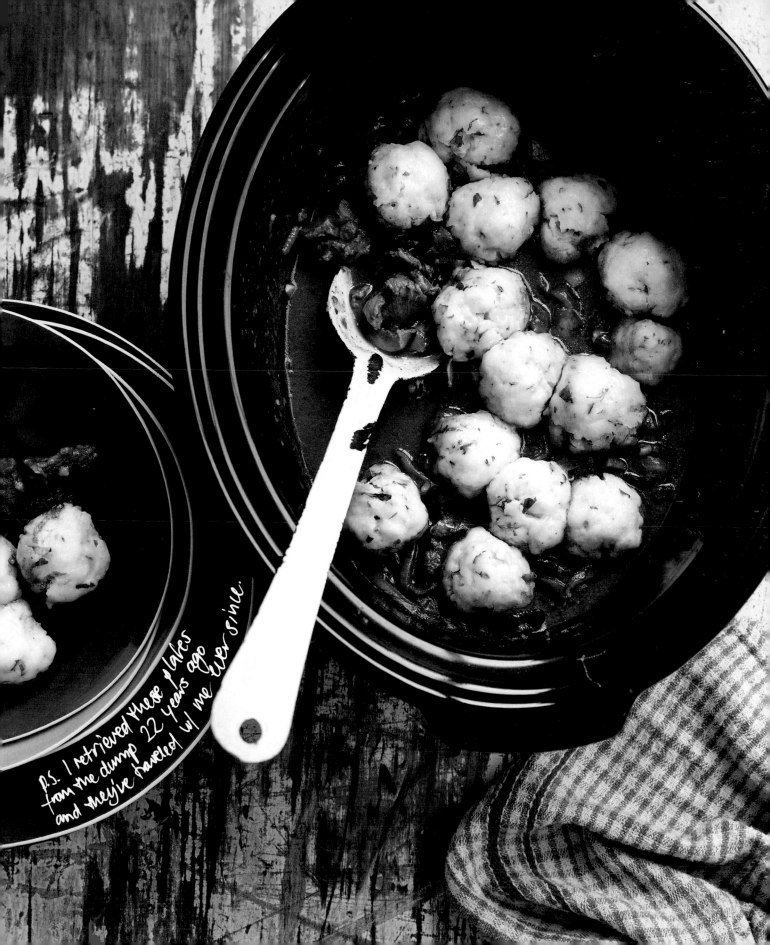

P.S. I retrieved these plates from the dump 22 years ago and they've traveled w/ me ever since.

BEGINNER'S COQ AU VIN PÂTÉ

MAKES 3 CUPS ———————————————————————————————————————

New to liver? This is the dish for you. Sexify your first time (or your fiftieth) with bacon and pad things out a tad with mushrooms. These particularly Frenchie flavors work mostly because, well, the French do flavor fabulously.

I wrap this pâté in a lettuce leaf or mustard leaf and have it for breakfast many mornings. True story.

Ask your butcher to do the cleaning. They'll probably be thrilled to help out a new liver-lovin' customer.

1¼ pounds cleaned chicken liver or duck liver (or a combo)

3½ ounces butter

1 slice bacon, chopped

1 small onion (or 1 leek or ¼ bunch green onions), chopped

½ pound mushrooms (any kind; I like portobello), chopped

2 cloves garlic, chopped

1 tablespoon chopped thyme

2 teaspoons chopped sage

sea salt and freshly ground black pepper

½ cup dry white wine (or vermouth, scotch or brandy)

This is wonderfully gruesome work. Revel in it.

Liver: the ONLY superfood
This stuff is the most nutrient-dense food on the planet. It contains more nutrients, ounce for ounce, than any other food:

* 3 times as much choline as an egg;
* 17 times more B^{12} than red meat;
* 1,400 times more vitamin A than red meat.

Trim the livers of any tough connective tissue and make sure the butcher hasn't left any green material (on chicken liver it's gallbladder and on duck liver it's bile).

Melt the butter in a skillet over medium heat. Add the bacon and onion, leek or green onions and cook, stirring occasionally, until they start to turn lovely and golden. Add the mushrooms, liver, garlic and herbs and season to taste with salt and pepper. Cook, stirring occasionally, until the livers have browned and are only slightly pink on the inside (about 5 minutes). Transfer the lot to a blender (or an immersion blender beaker).

Add the wine to the skillet and bring to a boil, scraping up the browned bits. Boil for about 1 minute to reduce slightly, then pour into the blender with the liver mixture. Process until very smooth.

Spoon the pâté into a bowl or jar. Allow to cool, then cover with plastic wrap, pressing the wrap against the surface of the pâté so that it doesn't oxidize. Serve with raw veggie sticks or crackers, or simply roll it up in a green leaf. The pâté will keep in the fridge for up to 3 weeks and in the freezer for up to 3 months.

You can cover the top of the pâté with a little melted butter to prevent it browning if you like, but I don't bother.

½ SERVING VEG + FRUIT PER SERVING

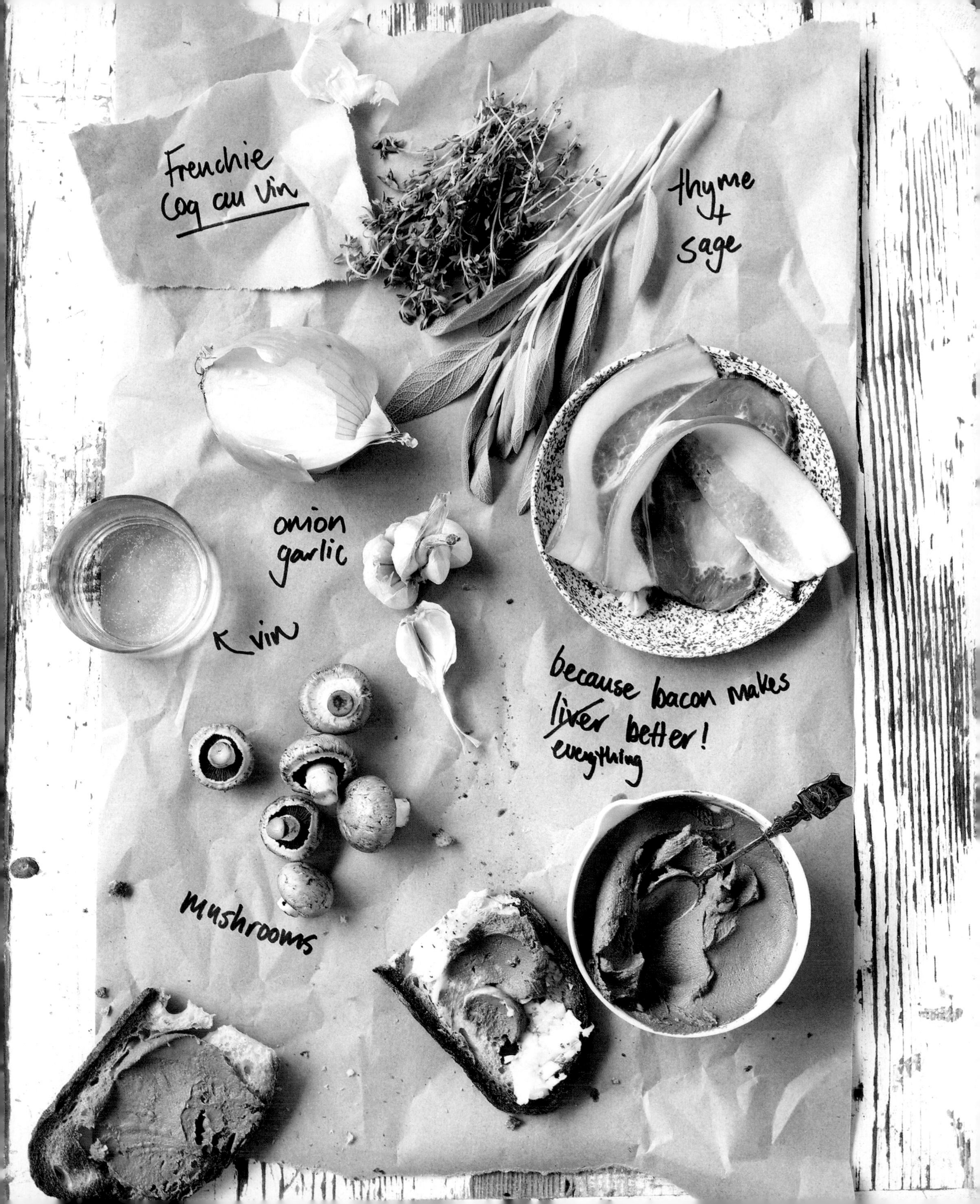

Frenchie
Coq au vin

thyme
+
sage

onion
garlic

← vin

because bacon makes
liver better!
everything

mushrooms

CHINESE
BEEF CHEEKS

This dish is super rich and loaded with flavor, turbo charged by being marinated in the fridge overnight. Serve it with rice or quinoa and plenty of steamed green veggies to balance out the richness.

Beef cheeks are brimful of gelatin—really good for gut health.

5 beef cheeks (2–3 pounds)

1 bunch green onions, finely chopped (reserve several green tops for garnish)

5 cloves garlic, thinly sliced

1½-inch knob of ginger, grated

1 red bird's-eye (Thai) chili, thinly sliced

1 teaspoon five-spice mix

½ teaspoon granulated stevia (optional)

¼ cup Chinese rice wine or dry white wine

¼ cup soy sauce or tamari (preferably low-salt)

2 cups sliced mushrooms (shiitake or portobello)

½ cup Homemade Beef Stock (page 42)

Cooked Quinoa (page 26) or steamed rice, to serve

6 cups steamed greens

The night before: Trim the fat from the outside of the beef cheeks (it can be quite thick) and cut each cheek into two or three even-sized pieces. Place in the insert of the slow cooker along with all the ingredients except the mushrooms, stock, greens and reserved green onion tops, and toss to combine. Cover and refrigerate overnight.

In the morning: Place the mushrooms on top and pour over the stock along with 1½ cups of water. Cook on low for 7 hours or on high for 3½ hours.

Just before serving, slice the reserved green onion tops into long, thin strips and plunge into ice water for a minute to make them curly (if desired). Garnish the beef with the green onions, and serve with quinoa or rice and steamed greens.

🍴 2½ SERVINGS VEG + FRUIT PER SERVING

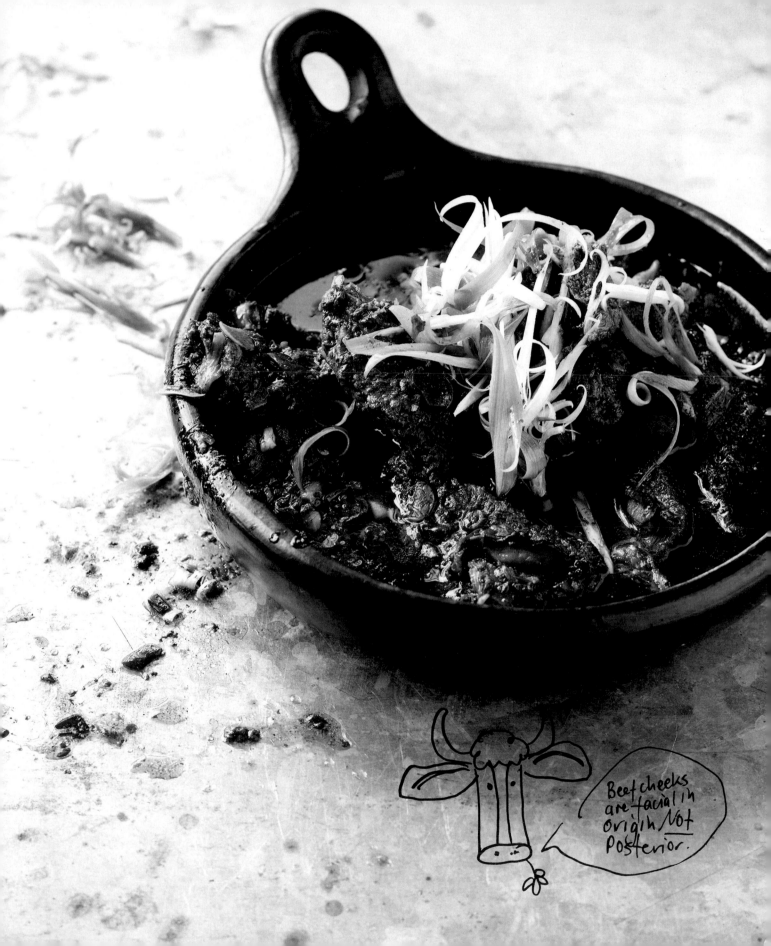

"SWEET" TACOS WITH EASY SLAW

These use sweetbreads, the culinary name for the pancreas and thymus glands of various animals. (No need to tell the kids this.) Sweetbreads are definitely sweet and very moist and add great flavor and bulk to robust, salty dishes like tacos. Most good butchers sell them, or will get them in for you.

Sweetbreads

These morsels are rich in trace minerals such as zinc and selenium, said to reduce inflammation and to improve immunity, digestive processes and blood sugar signaling. Sweetbreads cook quickly and actually are quite forgiving since they can't really be overcooked. To counteract the richness of the meat, many recipes serve sweetbreads with an acidic sauce featuring lemons or capers.

2 onions, finely chopped

4 cloves garlic, crushed

1 green bell pepper, chopped

1 bunch cilantro stems, finely chopped (reserve the leaves for garnish)

2 pounds beef brisket

14 ounces sweetbreads, cut into ½-inch cubes

1½ tablespoons tomato paste

1 teaspoon cayenne pepper

1 teaspoon dried oregano

1½ teaspoons ground cumin

¾ cup Homemade Beef Stock (page 42)

2 zucchini, grated — *or use zucchini ice cubes (see page 24)*

12 taco shells or burrito wraps

TO SERVE

sliced avocado

Easy Slaw (see below)

sour cream, full-fat organic plain yogurt or grated cheese

Place the vegetables and cilantro stems in a slow-cooker insert. Place the brisket and sweetbreads on top. Add the tomato paste, cayenne pepper, oregano and cumin, then pour the stock over the lot. Cover and cook on low for 8–9 hours or on high for 4–5 hours.

Remove the brisket and shred. Return the shredded meat to the slow-cooker insert with the zucchini and cook on high, lid off, for 20 minutes. Place the meat, avocado, slaw, sour cream and cilantro leaves (or whatever sides you prefer) in serving dishes in the center of your table. Heat the tacos (or warm the burritos) and have everyone "load" their own.

EASY SLAW

18 ounces coleslaw mix or 2 large carrots and ½ red or white cabbage, grated

½ cup dressing (Whey-Good Mayo [page 50], Powerhouse Dressing [page 53] or whatever you have)

Mix together and off you go.

MAKE IT WITH GOAT:

Use a 2-pound goat leg or shoulder, brown all over in a skillet and add to the slow cooker as you would the beef brisket.

2 SERVINGS VEG + FRUIT PER SERVING

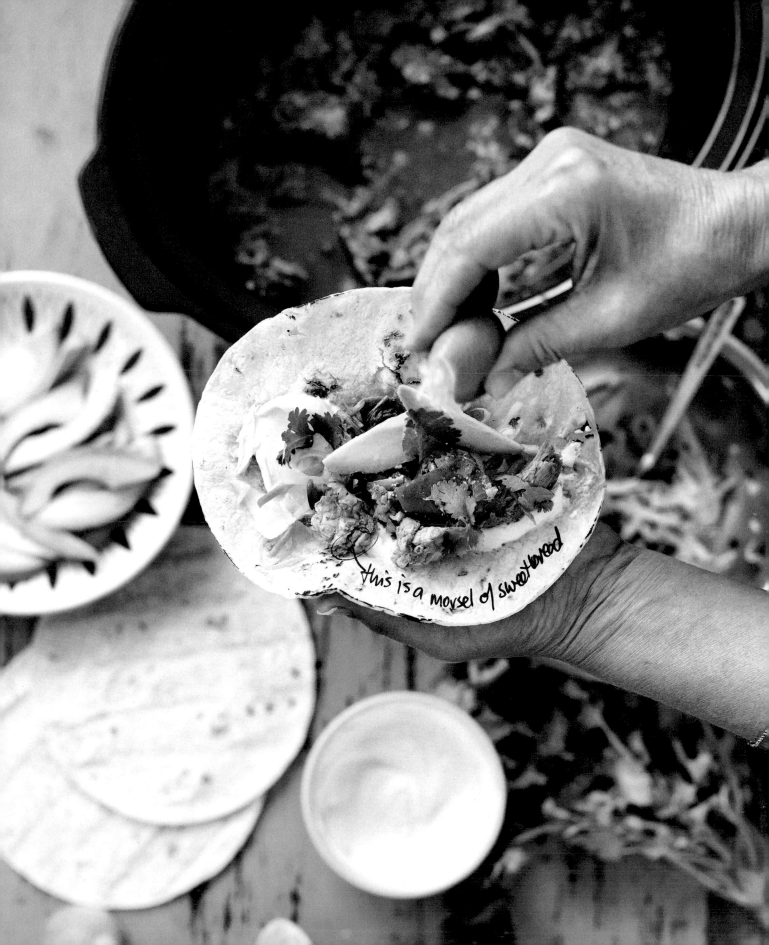

this is a morsel of sweetbread

LAMB'S FRY AND PEAR MEATLOAF

SERVES 6

Mum used to make us lamb's fry (livers cooked with bacon and mushrooms) on weekends. I really rather loved it. Livers need to be cooked quickly or they get feathery, which means they often have to be eaten by themselves (that is, as a slab of offal). If that sounds off-putting, try a tip my butcher gave me: he grinds some lamb and lamb liver together, fresh. Yours will do the same, I'm sure. And then you can package it all up into this derivative loaf.

Be mindful we're talking about lamb's livers here. In the US, "lamb fries" (note the absence of the possessive apostrophe) refers to lamb testicles; in the UK "lamb's fry" refers to a mixture of all kinds of entrails. Got it?

Awfully good offal

* Organ meats are 10 to 100 times higher in nutrients than muscle meats.
* Those claims that meat is linked to cancer and early death? It's the methionine in muscle meat (bone- and organ-free cuts) that such grimness is linked to. Offal (as well as meat bones and skin), however, has high levels of glycine, which effortlessly balances the excessive methionine in muscle meats.
* Offal is also super-high in vitamins B^6 and B^{12}, folate, betaine and choline, which work together synergistically to balance methionine.
* Eat the whole beast is the lesson here, people.

If your mixture is quite moist (my team's least favorite word) add 1–2 tablespoons of chia seeds (or extra almond meal) and allow to sit for 10 minutes to let the seeds do their soaking-up thing.

butter or ghee, for greasing

2 tablespoons almond meal

1 pound lamb's livers ground with 1 pound lamb or pork

1 zucchini, grated and squeezed in a clean tea towel to remove moisture

1 pear or apple, peeled, cored and grated, plus extra slices for garnish

1½ cups diced mushrooms (any kind)

1 onion, finely diced

1 tablespoon chopped sage or thyme, plus extra sage leaves for garnish

1 teaspoon ground mustard seeds or 1 tablespoon 'Bucha Mustard (page 336) or Dijon mustard

2 cloves garlic, minced

2 large eggs

sea salt and freshly ground black pepper

4 slices bacon

Shaved Sprouts and Pecorino Salad (page 305) or any leafy salad, to serve

Preheat the oven to 400°F and lightly grease a 9 × 5-inch loaf pan.

Place all of the ingredients except the bacon in a large bowl and mix well. Press the mixture into the greased loaf pan. Lay the bacon slices across the top, tucking them in at the ends if they are too long. Arrange the extra sliced pear or apple on top, and sprinkle over the extra sage leaves. Bake for 45 minutes. Serve hot or cold with Shaved Sprouts and Pecorino Salad (or any green salad from this book). Freeze leftover slices of meatloaf between pieces of parchment paper for up to 3 months.

MAKE IT FOR LATER:

Double the mixture and place it in two loaf pans. Freeze one of the pans (covered with a freezer-proof bag) for up to 3 months. When ready to use, simply bake in your preheated 400°F oven for 1–1½ hours.

2 SERVINGS VEG + FRUIT PER SERVING

After cooking + shooting this
I ate the skin chips wrapped
in radicchio with sprigs of
CARROT TOPS and it was a
Taste sensation

sweet potato
skin chips
(page 23)

carrot tops are
a boon of a garnish.

CHICKEN CRACKLE SALT

MAKES 1 CUP

In my quiet moments I sometimes wonder, "What the hell happens to all that chicken skin that's criminally removed from chickens in poultry shops for all those folk insisting on skinless breasts?" Sadly, it's tossed. Happily, however, I have a fix for this travesty. My friend Aaron from the ethical catering company Studio Neon in Sydney got me onto this when he made some for my 40th birthday. Gosh it made me happy . . . fat, salt and leftovers all in one mix! The other thing I like about this recipe is that it entails going to your butcher or local chicken shop and asking them to do you a favor—to set aside some skin. Forced mindful human engagement: this is what real food and real eating are about.

7 ounces chicken skin

7 ounces good-quality sea salt

Bring a small saucepan of water to a boil over high heat. Add the chicken skin, reduce the heat and simmer for 10 minutes. Drain, and allow the skin to cool slightly. While it's still warm use a spoon or a butter knife to scrape off any excess fat that may be on the underside.

 Stretch and flatten the chicken skin on a wire rack placed over a baking sheet. Place another wire rack on top of the chicken skin (this stops it from flying around as it crisps up if you have a convection oven). Bake for 10–15 minutes or until brown and crispy. The skin will continue to crisp up as it cools.

Slightly break up the chicken skin and crush it with the salt using a large mortar and pestle (or use an immersion blender, though be careful not to turn it into a fine powder—we want texture). Place in a sealable glass or plastic container and store in the pantry for up to 2 weeks.

MAKE IT A SOUP TOPPER:
Skip the salt-and-crush stage and serve broken shards atop a soup or salad.

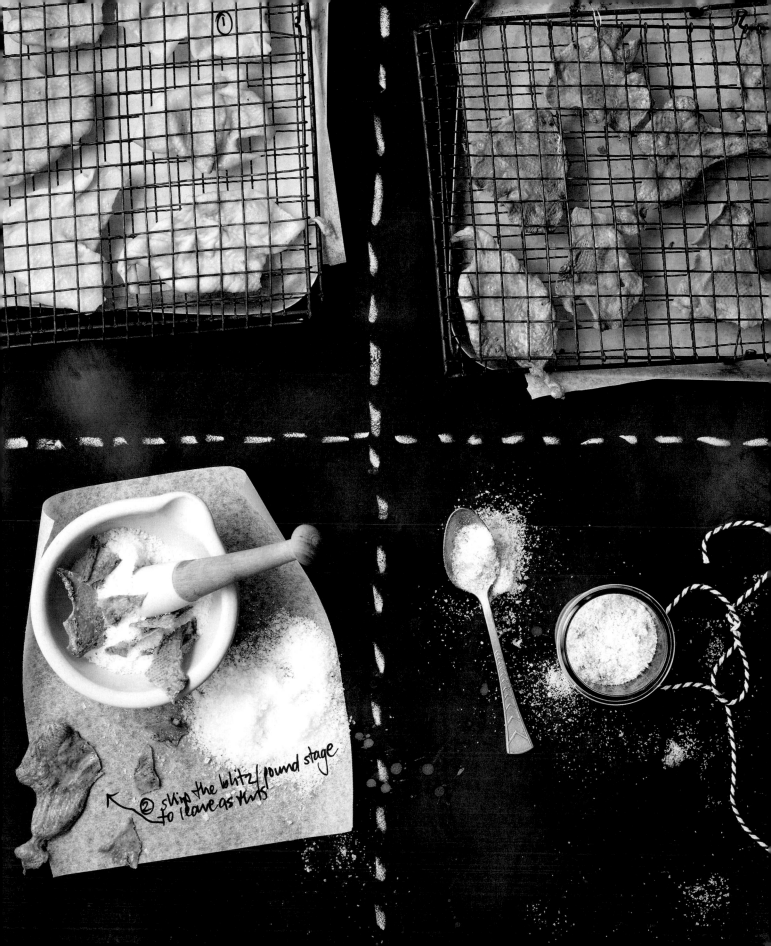

② skip the blitz/pound stage
to leave as this!

BLOKE BEEF 'N' BEER WITH MASH

SERVES 6 —————————————————————————————————————

The local pub on a plate, brewed masterfully in the one pot
(2½ minutes of washing up entailed).

Beer + Meat = Good
A recent study has found
that when you marinate meat
with beer, it greatly reduces
the carcinogens that are
produced (yes, really) in the
cooking process.

1 pound and 6 ounces parsnips (or
potatoes or sweet potatoes), peeled and
chopped into 1½-inch chunks

2 onions, finely diced

2–3 pounds beef brisket,
excess fat trimmed

1½ tablespoons Dijon mustard

good pinch of sea salt

freshly ground black pepper

3 sprigs thyme

2 bay leaves

½ cup beer (preferably one with a
malty flavor)

3 big handfuls of string beans, trimmed

large knob of butter

Place the parsnips, potatoes or sweet potatoes and the onions in the base of your
slow-cooker insert. Coat the brisket in the mustard, season with salt and pepper
and place on top of the veggies. Add the thyme and bay leaves and pour over the
beer. Cover and cook on low for 8–10 hours or high for 4–5 hours.

In the last 15 minutes of cooking, place the beans on top of the meat. Cover
again and cook on high until the beans are tender.

*Feel free to thicken the
sauce by heating it in
a small saucepan and
stirring in 1 tablespoon
of arrowroot or other
flour.*

Remove the meat and the steamed beans from the slow cooker and set aside.
Using two forks, shred ("pull") the brisket. Drain most of the sauce from the insert
and set aside.

Add the butter to the insert and season with salt and pepper. Use a potato masher
to mash the veggies until smooth, adding extra sauce as needed. Serve the meat
with the mash and steamed beans. Drizzle the remaining sauce over the top.

MAKE IT WITH GOAT:
Use a 2–3-pound goat leg
or shoulder and follow the
recipe above.

2 SERVINGS VEG + FRUIT PER SERVING

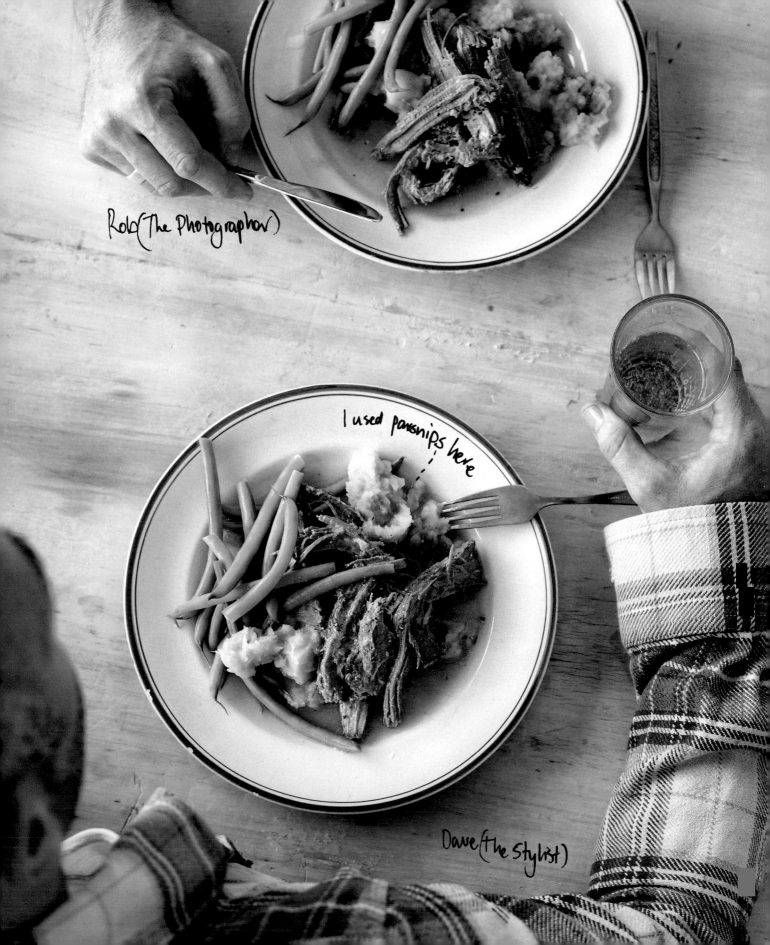

Rob (The Photographer)

I used parsnips here

Dave (the Stylist)

HOMEMADE BACON

MAKES 800 G

Some people get upset about nitrates in their bacon. The science says it's not really doing any harm. Similarly, some get upset about the sugar used to cure bacon. Don't. It's generally rinsed off. So why make your own? It saves money and gets your hands dirty! Plus it means you can experiment with flavors.

Nitrates in bacon
The nitrite in our saliva accounts for 70–90% of our total nitrite exposure; your spit contains far more of the stuff than anything you could ever eat. Also, the study that originally linked nitrates and cancer risk has since been discredited after being subjected to a peer review. And, indeed, more recent research suggests that nitrates and nitrites may not only be harmless, they may be beneficial, especially for immunity and heart health.

2½–3 pounds pork belly, rind left on

3 tablespoons sea salt

1 tablespoon freshly ground black pepper

1 tablespoon coriander seeds, fennel seeds or dried rosemary (or a combo)

½ teaspoon ground cinnamon or ground nutmeg

1 clove garlic, minced

Rinse the pork belly and pat it dry. Combine the remaining ingredients in a small bowl and rub all over the pork. Place the pork and any remaining seasoning in a big re-usable plastic bag on a flat pan with a weight on top. Refrigerate for 1 week, flipping the bag every day or so. Liquid will build up—don't fret (it's the salt drawing moisture from the meat); throw it out.

Preheat the oven to 200°F. Rinse the pork, pat it dry and place in a baking dish. Roast uncovered for 2 hours. Remove from the oven and once cool to the touch, transfer the bacon to a chopping board and slice off the skin. Let the bacon cool to room temperature, then wrap it in wax paper and refrigerate. Slice as you need it. It will keep for 2 weeks in the fridge. Or cut it into cubes and freeze for 3–6 months.

USE THE LEFTOVER RIND:
Add it to any of your freezer stock bags (see page 32) to make a tastier stock.

SOME BEEFIN' GOOD JERKY

MAKES 1½ POUNDS

This jerky is seriously easy to make and will leave you feeling a little bit "frontier." It's great for lunchboxes. I fiddled around with this recipe to get a smoky-sweet "processed meat" vibe. Here she goes . . .

Beef is best, and ensure it's lean in just this instance!

2 pounds ground meat

1½ teaspoons sea salt

½ teaspoon black pepper

1 teaspoon garlic powder
(or 3 cloves garlic, finely minced)

1 teaspoon ground cumin

1 teaspoon smoked paprika

If your oven only goes down as far as 200°F that's dandy, but note the different cooking time.

Preheat the oven to 150°F and line two baking sheets with parchment paper. Use your hands to mix all the ingredients together in a big bowl. Take half the mixture and press it out on the first tray to 2 inches thick (use a rolling pin or bottle). You can work to a neat rectangle (though I like to keep it an organic shape and then break it into shards later). Repeat with the rest of the mixture on the second tray.

Dry for 6 hours in the oven (about 4 hours if using a 200°F oven), pouring the juices into a jug every hour or so. (Keep the jug in the fridge—see below.)

Flip the jerky in the final hour. The stuff is done when you break off a piece, let it cool and it no longer leaks any moisture when squeezed.

Once done, allow the jerky to cool completely on a wire rack, then snap into shards (or cut with scissors) and store in an airtight container in the fridge for up to 2 months.

USE THE LEFTOVER MEAT JUICES:
Pour the juices into an ice-cube tray, freeze and use them to braise vegetables, add to soups or stews, or to make gravy.

While the oven is on at this low temperature it's a good time to make Good for Your Guts Garlic (page 340) or to dry some activated nuts (see page 28), if you don't mind them infused with a meaty flavor. If your oven only goes to 200°F, why not make Homemade Bacon (opposite) at the same time?

A BUNCH OF
SUNDAY COOK-UPS

BIG COZY MEALS

to **BULK-COOK** often using a slow cooker

on a

LAZY WEEKEND

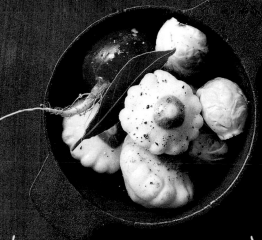

leaving you with leftover meat 'n' bits that extend for weeks.

THE CHEAPEST
STEW EVER

SERVES 6 + 8 PORTIONS OF LEFTOVER BEEF OR STOCK ─────────────

Seriously, this stew is drastically cheaper than chips. I've designed it so it can be served as a stew with leftover stock or a hearty soup with lots of leftover meat.

2 onions, chopped

2 large carrots, cut into 1½-inch chunks

2 large parsnips, cut into 1½-inch chunks

2 turnips or potatoes, cut into 1½-inch chunks

2 celery stalks, chopped, leaves reserved

2 bay leaves

½ teaspoon dried oregano

2 cups Homemade Beef Stock (page 42)

1 Parmesan rind (if you have one in your freezer)

3 pounds stewing beef (blade, chuck, brisket—whichever's cheapest), cut into 1-inch cubes

1 tablespoon English mustard

½ teaspoon sea salt

freshly ground black pepper

2 cups Parcooked 'n' Frozen chard or kale (page 22)

Place all the ingredients, except the chard or kale, into the slow-cooker insert. Cover and cook on low for 8–10 hours or high for 4–5 hours. Remove and discard the bay leaves and Parmesan rind (if using).

To serve as a stew: Remove half of the meat and 2 cups of stock from the slow-cooker insert and set aside (see below). Add the chard or kale and all but a few of the reserved celery leaves and heat through. Serve topped with the few remaining celery leaves and a big glug of olive oil.

To serve as a soup: Remove all of the meat from the slow-cooker insert, add the chard or kale and reserved celery leaves (keep a few for garnish) and heat to make soup. (Purée it with an immersion blender if you prefer.) Serve sprinkled with the remaining celery leaves and some sliced sourdough or Socca wedges (page 106) on the side.

USE THE LEFTOVER STOCK:
If you have reserved 2 cups of stock, either drink it as a broth or freeze it in 1-cup portions to make another soup.

USE THE LEFTOVER MEAT:
Divide any leftover beef cubes into ½-cup portions and freeze for up to 3 months.

MAKE IT AN AUTOIMMUNE STEW:
When I'm inflamed and my immune system is cranky with me, I amend The Cheapest Stew Ever a touch to make this cytokine pacifier. I swap the onions for 1 fennel bulb, chopped, ditch the potato and use turnip or sweet potato, and serve with steamed zucchini or asparagus and a HUGE glug of olive oil.

If you're really serious about adjusting your diet to help manage an AI disease, then you might like to try avoiding fructans (e.g., onion and garlic) and deadly nightshades (e.g., potato, tomato, eggplant, bell pepper and chili).

 2 SERVINGS VEG + FRUIT PER SERVING

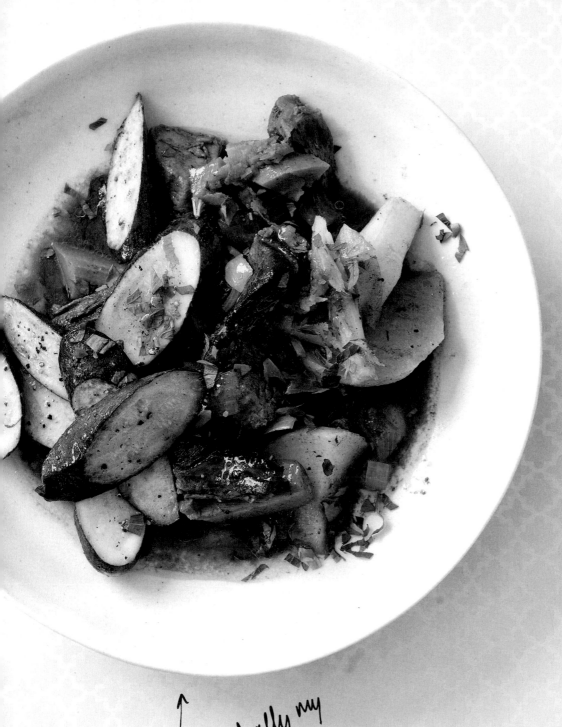

This is actually my
Autoimmune Stew
version here

THREE WAYS with CHICKEN POT AU FEU

This French classic ("pot on fire") sums up many things I love about French cooking + eating. It maximizes the potential of the meat + veg while also!! requiring a mindful eating ritual.

1. BASIC POT-AU-FEU

SERVES 6 + LEFTOVER SHREDDED CHICKEN + STOCK

1 whole chicken

1 teaspoon peppercorns (black or white)

2 teaspoons sea salt

2 bay leaves

5 sprigs thyme

1 bunch Dutch carrots, trimmed (or 3 large ones, halved lengthwise, then cut into 2-inch-long batons)

6 small parsnips, halved lengthwise

2 turnips, scrubbed and cut into 6 wedges

1 fennel bulb, trimmed and cut in half lengthwise, or 2 celery sticks, cut into 2-inch lengths

2 onions, peeled and quartered

1 head garlic, halved crosswise, outer leaves peeled

TO SERVE

Homemade Aioli (page 50)

'Bucha Mustard (page 336; optional)

Leftovers Pesto (page 55; optional)

Investing in an organic one is non-negotiable for this dish as we'll be boiling the bones.

Remember to reserve all the veggie scraps for the second batch of stock.

Plonk the chicken, leg side down, in a big stockpot. Sprinkle over the peppercorns, salt and herbs. Cover the whole lot with water. Place the lid on the pot and bring to a gentle boil. Reduce to a simmer and cook for 45–60 minutes, skimming off the gray "scum" a few times. Once the chicken is cooked (the legs pull away easily and the juices run clear when you cut into it), transfer to a chopping board to cool a little.

Add all the vegetables to the pot, cover and cook until soft (about 20–30 minutes).

Meanwhile, carve the chicken into portions, reserving some for shredding (see below) and keeping the carcass and any excess skin.

To serve, divide the veggies between large serving bowls and top with the chicken pieces. Ladle over some stock, avoiding the herbs floating about. Serve with bowls of aioli, mustard and/or pesto in the center of the table.

USE THE LEFTOVER CARCASS, BONES AND VEGGIE SCRAPS:
Make Homemade Chicken Stock (page 42).

USE THE LEFTOVER CHICKEN SKIN:
Make Chicken Crackle Salt (page 204).

USE THE LEFTOVER CHICKEN STOCK:
Drink it as a broth, or freeze it in 1-cup batches for up to 3 months.

SHREDDED CHICKEN

Shred any leftover chicken, divide it into ½-cup portions and freeze for up to 3 months.

2½ SERVINGS VEG + FRUIT PER SERVING

aioli

'bucha
mustard

leftovers pesto

Pot au Feu

Fini!

Use leftover chook skin to make chicken
Salt + drink the leftover stock for
lunch tomorrow

2. SOOTHING ASIAN POACHED POT

SERVES 6 + LEFTOVER SHREDDED CHICKEN + STOCK

1 whole chicken (yep, organic)

1 small (or ½ large) napa cabbage, cut into 6 wedges (don't remove the core as this will keep the wedges intact)

4 celery stalks, cut into 4-inch lengths

1 bunch green onions, cut into 4-inch lengths

12 shiitake mushrooms, stems removed and sliced (or dried ones, soaked in boiling water for 20 minutes, the soaking liquid reserved)

½ bunch cilantro, leaves picked, roots and stems left intact

4 cloves garlic, peeled and left whole

4 star anise

1 cinnamon stick

2-inch knob of ginger, sliced

dash of tamari or soy sauce (or a big shake of dulse flakes)

1 teaspoon peppercorns (preferably white)

2 teaspoons sea salt

Follow the instructions for Basic Pot-au-Feu (page 214), using the ingredients here, but add the cilantro roots and stems only to the stockpot— the cilantro leaves are for serving.

3. PRETTY SPRING POT

SERVES 6 + LEFTOVER SHREDDED CHICKEN + STOCK

1 whole chicken (organic once again)

2 bay leaves

5 sprigs thyme

1 teaspoon peppercorns (black or white)

2 teaspoons sea salt

rind of ¼ lemon, sliced

4 cloves garlic, peeled and left whole

1 leek, halved lengthwise and cut into 2-inch lengths

3 baby yellow beets, quartered (or 1 bunch Dutch carrots, trimmed)

1 fennel bulb, trimmed and cut into 6 wedges lengthwise, fronds reserved

1 bunch asparagus, trimmed

2 cups peas (snow peas or sugar snap peas, podded; or fresh broad beans, double-podded)

After podding, blanch them in boiling water to slip them out of their skins.

TO SERVE

6 poached eggs

You can cook your poachies in the stock after you've removed the veggies, rather than pulling out a new pot. Follow the instructions on page 44.

Follow the instructions for Basic Pot-au-Feu (page 214), adding the lemon rind with the herbs, salt and pepper. Add the garlic, leek, beets or carrots and fennel after removing the chicken. Add the asparagus just 5 minutes before serving, and the peas or broad beans only 1 minute before. Serve with a poachie on top and a sprig or two of fennel frondage.

1 SERVING VEG + FRUIT PER SERVING

2 SERVINGS VEG + FRUIT PER SERVING

SLOW-COOKED GREEN PEAS AND HAM

SERVES 6 + LEFTOVER HAM HOCK CHUNKS

This singular slow-cooked effort stretches to 10–12 portions. Eat it as a ham-flavored soup and reserve the meat for later, or as a dense meaty stew, reserving the lush stock for later. It's best made in a slow cooker. Slow and low will better extract the collagen-y goodness from the ham.

Why ham on the bone?
It's cheaper, even bearing in mind the extra weight of the bone, and more gelatinous, and it can be used for making a second batch of stock.

Unsmoked is better, but smoked is okay, too.

3–4 pounds ham bone/hocks

1 pound green split peas (or any legume, though peas are best), soaked overnight

3 carrots, finely chopped

3 celery stalks, finely chopped (keep a few leaves for garnish)

1 onion, finely chopped

I soak all beans, even split peas (see page 28).

3 cloves garlic, minced

2 bay leaves

2 tablespoons chopped thyme or 2 teaspoons dried thyme

2 big crunches each of sea salt and black pepper

Place everything in a slow-cooker insert with 2 quarts of water. Cook for 8–10 hours on low or 6–7 hours on high. Chuck out the bay leaves. Remove the ham hocks and reserve to make Ham Hock Chunks (see below).

Because of the gelatinous nature of the ham, your soup will solidify when cooled. This is a glorious thing. Simply heat to liquefy.

Purée the soup using an immersion blender or leave it as is if you like to keep things chunky. Serve with a few chunks of ham and some celery leaves on top.

HAM HOCK CHUNKS

Once the ham hocks are cool enough, pull the meat from the bones and chop it into chunks. Divide into ½-cup portions and freeze for up to 3 months.

MAKE IT ON THE STOVETOP:
In a large saucepan, gently sauté the carrots, celery, onion and garlic in 1 tablespoon of olive oil for 10 minutes. Add the rest of the ingredients. Cover and bring to a boil, then reduce the heat and simmer for 1½–2 hours.

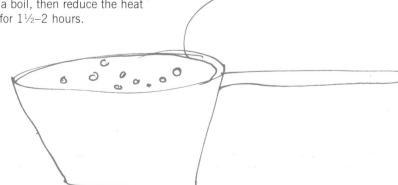

 1½ SERVINGS VEG + FRUIT PER SERVING

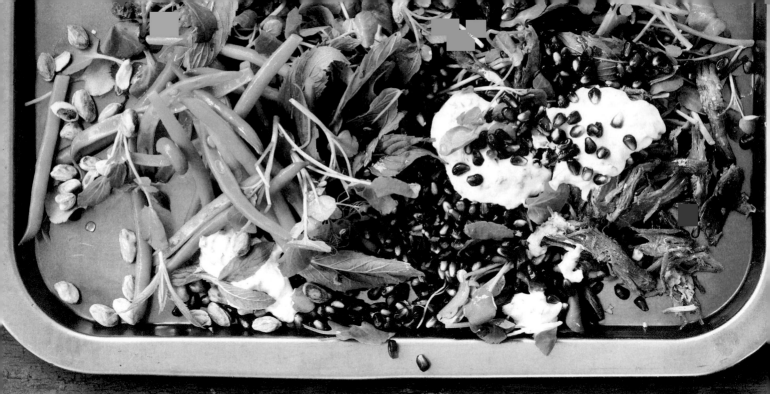

PERSIAN LAMB SALAD

CHEAT ROAST DINNERS
→ Pork, lamb, beef + shredded leftovers.

Roasts are great one-panners, but they can be temperamental, requiring thermometers to ensure a quality result, and I find them fiddly to serve (crooked carving can create carnage). Plus, they tend to rely on primary cuts of meat. I get around all this by using secondary cuts that are foolproof to cook, and can be served as a "pulled" roast. (no carving!).

The recipes herewith are designed to leave you with leftover pulled meats for later. Yeah, thank me later.

GREEK LAMB SALAD

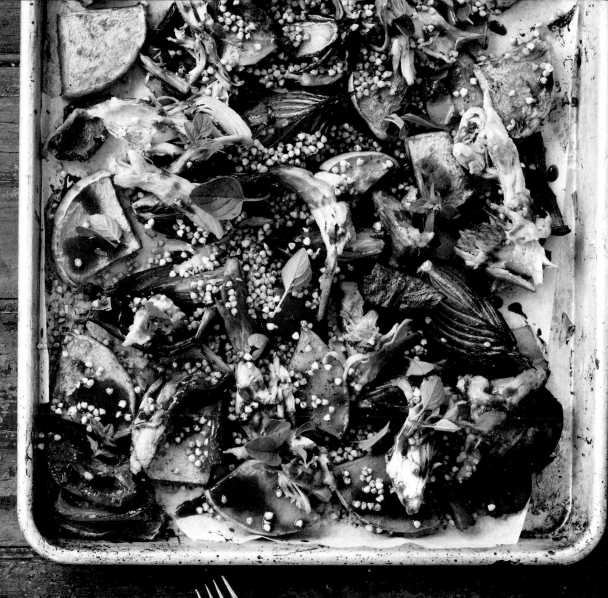

JERK PORK
SHOULDER ROAST

I QUIT SUGAR

SUGAR FREE

FOOD FREEDOM

I garnished this with carrot tops.

a reader made these forks for me!

head on over for recipes

ROAST LAMB SHOULDER *with Shredded Lamb* ↘

SERVES 6 + LEFTOVER SHREDDED LAMB

A versatile summer roast that can be
served as a variety of salads.

4-pound lamb shoulder, bone in,
fat trimmed

5 cloves garlic, sliced

5 sprigs oregano or 1 tablespoon
dried oregano

¼ cup olive oil

juice of 1 lemon

sea salt and freshly ground
black pepper

1 onion, cut into wedges

¼ cup Homemade Beef Stock (page 42)
or water

2–3 tablespoons arrowroot (for
gluten-free and paleo) or cornstarch,
mixed to a paste with cold water

**Eating meat on the bone
(and with the skin)**
This will provide your body with
the amino acid glycine, which
neutralizes the methionine
in muscle meat—the bit that
gives meat eating its bad
carcinogenic rap.

Make about twenty ⅜-inch-deep cuts all over the lamb shoulder and place in the
slow-cooker insert. Poke the garlic and oregano into the slits and rub the lot with
the olive oil, lemon juice, and salt and pepper. ↖

Put the onion in the slow-cooker insert and plonk the lamb on top. Pour over
the stock, then cover and cook on low for 8–9 hours, or high for 4–5 hours.

*Feel free to
marinate it for
a few hours or
overnight.*

Remove the meat, cover and leave to rest before shredding (see below).
Meanwhile, make a chunky gravy from the juices and onion by adding the flour
slurry to the insert. Stir it well, leave the lid off and cook on high for 20 minutes,
or until the sauce thickens into a gravy. Serve as a salad (see right) with the gravy
on the side.

SHREDDED LAMB

When the meat has cooled, place in a bowl and shred with two forks.
Divide leftovers into ½-cup portions and freeze for up to 3 months.

*You could marinate
your lamb in the
same dish to save
washing up.* →

MAKE IT IN THE OVEN:
Preheat the oven to 400°F. Heat a dash
of oil in a large, deep ovenproof dish on
the stovetop over medium-high heat.
Add the marinated lamb and sear for
5 minutes on each side. Add the onion,
half the stock and any marinade juices
and cover with foil. Place in the oven,
reduce the heat to 325°F and cook,
covered, for 3–4 hours, until the meat
falls away from the bone. Remove the
meat and make the gravy with the
remaining stock.

MAKE IT WITH GOAT:

Use a 2–2½-pound goat leg or
shoulder and follow the recipe
above.

GREEK LAMB SALAD

SERVES 6

1 bunch Massaged Kale (page 23)
or 6 cups baby spinach leaves

⅓ cup kalamata olives

3½ ounces feta, cubed

½ red onion, finely chopped

½ pound cherry tomatoes, halved

⅓ cup olive oil

2 tablespoons lemon juice

sea salt and freshly ground black pepper

3 cups Shredded Lamb (see left)

full-fat organic plain yogurt
or Quick Zucchini Tzatziki (page 188), to serve

Combine all of the ingredients in a large bowl. Toss gently and top with the yogurt or tzatziki.

PERSIAN LAMB SALAD

SERVES 6

1 bunch watercress

3 cups string beans, steamed
(or blanched)

½ cup mint leaves

seeds from ½–1 pomegranate

¼ cup pistachios

3 cups Shredded Lamb (see left)

DRESSING

1 cup full-fat plain organic yogurt

2 tablespoons lemon juice

1 tablespoon tahini

½ teaspoon brown rice syrup
or a tiny pinch of granulated stevia

½ teaspoon ground cumin

To make the dressing, combine the ingredients in a small bowl and mix well. Toss the watercress, beans, mint leaves, pomegranate seeds, pistachios and lamb in a large serving bowl. Dollop the dressing on top.

1½ SERVINGS VEG + FRUIT PER SERVING

1½ SERVINGS VEG + FRUIT PER SERVING

JERK PORK
SHOULDER ROAST *plus Pulled Pork ↓*

SERVES 6 + LEFTOVER PULLED PORK

A full Caribbean meal with all the trimmings in one fell swoop. I like to make this one in the oven (see below).

JERK MARINADE

1 tablespoon ground allspice

2 teaspoons ground nutmeg

1 small red chili, roughly chopped

6 green onions, roughly chopped

4–5 sprigs thyme, leaves picked, or 1 tablespoon dried thyme

⅓ cup apple cider vinegar

4 cloves garlic, peeled

2 tablespoons brown rice syrup

2 tablespoons olive oil

good pinch of sea salt

freshly ground black pepper

juice of 3 limes

3¾-4½ pounds pork shoulder, bone in, fat trimmed

14 ounces pumpkin, cut into small wedges (roughly the size of the onion quarters), skin on

2 red onions, quartered

2 large bell peppers (red, yellow or green), seeds removed, cut into eighths

mint or oregano leaves, to garnish

steamed string beans or okra, to serve

Cooked Quinoa (page 26) or Cooked Buckwheat (page 27), to serve

For the marinade, place all of the ingredients in a small blender or food processor and blitz until combined (or grind them to a paste using a large mortar and pestle).

Make about ten ⅜-inch-deep cuts all over the pork shoulder and place in the slow-cooker insert. Pour over three-quarters of the marinade and massage into the pork, ensuring it gets into the cuts. Cover and place in the fridge for at least 2 hours (preferably overnight).

Toss the pumpkin, onions and bell peppers in a large bowl with the remaining marinade. Cover and place in the fridge—also for 2 hours (or overnight).

Cook the pork for 7 hours on low or 4 hours on high. Lift the pork out of the slow cooker, place the vegetables in, then turn the pork over and place it on top of the veggies. Cover and continue cooking on high for 2 hours, or until the meat falls away from the bone.

Remove the pork and shred (see below). Return half of the meat to the slow cooker and mix it in with the vegetables. Serve with mint or oregano leaves, string beans or okra and a side of cooked quinoa or cooked buckwheat.

I like to toss a few Activated Groaties (page 27) over the top.

PULLED PORK

Place the pork in a bowl and, using two forks, shred ("pull") the meat, discarding the bone. Divide any leftover meat into ½-cup portions and freeze for up to 3 months.

MAKE IT IN THE OVEN:
Preheat the oven to 400°F. Place the marinated pork in a baking dish and cover with foil. Place in the oven, reduce the heat to 325°F and cook for 3–4 hours, until the meat falls away from the bone. In the last 30–40 minutes, scatter the marinated vegetables in another baking dish and bake until done (feel free to pop the pumpkin in earlier to cook a little longer than the other veggies).

¾ TEASPOON ADDED SUGAR PER SERVING

2 SERVINGS VEG + FRUIT PER SERVING

COFFEE- AND CACAO-CURED PULLED BEEF

SERVES 6 + LEFTOVER PULLED BEEF _____

This "roast" will leave you with some smokin' Texan brisket to play with.
Use it in salads, sandwiches, tacos and so on. To eat as a meal, serve
with a medley of sides (see below).

4–4½ pounds beef brisket

SPICE RUB

2 tablespoons finely ground dark roast
instant coffee

2 tablespoons brown rice syrup

1½ tablespoons raw cacao powder

1 tablespoon sweet smoked paprika

1 tablespoon garlic powder

2 teaspoons ground cumin

2 teaspoons chili powder

2 teaspoons sea salt

Place the brisket in the base of the slow-cooker insert. Combine the spice-rub
ingredients and pour over the top. Massage into the beef, ensuring every part is
coated. Cover and refrigerate for at least 2 hours (preferably overnight).

Cook the brisket on low for 9 hours or high for 5 hours, or until the meat is
tender. Shred the brisket (see below). Serve with your choice of Easy Slaw
(page 200), Blaukraut (page 182), Crunchy Broccoli Buckwheat Tabouli
(page 187) and/or some sliced avocado.

PULLED BEEF

Place the brisket in a bowl and shred ("pull") with two forks. Divide leftover
meat into ½-cup portions and freeze for up to 3 months.

¾ TEASPOON ADDED SUGAR PER SERVING

SWEET PERSIAN TAGINE
and Shredded Lamb or Pulled Pork !

SERVES 6 + LEFTOVER SHREDDED LAMB OR PULLED PORK

This is a great all-in-one meal for the cooler months, or if you're a Vata type. Again, we cook up extra meat to freeze and use later.

4½ pounds lamb or pork shoulder, bone in

1½ tablespoons Ras el Hanout Mix (page 45) or 2 teaspoons each of sweet paprika, ground cumin and ground cinnamon

2 teaspoons ground turmeric

2 teaspoons ground ginger

pinch of granulated stevia (optional)

1 cup dried chickpeas

1 onion, thinly sliced

½ can (7 ounces) diced tomatoes

2 pounds sweet potatoes or carrots, chopped into 1½-inch chunks

1 cup Homemade Stock (page 42) or water

1 tablespoon harissa paste

2 handfuls of string beans, halved

4 apricots, quartered and stones removed

2 tablespoons lemon zest or 3 tablespoons chopped leftover lemon from Lemon and Turmeric Tonic-ade (page 347)

½ cup pitted green or black olives

TO SERVE

mint leaves, torn

⅓ cup whole blanched almonds

Moroccan Cauliflower, Chickpea and Quinoa Bake (page 238)

Place the lamb or pork in a slow-cooker insert. Sprinkle over the spices and stevia and rub into the meat, making sure it is well coated. Cover and leave overnight in the fridge. Place the chickpeas in a bowl with plenty of water and leave overnight on the counter.

Drain and rinse the chickpeas and add to the slow-cooker insert with the onion, tomatoes, sweet potato or carrot, stock or water and harissa paste. Cover and cook on low for 8 hours or high for 5 hours.

Forty-five minutes before serving, remove half of the lamb or pork, then shred (see below). Add the string beans, apricots, lemon and olives to the slow cooker and cook for 30 minutes or until the apricots have softened. Serve topped with mint leaves and almonds, with a side of Moroccan Cauliflower, Chickpea and Quinoa Bake.

SHREDDED LAMB OR PULLED PORK

Transfer the lamb or pork to a large bowl and shred the meat with two forks, discarding the bone. Return half to the cooker and divide the remaining lamb or pork into ½-cup portions and freeze for up to 3 months.

MAKE IT WITH GOAT:
Use a 4½-pound goat leg or shoulder, with the bone in, and follow the recipe above.

3 SERVINGS VEG + FRUIT PER SERVING

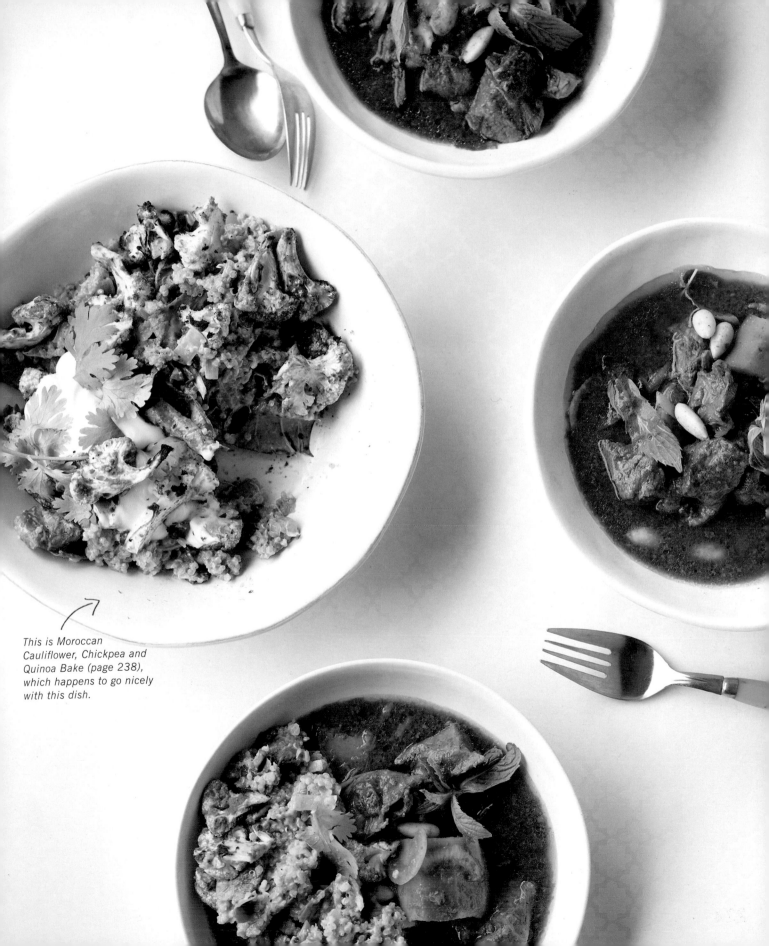

This is Moroccan Cauliflower, Chickpea and Quinoa Bake (page 238), which happens to go nicely with this dish.

MIDWEEK
ONE-PAN
WONDERS

very fun, complete meals made using [one] pot,
Dinner done.

[one] baking sheet, or [one] skillet.

DINNER-FOR-TWO EGGPLANT PARMIGIANA

SERVES 2

2 eggplants, each cut
into 5 rounds

¼ teaspoon sea salt

7-ounce ball fresh buffalo mozzarella,
sliced

1½ cups Nomato Sauce (page 51)
or sugar-free tomato purée

½ cup grated Parmesan

1 bunch broccolini (or 1 small head
broccoli, cut into florets)

Preheat the oven to 400°F and line a baking sheet with parchment paper.

Lightly season the eggplant with salt and place on the sheet in a single layer.
Bake for 15 minutes, or until the eggplant is beginning to turn golden brown.
Remove from the oven. Select the two largest eggplant slices and turn them over.
Layer with some mozzarella, Nomato Sauce and Parmesan. Take the two next-
largest slices and repeat the layering, finishing with the sauce and a sprinkle of
Parmesan. Arrange the broccolini or broccoli around the stacks. Return to the oven
and bake for 20 minutes or until the cheese is melted and golden.

MAKE IT MEATY:
Add a cooked Basic Meatball or two (page 144),
squashed, between the layers.

4 SERVINGS VEG + FRUIT PER SERVING

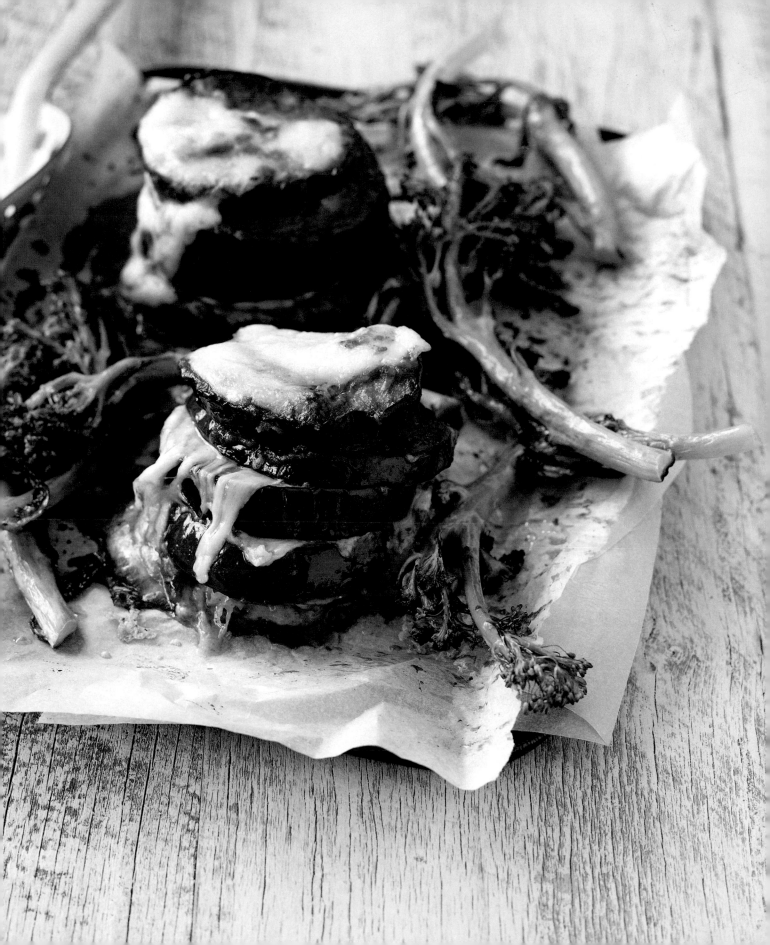

SWEET POTATO NACHOS

SERVES 2 ──────────────────────────────

1 large sweet potato or 2 small
(about 8–9 ounces), halved lengthwise

1 cup Pulled Pork (page 222),
Shredded Chicken (page 214)
or Cooked Beans (page 28)

¼ teaspoon sweet paprika

¼ teaspoon ground cumin

½ avocado, chopped

1 lime, halved

1 long red chili, sliced

2 ounces cheddar, grated

1 small red onion, thinly sliced

1 ear corn on the cob, cut into 6 pieces

6 cherry tomatoes

9 ounces coleslaw mix
or ¼ red cabbage, grated
(or a handful of string beans)

olive oil, for drizzling

sour cream or yogurt, to serve

cilantro leaves, to serve

corn chips or Sweet Potato Skins
(page 23), to serve

Preheat the oven to 400°F. Line a baking sheet with parchment paper. Place the sweet spuds cut side up on the sheet and bake for 1 hour or until soft.

Meanwhile, in a small bowl combine the meat or beans, spices and avocado with a squeeze of lime juice. Mix well.

Remove the spuds from the oven and crank the heat up to 425°F. Scoop out some of the flesh from the center of the potato (reserve for Sweet Potato Purée; page 23) and fill with the avocado mixture. Sprinkle over the chili and top with the cheddar. Arrange the onion, corn, tomatoes and coleslaw (or cabbage or beans) on the baking sheet and drizzle over plenty of olive oil. Return the sheet to the oven and bake for 10–15 minutes until everything is golden.

To serve, dollop with sour cream or yogurt, sprinkle with the cilantro and top with the corn chips or Sweet Potato Skins.

4 SERVINGS VEG + FRUIT PER SERVING

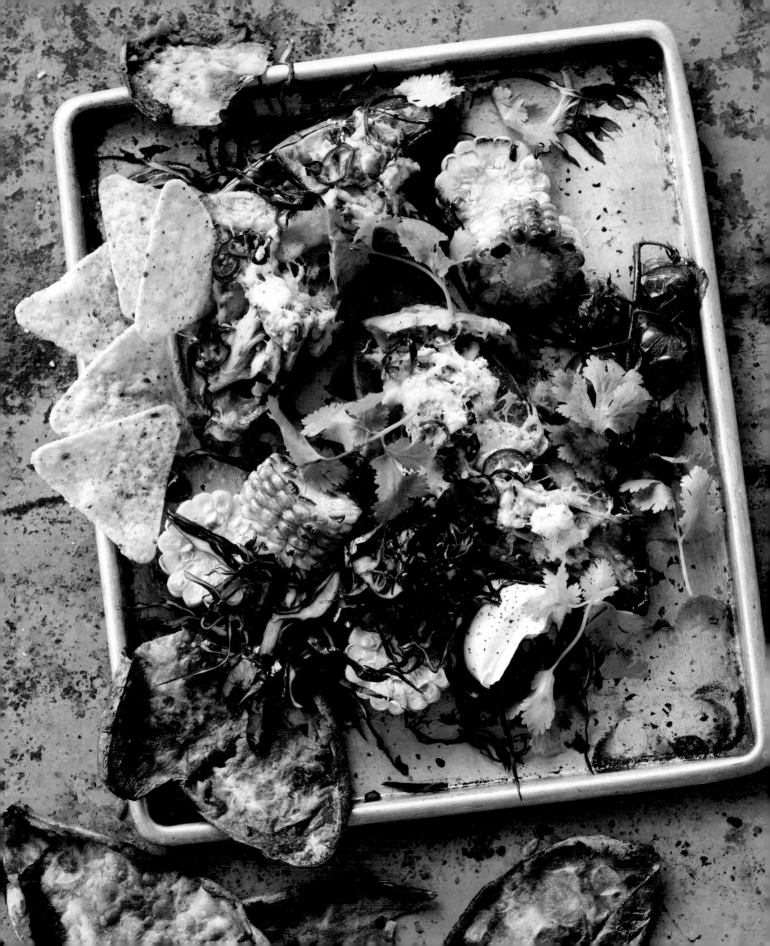

CRUNCHY CHICKEN
SATAY IN A PAN

½ cup crunchy natural peanut butter

1 tablespoon coconut oil, melted

2 tablespoons tamari

1 teaspoon chili flakes

1 clove garlic, minced

¾-inch knob of ginger, minced

6 chicken thighs or drumsticks
(or a combo)

10 ounces sugar snap peas, trimmed

1 bunch asparagus, ends snapped,
spears halved

2 green onions, thinly sliced

¼ cup peanuts

1 lime, cut into wedges

2 tablespoons white sesame seeds

Preheat the oven to 400°F. Combine the peanut butter, coconut oil, tamari, chili, garlic and ginger in a baking dish and mix well. Add the chicken and toss around to coat. Place in the oven and bake for 15 minutes.

Remove from the oven and artfully arrange the green veggies, onions, peanuts, lime wedges and sesame seeds around and over the chicken. Return to the oven and cook for another 10 minutes, or until the chicken is browned.

1 SERVING VEG + FRUIT PER SERVING

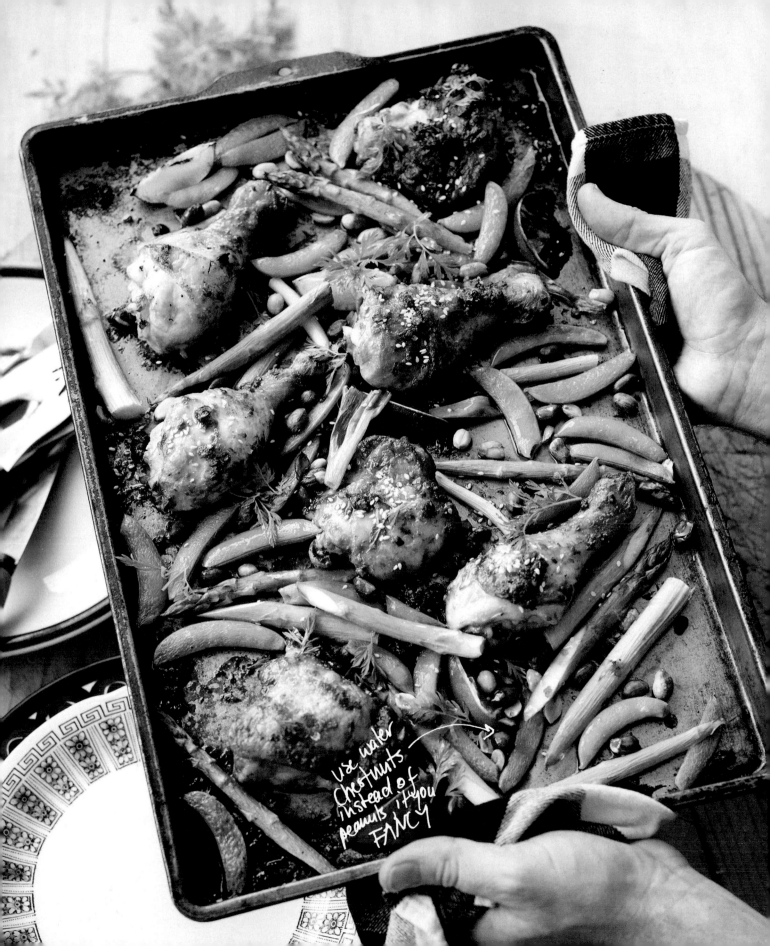

use water
chestnuts
instead of
peanuts if you
FANCY

MY RECALIBRATING PORK MEAL

When I've been traveling or eating a little too much sugar (you heard right) or I'm just a breathing picture of average-ness (autoimmune inflammation and the like), this is the meal I turn to, generally with a dignified glass of preservative-free red wine.

Go for free-range (outdoor reared) organic pork to ensure they're not fed recycled food waste (which risks bacterial contamination).

Why get pork on your fork?
My work with *National Geographic*'s Blue Zones longevity team revealed that pork is one of the foods common to all of the Blue Zones (regions and countries boasting the most centenarians). One Japanese study has suggested that the link between eating pork and longevity may have something to do with the fact that pigs are genetically similar to humans and that there may be something in pork protein that helps repair arterial damage. An interesting hypothesis only.

Sustainable cheap cuts:
Where possible, choose pork shoulder chops (also known as blade chops, blade steak, pork shoulder steaks, pork shoulder blade steaks).

2 bone-in pork chops, each about ¾-inch thick (about 14 ounces in total)

1 sweet potato, cut in half lengthwise and sliced into rounds (¼-inch thick)

sea salt and freshly ground black pepper

2 teaspoons coconut oil

1 fennel, sliced lengthwise into 8 wedges (the whole lot, including stems and fronds)

1 bunch asparagus, ends snapped, spears halved

1 firm peach or apple, cut into eighths

1 teaspoon chopped sage, rosemary or thyme

2 tablespoons apple cider vinegar or sauerkraut brine (see page 337)

big splash of Homemade Chicken Stock (page 42) or 2–3 frozen stock cubes (see page 25)

1 teaspoon Dijon mustard

Preheat the oven to 400°F. Season the pork and sweet potato with salt and pepper. Heat the coconut oil in an ovenproof skillet over medium-high heat. Brown the chops and sweet potato, turning once (about 3 minutes each side). Lift the chops out briefly, adding the fennel, asparagus, peach or apple, and herbs to the pan. Stir to combine, then return the chops to the pan, placing them on top of the veggies, fruit and herbs. Mix the vinegar, stock and mustard together and pour over the lot. Place in the oven and cook for 15 minutes.

MAKE IT SERVE 6:
After searing 6 chops in the skillet, transfer to a large baking dish with triple the amount of each of the remaining ingredients and cook the lot for 20 minutes.

MAKE IT IN A SKILLET:
Alternatively, you can cook the lot in your pan—simply cover with a plate and simmer for 10 minutes.

2½ SERVINGS VEG + FRUIT PER SERVING

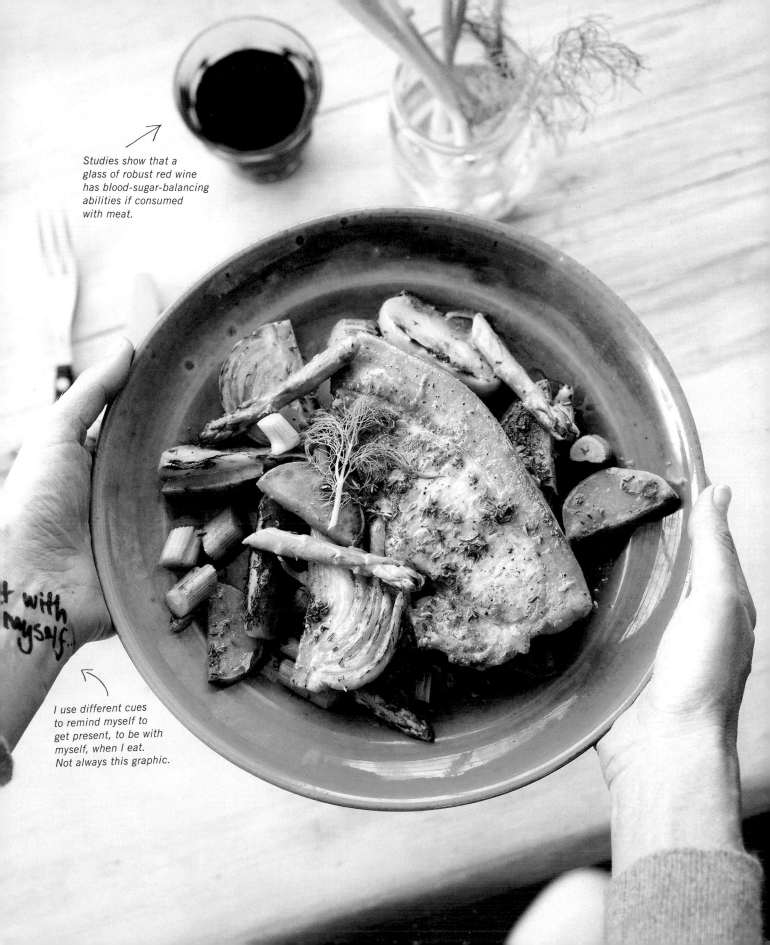

Studies show that a glass of robust red wine has blood-sugar-balancing abilities if consumed with meat.

t with mysuf.

I use different cues to remind myself to get present, to be with myself, when I eat. Not always this graphic.

SLOW-COOKER APPLE CIDER CHICKEN

SERVES 6

2¼ pounds chicken thighs
(skin left on, bones intact)

2–3 cloves garlic, crushed

2 green onions, thinly sliced

2 bay leaves

¼ cup tamari or soy sauce

¼ cup apple cider vinegar

juice of ½ lemon

1 cup quinoa, rinsed twice

1½ cups Homemade Chicken Stock
(page 42)

2–3 bunches baby bok choy
(or 4 cups any Asian greens)

If the chicken has started to fall off the bone (nice!) feel free to shred it, discarding the bones, before returning it to the slow cooker. →

Place the chicken in the bottom of a slow-cooker insert. Add the garlic, green onions, bay leaves, tamari or soy sauce, vinegar and lemon juice, and toss to coat the chicken. Cover and cook on low for 5½ hours or on high for 2½ hours. Remove the chicken from the slow cooker and set aside.

Add the quinoa and stock to the slow-cooker insert and stir. Cover and cook on high for 40 minutes, or until the quinoa is cooked (it should have "tails" sprouting). Return the chicken to the slow cooker. Add the greens, then cover and cook for a further 20 minutes, or until tender. To serve, arrange the greens on serving plates. Stir the quinoa and chicken, and spoon over the greens.

1 SERVING VEG + FRUIT PER SERVING

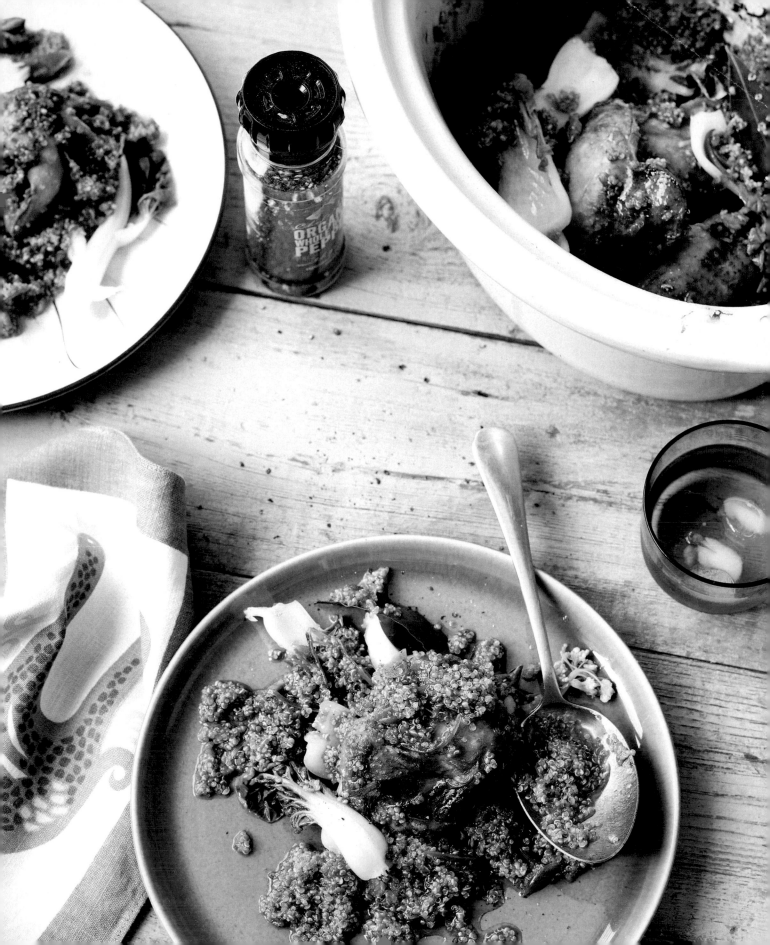

MOROCCAN CAULIFLOWER, CHICKPEA AND QUINOA BAKE

SERVES 6

This one is pictured on page 225.

1 head cauliflower, chopped into florets

1 onion, finely diced

2 cups Cooked Quinoa (page 26)

2 cups cooked chickpeas (see page 28) or 14-ounce can chickpeas, drained and rinsed

½ cup almonds, chopped (optional)

2 teaspoons curry powder

1 teaspoon ground turmeric

2 teaspoons ground cumin

sea salt and freshly ground black pepper

juice of 2 lemons

¼ cup coconut oil, melted

⅔ cup full-fat organic plain yogurt, mixed with a big pinch of ground cumin

cilantro or flat-leaf parsley leaves, to serve

Preheat the oven to 350°F. Combine all of the ingredients except the yogurt in a large baking dish and toss well until the cauliflower is evenly coated in spices and coconut oil. Roast for 20 minutes or until the cauliflower is crispy and brown on top.

Remove from the oven and serve with a dollop of cumin yogurt and a sprinkle of cilantro or parsley leaves.

MAKE IT A MOROCCAN CHICKEN AND CAULIFLOWER BAKE:
Omit the chickpeas and replace with 2 cups of Shredded Chicken (page 214).

1½ SERVINGS VEG + FRUIT PER SERVING

STEAK 'N' FIVE VEG

This recipe works equally well with lamb chops, pork chops or even sausages.

Know your sustainable steak

Inside skirt steak (called hanger steak in the US or butcher's steak 'cos butchers liked to keep it for themselves) is from the diaphragm and is a relatively tender piece of meat on its own. (None of these muscles get much of a workout!) It is best cooked in a cast-iron skillet or grilled until medium-rare.

Flat iron steak is a flat muscle off the shoulder blade. It's super-tender considering it's so close to a joint. Also best cooked in a cast-iron skillet or grilled.

1 sweet potato

1 parsnip

2 tablespoons coconut oil, melted

sea salt and freshly ground black pepper

2 x 5-ounce sustainable beef steaks

1 small red onion, thinly sliced

1 small clove garlic, crushed

8 brussels sprouts, trimmed and thinly sliced

1 cup thinly sliced red cabbage

1 cup thinly sliced kale or chard

juice of 1 lemon

pinch of chili flakes

If brussels sprouts aren't in season, use 1 cup coarsely chopped broccoli or cauliflower florets.

Preheat the broiler and place the rack about 6 inches below the element. Using a vegetable peeler, slice the sweet potato and parsnip lengthwise into ribbons and place on a baking sheet. Toss with half the coconut oil and a sprinkle of salt. Season the steak and place on top.

In a separate bowl, toss the onion, garlic, brussels sprouts, cabbage and kale or chard in the rest of the coconut oil, the lemon juice and chili until well coated. Add to the baking sheet, around the steaks, and grill for 1–2 minutes. Remove from the heat, turn the steaks and veggies and grill for another 1–2 minutes, or until the steaks are browned.

Remove the meat and let it sit, covered, for 5–10 minutes. Meanwhile, continue to grill the veggies until they are cooked through. Serve immediately.

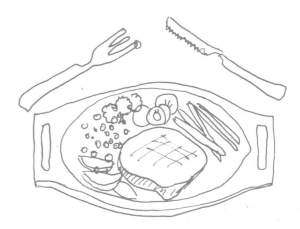

 4½ SERVINGS VEG + FRUIT PER SERVING

LAMB ROAST FOR TWO

WITH MINTED PEA PISTOU

SERVES 2

Which lamb chops are best?
From a planetary and hip-pocket perspective, go for leg/forequarter over loin chops. Lamb breast can also be used.

1 tablespoon olive oil, plus extra for drizzling

2 teaspoons chopped oregano or ½ teaspoon dried oregano

juice of ½ lemon (use the other half for the Minted Pea Pistou, below)

2 small cloves garlic, crushed

4 lamb chops

2 small onions, skin left on, sliced into wedges (not quite right down to the root, waterlily-like) or 1 small red onion, cut into wedges

1 red bell pepper, cut into chunks

2 small zucchini, sliced into rounds

sea salt and freshly ground black pepper

6 cherry tomatoes

¼ cup olives

¼ cup cubed feta

TO SERVE

Minted Pea Pistou (optional; see below)

mint or oregano leaves

Preheat the oven to 400°F.

Combine the oil, oregano, lemon juice, garlic and lamb in a bowl. Cover and refrigerate for at least 25 minutes (all day is fab).

Place the onion, bell pepper and zucchini in a large baking dish with a good drizzle of olive oil and season with salt and pepper. Bake for 25 minutes.

Add the lamb, cherry tomatoes, olives and feta to the baking dish and cook for another 20 minutes, turning the chops after 10 minutes. Serve with Minted Pea Pistou (if using) and a sprinkling of mint or oregano leaves.

MINTED PEA PISTOU

½ cup frozen peas, blanched in some boiling water and cooled

½ cup mint leaves

zest and juice of ½ lemon

¼ cup extra-virgin olive oil

Combine all the ingredients in a blender or food processor and blend until smooth.

Or simply blend ½ cup Leftovers Pesto (page 55) with the peas.

2 SERVINGS VEG + FRUIT PER SERVING

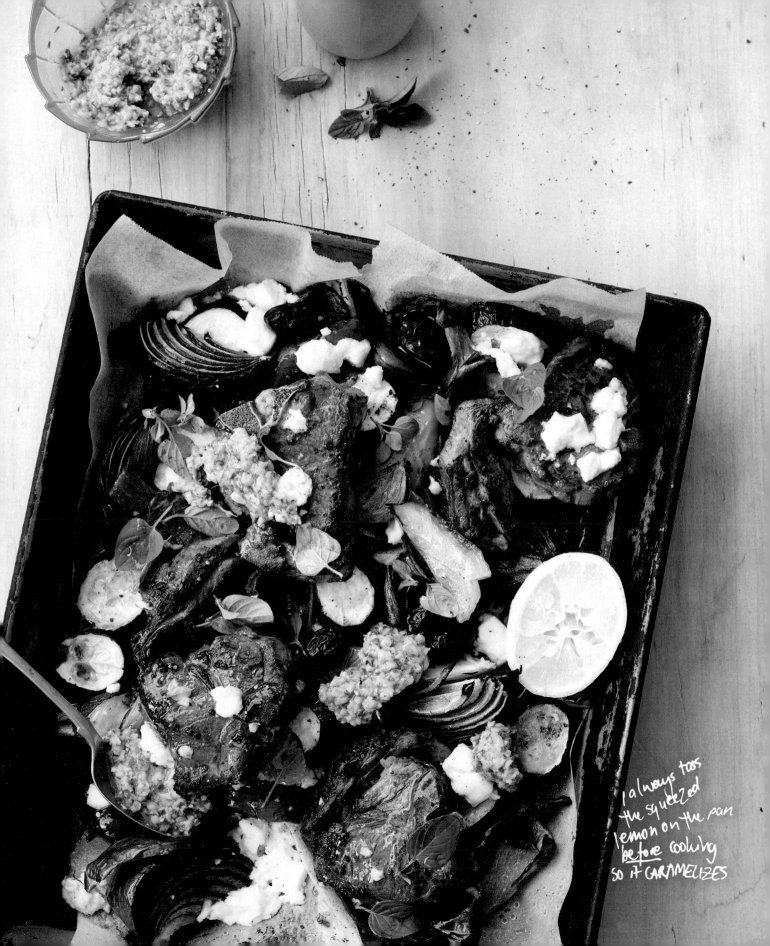

I always toss
the squeezed
lemon on the pan
before cooking
so it CARAMELIZES

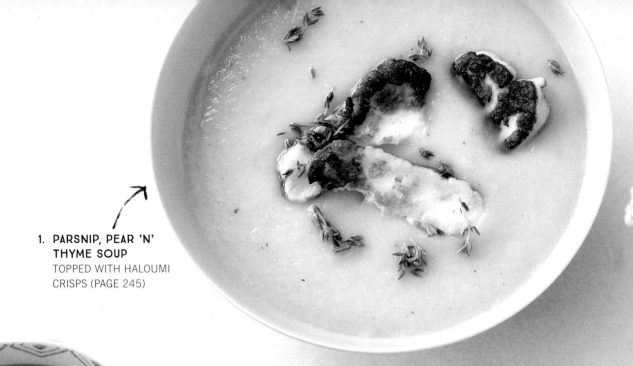

1. PARSNIP, PEAR 'N' THYME SOUP
TOPPED WITH HALOUMI CRISPS (PAGE 245)

A "ROOT 'N' A SHRUB" SOUPS

three ways, using a root veggie + blending it with some lovely herbaciousness

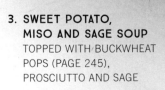

2. BEET, BEET LEAF 'N' APPLE BORSCHT
TOPPED WITH A POACHED EGG FLOATER (PAGE 245)

3. SWEET POTATO, MISO AND SAGE SOUP
TOPPED WITH BUCKWHEAT POPS (PAGE 245), PROSCIUTTO AND SAGE

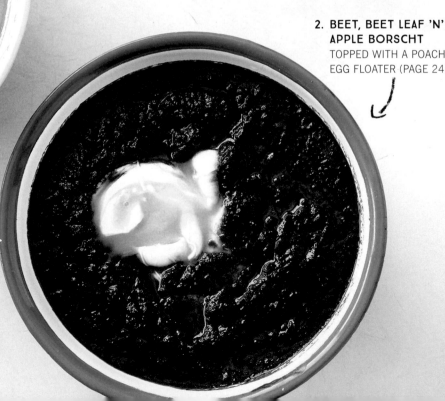

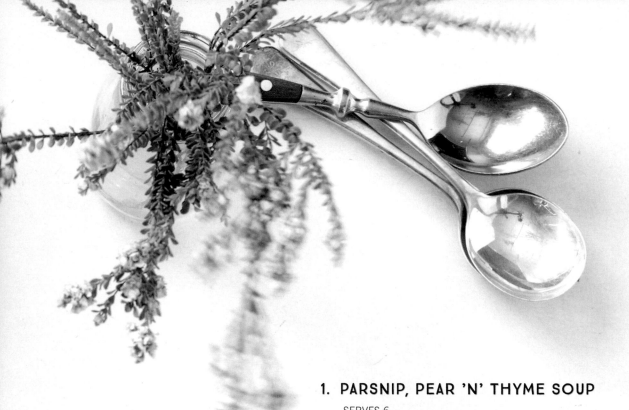

1. PARSNIP, PEAR 'N' THYME SOUP

SERVES 6

2 tablespoons coconut oil, olive oil, butter or ghee

2 onions, diced

4 large parsnips, roughly chopped

2 small pears, peeled, cored and roughly chopped

1 teaspoon sea salt

freshly ground black pepper

1½ quarts Homemade Vegetable Stock (page 42)

4 sprigs thyme, leaves picked, plus extra sprigs to serve

cream or full-fat organic plain yogurt, to serve

Heat the oil, butter or ghee in a large saucepan over a medium-high heat. Add the onion and cook gently for 8–10 minutes, until soft and translucent. Add the remaining ingredients and bring to a boil. Reduce the heat and simmer for about 20 minutes, or until all of the vegetables are cooked through. Pour the soup into a blender and blend to a purée. Serve with extra thyme sprigs and a dollop of cream or yogurt.

recipes continue . . . .

1 SERVING VEG + FRUIT PER SERVING

2. BEET, BEET LEAF 'N' APPLE BORSCHT

SERVES 6

1 tablespoon butter or ghee

3 cloves garlic, minced

1 large onion, roughly chopped

1 celery stalk, roughly chopped

1 carrot, roughly chopped

1 bunch beets (about 1¾ pounds), trimmed, scrubbed and cubed, leaves finely chopped

2 apples, peeled, cored and cut into large cubes

1½ quarts Homemade Vegetable Stock (see page 42)

sea salt and freshly ground black pepper

full-fat organic plain yogurt or Homemade Cream Cheese (page 46), to serve

Heat the butter or ghee in a flameproof casserole dish or large saucepan over low heat. Add the garlic, onion, celery and carrot and cook for 15 minutes, or until the vegetables have softened. Add the beets, chopped beet leaves and apple to the pan and cook for 5 minutes more, stirring to soften slightly. Add the stock and season to taste with salt and pepper. Cover and simmer for 45 minutes, or until everything is tender. Serve the soup chunky, or cool it slightly and purée it in a blender. Spoon into bowls and top with a swirl of yogurt or a dollop of cream cheese.

MAKE IT SUMMER PROBIOTIC BEET SOUP:
Use 1 cup of stock only. Once cooked, allow to cool and add 2 peeled and chopped cucumbers, ½ cup of sauerkraut brine (see page 337) or Grounding Crimson Tonic (page 347) and ½ cup of yogurt. Stir or purée and chill for 4 hours or overnight.

3. SWEET POTATO, MISO AND SAGE SOUP

SERVES 6

1 tablespoon coconut oil

2 onions, roughly chopped

2 cloves garlic, minced

3 medium-large sweet potatoes, peeled and roughly chopped

2 tablespoons red miso paste

1½ quarts Homemade Vegetable Stock (see page 42)

2 tablespoons chopped sage leaves

sea salt and freshly ground pepper

Caesar Salad Boats (opposite), to serve

Feel free to throw in any orange- or white-hued roast veggies you have lying around to fill out the soup.

Heat the coconut oil in a flameproof casserole dish or large saucepan over low heat. Add the onions and garlic and sauté for 5 minutes. Add the sweet potatoes and continue cooking until slightly softened, then add the miso paste. Add the stock and bring to a boil. Cover, then reduce the heat and cook for 20 minutes, or until the sweet potato is cooked through. Season to taste. Allow the soup to cool slightly, then blend in batches to your desired consistency. Serve with Caesar Salad Boats.

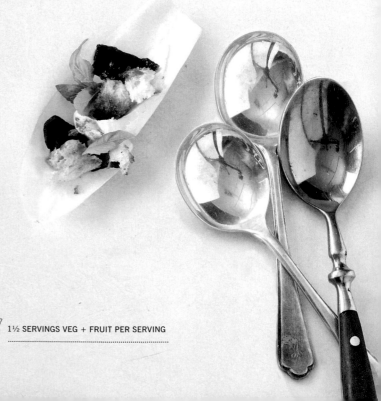

1 SERVING VEG + FRUIT PER SERVING

1½ SERVINGS VEG + FRUIT PER SERVING

A PAGE OF SOUP TOPPERS

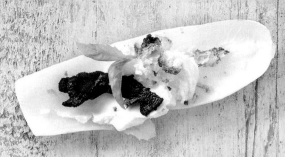

A soup can easily be turned into a weekday meal by sprinkling it with some nutritious and filling fairy dust. Most of the combos below will also jazz up my Leftover Mishmashes (pages 246–65) and Abundance Bowls (pages 126–37) perfectly.

BUCKWHEAT POPS

Toast 1 cup of Activated Groaties (page 27) in 1 teaspoon of coconut or olive oil over a medium heat. Sprinkle with salt, pepper, chili flakes, garam masala or ground cumin, to taste.

BONE MARROW BOMBS

This idea comes directly from my friend Matt Preston. (I asked first!)

5 x 2-inch lengths of bone marrow, removed from the bone (ask your butcher to do this)

lots of cornstarch or plain flour, for dusting

3 tablespoons butter

To prep the marrow, you'll need to soak it in cold, slightly salty water for 24 hours. Next day, remove the soaked marrow and pat dry. Pour the cornstarch or flour into a cereal bowl and roll each length of marrow in the flour, coating the whole lot. Melt the butter in a skillet over medium heat. When the butter is starting to get foamy, slip four bone marrow "bombs" into the pan and fry until all sides are crunchy. Repeat with the remaining marrow pieces.

HALOUMI CRISPS

Pan-fry strips of haloumi in a skillet, or grill them in a sandwich press. Allow to cool, then crumble or break into chunks.

BACON GRANOLA

See page 108.

SWEET POTATO CROUTONS

Cut a scrubbed (not peeled) sweet potato into ½-inch cubes and pan-fry in coconut oil in a skillet. Sprinkle with sea salt (this will speed up the cooking time) and a little ground cumin and cinnamon. Cook until dark golden.

POACHED EGG FLOATER

Break an egg or two into a teacup. Bring your soup to a gentle boil in a small saucepan over medium heat (you'll need the soup to be at least 2 inches deep). Gently tip the egg(s) into the soup, turn off the heat immediately and cover the pan lightly. Leave for 3–4 minutes, or until the eggs are cooked.

HARISSA CREAM CHEESE BOMBS

Swirl 1 tablespoon of harissa paste through 1 cup of Homemade Cream Cheese (page 46).

CAESAR SALAD BOATS

Pull apart a head of Belgian endive and line individual leaves with Homemade Cream Cheese (page 46). Top with Bacon Bits (page 44), an anchovy fillet and/or leftover Shredded Chicken (page 214).

MY LEFTOVER

MISHMASHES

Officially my favorite chapter where EVERYTHING comes ▷ together ◁ and you find yourself using up all your SCRAPS and dregs | and bobs + bits... and life makes a lot more flow-y SENSE.

I stand for

Or with a flurry of carrot tops

(Generally with an egg chucked in the middle)

GREEN SCRAPS SHAKSHOUKA

LEFTOVER GREENS + LEFTOVERS PESTO + SOME EGGS

SERVES 2 ——————————————————————————

A hipster (kale-ified) version of the classic Irish bubble 'n' squeak.

Use a few frozen cubes of zucchini (see page 24) if you like.

1 tablespoon butter

½ onion or leek (or use 3 green onions), thinly sliced

3 cups whatever green vegetables you have: sliced fennel (reserve the fronds), grated zucchini, thinly sliced snow peas and asparagus are all great

¼ teaspoon ground cumin

¼ teaspoon chili flakes (or a few drops of Tabasco)

juice of ½ lemon

2 handfuls of leafy greens and herbs (kale, beet leaves, spinach, flat-leaf parsley, basil, cilantro, fennel fronds, etc.)

sea salt and freshly ground black pepper

2 tablespoons Leftovers Pesto (page 55)

2–3 eggs

¼ cup whatever cheese you have, crumbled or grated

sliced olives, to serve (optional)

Melt the butter in a skillet over medium-high heat. Add the onion, leek or green onions, green vegetables and cumin. Sauté for 5–7 minutes. Add the chili, lemon juice and leafy greens and herbs and cook until wilted. Season with salt and pepper and stir in the pesto.

Create two or three divots in your mixture and break the eggs in one by one. Reduce the heat to low. Sprinkle with cheese. Cover (with a plate or lid) and cook for about 5–7 minutes, or until the eggs are set. To serve, toss in a few black olives and their brine, if you like.

4 SERVINGS VEG + FRUIT PER SERVING

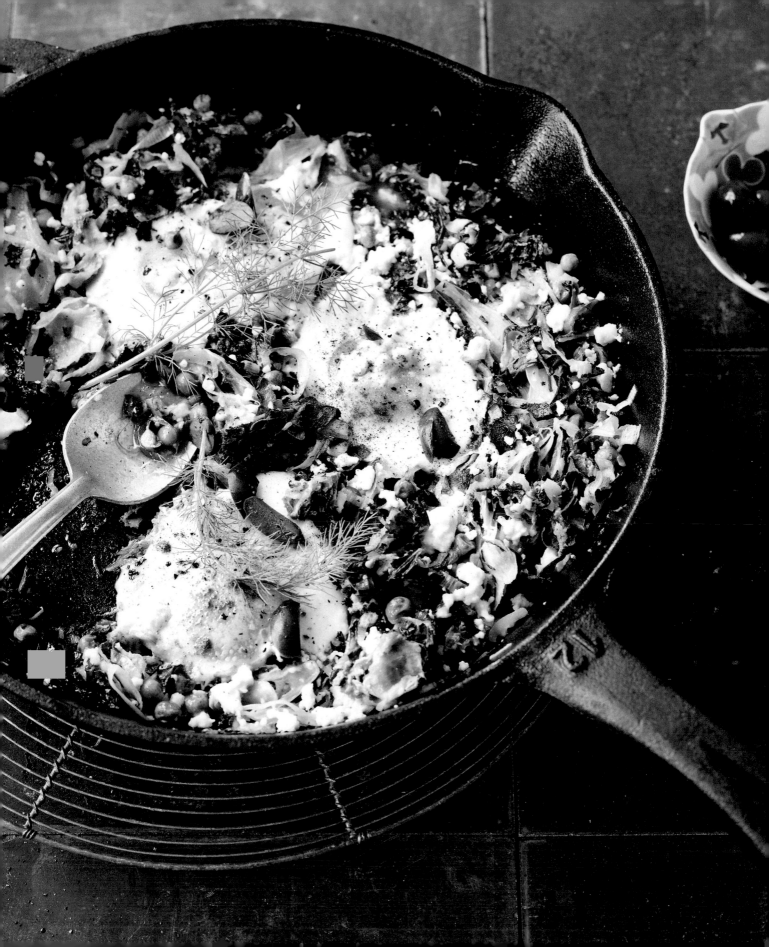

CRISP BIBIMBAP SKILLET PANCAKE

KIMCHI + LEFTOVER SHREDDED MEAT + COOKED QUINOA

SERVES 2

I love this Korean version of bubble 'n' squeak. It's regarded as a winter healing food in Korea and it's all about using leftovers. I've given it a spin by combining a few steps and abandoning a few pots. Oh, and refashioning the whole lot as a crisp pancake. You're welcome.

If you have a big paella pan, you can triple the recipe to feed the family.

1 tablespoon sesame oil or coconut oil

1 cup Cooked Quinoa (page 26)

1 cup "But the Kitchen Sink" Kimchi (page 337), including a little brine, plus extra to serve (or use 2 cups shredded leafy greens or cabbage tossed with a big splash of tamari)

3 green onions, finely chopped

1 tablespoon tamari, soy or fish sauce

2–3 eggs

½ cup leftover cooked meat (see any recipe in the Sunday Cook-Ups chapter)

2–3 separate mounds of different-colored cooked or raw vegetables, grated or thinly sliced (carrots, red cabbage, brussels sprouts, squash, zucchini, beans, peas, spinach, bean sprouts, etc.)

TO SERVE

a generous sprinkle of a crunchy, tasty thing (sesame seeds, dulse flakes, Seaweed Dukkah [page 45], etc.)

Simple "Gochujang" Sauce (see below; optional)

Heat the oil in a skillet over medium-high heat. Add the quinoa, kimchi (or greens), green onions and tamari, soy or fish sauce to the pan, stirring to combine, then press flat with a wooden spoon. Reduce the heat and cook for 5 minutes or until the mixture begins to crisp and caramelize on the bottom. Crack the eggs on top and swirl to cover. Reduce the heat to low, cover (with a plate or lid) and cook for 4–5 minutes, until the eggs are just set. Arrange the meat and colored veggies on top and heat through.

You can flip the pancake onto a plate before adding the toppings if you want a crunchy vibe.

The egg will spread through the pancake and crisp everything up even further.

Remove from the heat and serve with the extra kimchi (or greens, if using), a sprinkling of something crunchy and tasty and some "gochujang" sauce, if you like.

SIMPLE "GOCHUJANG" SAUCE

¼ cup Nomato Sauce (page 51)

pinch of chili flakes or a few drops of Tabasco

½ teaspoon brown rice syrup

Mix in a teacup. Done.

3 SERVINGS VEG + FRUIT PER SERVING

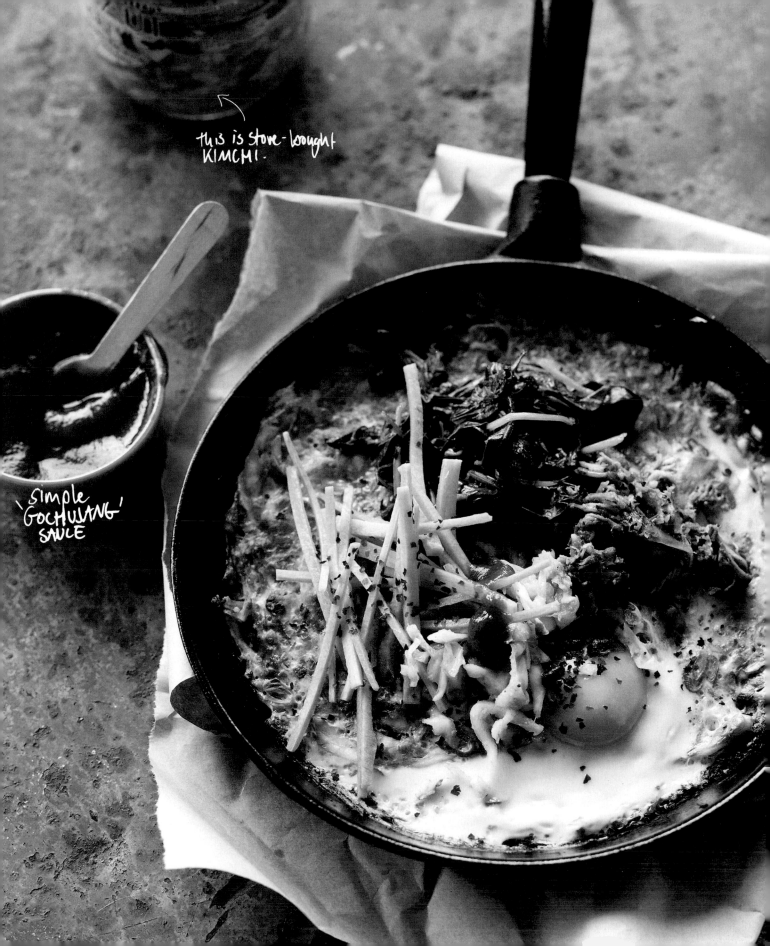

this is store-bought
KIMCHI.

'simple
GOCHUJANG'
SAUCE

MY SALAD of the SCOUNDREL

SERVES 2

Translated from the French *salade canaille*, this meal is made up of a "rabble" of bits and pieces, which are given some perk with the addition of fridge-door flavor bombs. Perfectly designed for Sunday-night floor picnics.

PICKLED ROAST VEGGIES

Combine 1–2 cups of leftover Roasted Roots (page 23) with ½ red onion that's been sliced and soaked in apple cider vinegar for 10 minutes. Sprinkle with celery leaves (optional), a pinch of sea salt and a drizzle of extra-virgin olive oil. Toss.

2 SERVINGS VEG + FRUIT PER SERVING

GRIBICHE SAUCE PLATE

Finely chop ¼ red onion and mix with 1–2 tablespoons of Whey-Good Mayo (page 50) and 1 teaspoon each of Dijon mustard and chopped capers. Dollop over 1 cup of leftover cooked meat (any kind; see Sunday Cook-Ups chapter), or 2–3 hard-boiled eggs, diced. Garnish with celery leaves.

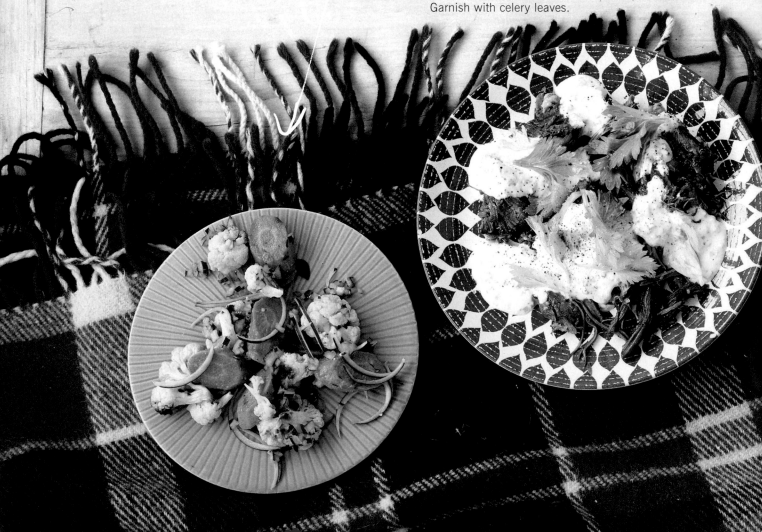

GOLDEN OATMEAL WEDGES

Combine 2 cups of leftover oatmeal, rice, lentils or Cooked Quinoa (page 26) with ⅓ cup of grated Parmesan and 1 tablespoon of chopped thyme, chives or other fresh herbs. If your mixture is a bit soggy, add 1 teaspoon of chia seeds. Line a plate with parchment paper. Scoop the oatmeal onto the plate and press it into a "pancake" the size of your skillet. Transfer it to the fridge for 30 minutes to firm. Heat 1½ tablespoons of butter in your skillet and fry the oatmeal cake on both sides until golden.

PINK DEVILISH GOOGIE EGGS

Marinate 12 peeled hard-boiled eggs in 1½ cups of leftover brine from the pink sauerkraut (see page 337) for at least 2 hours (or overnight) in the fridge. Pat the eggs dry and slice in half lengthwise. If you like, remove the yolks and mash with 1 tablespoon of Whey-Good Mayo (page 50), then spoon the mixture back in and sprinkle with curry powder.

If you don't have pink brine, slice 1 old beet and boil it in 1 cup of water and ½ cup of white vinegar for 20 minutes. Strain and cool.

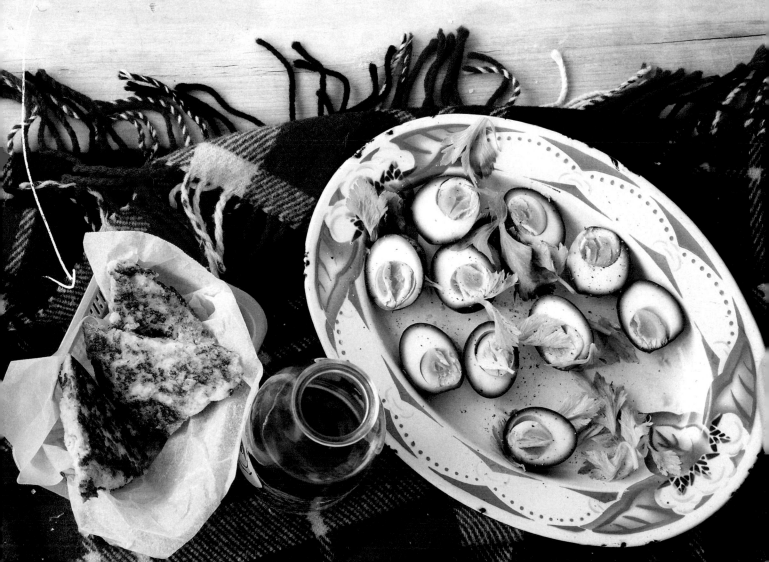

FRIDGE-DOOR TONNATO

MAKES 1½ CUPS

FIVE WAYS TO USE FRIDGE-DOOR TONNATO:

1. Pour over Shredded Lamb (page 220) and steamed beans and sprinkle with celery leaves to make Cheat's Vitello Tonnato (pictured).

2. Dollop on a grilled lamb chop with a side salad.

3. Toss through pasta and broccoli (cooked in the one pot).

4. Drizzle over a plate of boiled eggs.

5. Spoon over a wedge of iceberg lettuce.

15 ounces Italian canned tuna in olive oil, drained (reserve liquid; see below)

1 tablespoon capers

1 tablespoon chopped anchovies, or a splash of fish sauce

½ cup Whey-Good Mayo (page 50)

juice of ½ lemon

Combine all of the ingredients in a blender and purée. Store in the fridge and use within 2–3 days.

USE THE LEFTOVER TUNA BRINE OR OIL:
Use it to make a dressing, for sautéing or drizzling or freeze it in an ice-cube tray with herbs (see page 25).

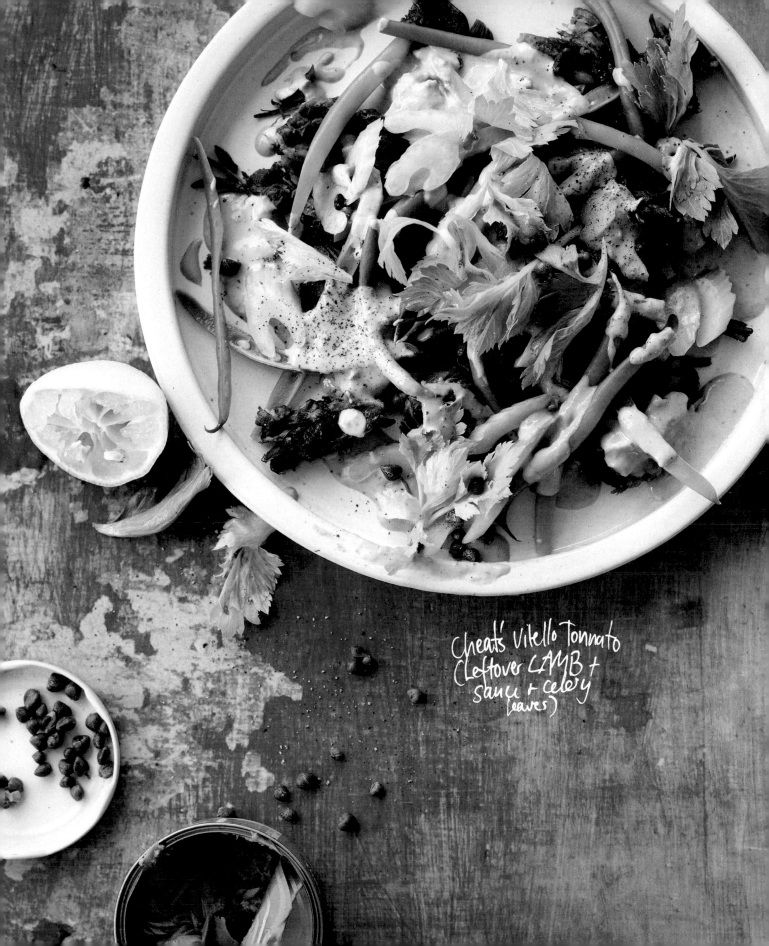

Cheat's Vitello Tonnato (Leftover LAMB + sauce + celery leaves)

LAST NIGHT'S DINNER
WITH AN EGG STUCK IN IT

LEFTOVER DINNER + HOMEMADE STOCK + EGG

SERVES 1

I call it "Doggie Bag Dinner the Next Day" or "Repurposed Stew." The French call it *oeufs en restes*, which lends things a little *élan*. Whatever. The idea entails putting a leftover meal in a pan—it can be a whole meal (chopped up), a soup, a pasta or a stew—adding a dash of broth and sticking an egg in the middle of it.

If you need to thicken a stew or soup, add ⅓ cup of grated potato or 1–2 teaspoons of chia seeds.

The 2:4 Doggie-Bag Rule
Don't be scared of food poisoning: simply get the meal to a fridge within 2 hours, and keep it there for no more than 4 days before eating. Oh, and reheat it in the microwave for at least 2 minutes, until it's steaming hot (above 170°F).

3 cups leftover dinner (chop up anything that doesn't have a goopy consistency)

¼ cup Homemade Stock (page 42) or 2–3 frozen stock cubes (see page 25)

1 egg

a good glug of olive oil

sea salt

Heat the leftovers in a skillet or a small saucepan with a little stock. Once they're hot and bubbling, create a divot in the middle of the mixture and crack in your egg. Cover (with a plate or lid), then reduce the heat and cook until the egg is set. Remove from the heat, drizzle with the olive oil and season with salt.

I add a small handful of peas: I believe a pea can improve most things.

3 SERVINGS VEG + FRUIT PER SERVING

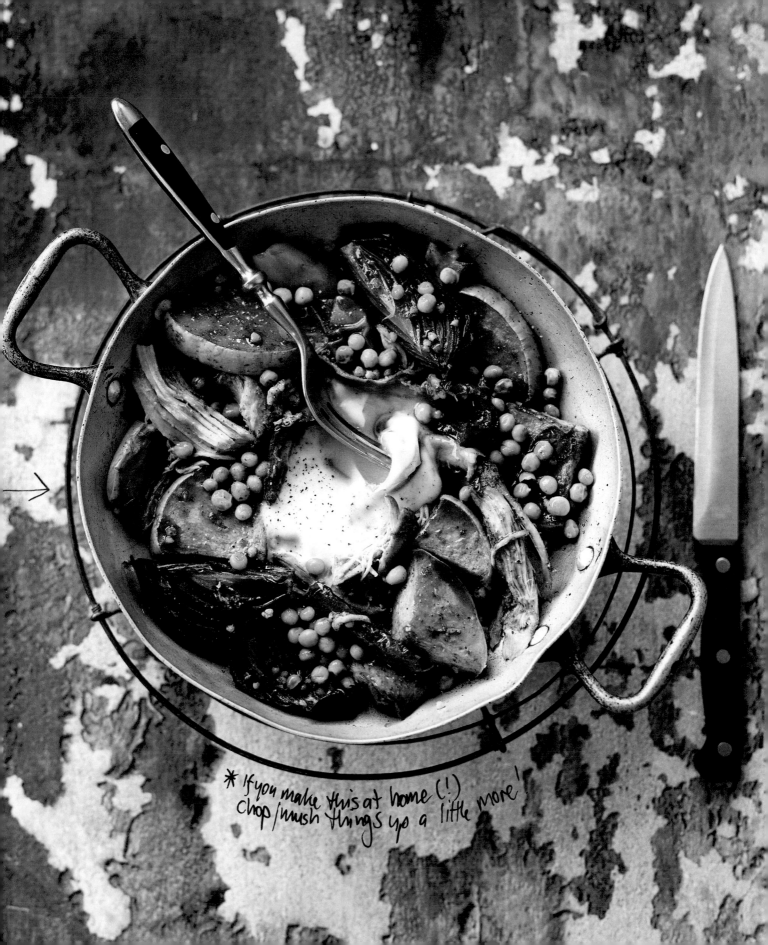

*If you make this at home (!)
chop/mush things up a little more!

SHORTCUT CHOUCROUTE

LEFTOVER MEAT + CABBAGE + OLD SAUERKRAUT

SERVES 2 ———

A great trick for using up 'kraut that's about to turn.

4 good-quality pork sausages
or 8 Basic Meatballs (page 144)

1 onion, cut into wedges

½ apple, cut into wedges

9 ounces coleslaw mix
or 3 cups shredded cabbage

1 cup Sauerkraut (page 337),
including juices

Preheat the oven to 400°F.

Place the sausages or meatballs and onion in a baking dish and roast for
10 minutes. Add the apple, coleslaw or cabbage and sauerkraut and cook
for a further 20 minutes, or until the sausages are plump and golden.

**MAKE IT KIMCHI CHICKEN
CHOUCROUTE:**
Use chicken sausages or meatballs
instead of pork and "But the Kitchen
Sink" Kimchi (page 337) instead of
sauerkraut.

*You can also finish the
cooking under the broiler
if things aren't browned
to your liking.*

3 SERVINGS VEG + FRUIT PER SERVING

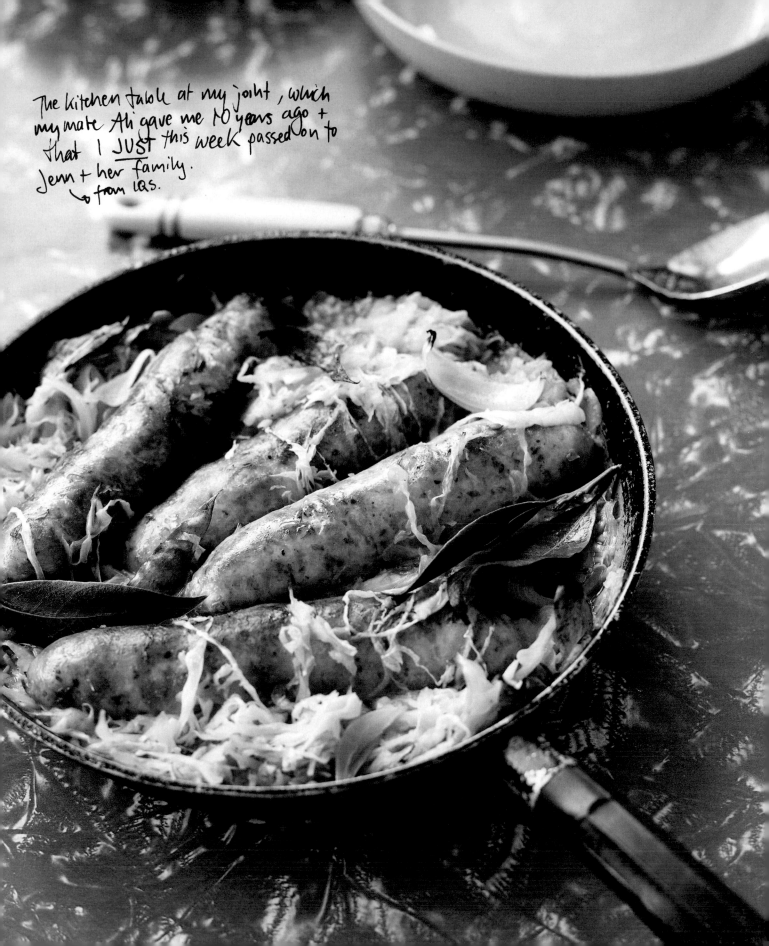

The kitchen table at my joint, which my mate Ali gave me 10 years ago + that I JUST this week passed on to Jenn + her family.
↳ from LQS.

VEGAN WHATCHAGOT QUICHE

LEFTOVER VEGGIES + MORE LEFTOVER VEGGIES + CHIA

SERVES 6 ————————————————————————————————————

You might not be vegan, but you might run out of eggs sometimes . . .

No leftover cooked cauli? Throw 4 cups of chopped raw florets (and the red onion) into a baking dish with some coconut oil and roast for 20 minutes in an oven preheated to 375°F.

coconut oil, for greasing

3 cups leftover roasted cauliflower, chopped

1 red onion, finely chopped

3 cups grated veggies (e.g., a mix of 1 large zucchini, 1 sweet potato or turnip and 1 parsnip or carrot)

½ cup pitted black olives, chopped

¼ cup chia seeds, stirred into 1 cup cold water

2 teaspoons chopped thyme, sage or rosemary, plus extra whole sprigs and leaves to serve

¼ cup gluten-free flour (buckwheat flour or chickpea flour is great)

mixed seeds (e.g., flaxseeds, pepitas, sunflower seeds), to serve

lemon zest, to serve

Sweet Paprika Stem Chips (see below), to serve (optional)

Grease a large quiche dish or springform cake pan with coconut oil. Combine all the ingredients in a large bowl and mix well. Pour into the dish or pan. Cover and refrigerate for at least 2 hours (or overnight) to allow the ingredients to bind.

Preheat the oven to 375°F. Bake the quiche for 40–45 minutes, or until the top is nicely browned. To serve, sprinkle with the seeds, lemon zest and extra herbs.

SWEET PAPRIKA STEM CHIPS
LEFTOVER BROCCOLI AND CAULIFLOWER STALKS

MAKES 2–3 CUPS

This is a great way to use up the stalks of your broccoli and cauliflower.

stalks of 3–4 heads of broccoli or cauliflower

1 tablespoon coconut oil

½ teaspoon salt

½ cup grated Parmesan

pinch of sweet paprika

Whenever I cook with broccoli and cauli, I cut the stalks into sticks and store them in the freezer ready for this cause.

Cut the broccoli and cauli stalks into chips ½ inch wide and toss with the oil and salt. Line a baking sheet with parchment paper and lay the chips out evenly. Bake for 10 minutes, then turn, sprinkle with Parmesan and paprika and bake for another 10–15 minutes. Serve as a side or with The Whole Brassicus Hummus (page 187).

MAKE IT VEGAN:
Use ¼ cup of nutritional yeast powder instead of Parmesan.

2 SERVINGS VEG + FRUIT PER SERVING

THE FISH THAT
GOT AWAY PIE

LEFTOVER FISH + LEFTOVER VEGGIES + EGGS

SERVES 6 ————————————————————————————————————

Sometimes I realize I have some whitefish in the freezer or in the fridge that's been there a touch too long. When this is the case, I make this pie or my Sustainable Sweet Fish Curry (page 164). You can also use leftover Shredded Chicken (page 214).

3½ tablespoons butter

1 oniony thing (1 onion, 1 leek or 6 green onions), thinly sliced

2 tablespoons all-purpose flour

1½ cups milk

22 ounces leftover whitefish or offcuts, cut into bite-sized pieces

2–3 hard-boiled eggs, quartered (optional)

3 cups chopped veggies (use any frozen or leftover veggies, such as cauliflower, zucchini or carrot—I always include frozen peas)

1 tablespoon Dijon mustard

½ cup finely chopped flat-leaf parsley

GREEN NUTTY CRUST

3–4 cups raw broccoli or cauliflower, grated or chopped finely in a food processor

⅓ cup finely grated Parmesan

¼ cup sunflower seeds

Preheat the oven to 350°F. Melt the butter in a saucepan over medium heat. Add the oniony thing and cook for 1 minute, or until softened. Add the flour and cook, stirring, for 1–2 minutes. Gradually add the milk, whisking to remove any lumps. Bring the mixture to a boil and simmer, stirring constantly, for 3–4 minutes. Reduce the heat to low-medium and stir in the fish, eggs (if using), veggies, mustard and parsley. Dump the lot into a large baking dish.

To make the crust, combine the ingredients in a bowl and mix well. Spoon the crust mixture over the fish and veggies and bake for 20–25 minutes, until golden and bubbling at the edges.

MAKE IT AN ORANGE NUTTY CRUST:
Use grated root veggies (sweet potato, carrot, etc.) instead of the broccoli or cauliflower and 2 tablespoons of butter instead of the Parmesan.

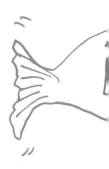

2½ SERVINGS VEG + FRUIT PER SERVING

"PIZZA" BREAD-AND-BUTTER CRUMBLE

LEFTOVER MEAT + LEFTOVER VEGGIES + NOMATO SAUCE

SERVES 2

2–3 cups Parcooked 'n' Frozen kale or chard (page 22)

1 cup leftover meat (any kind; see Sunday Cook-Ups chapter, pages 210–25)

1–2 frozen stock cubes with herbs (see page 25) or ¼ teaspoon dried herbs

½ cup Nomato Sauce (page 51) or sugar-free purée

BREAD AND BUTTER CRUMBLE

1 tablespoon butter, melted

1 cup Cooked Quinoa (page 26) or Cooked Buckwheat (page 27)

2 tablespoons grated cheese (any hard cheese is fine)

Preheat the oven to 400°F. Combine the kale or chard, meat, stock or herbs, and Nomato Sauce or purée in a small baking sheet or skillet.

To make the crumble, combine the ingredients in a small bowl and mix well. Spoon the crumble over the meat-and-vegetable mixture and bake for 15–20 minutes, until golden and bubbling.

MAKE IT A CREAMY GRATIN:
Use cream instead of Nomato Sauce.

I actually prefer this "white" version. But it meant ditching the catchy "pizza" title.

2 SERVINGS VEG + FRUIT PER SERVING

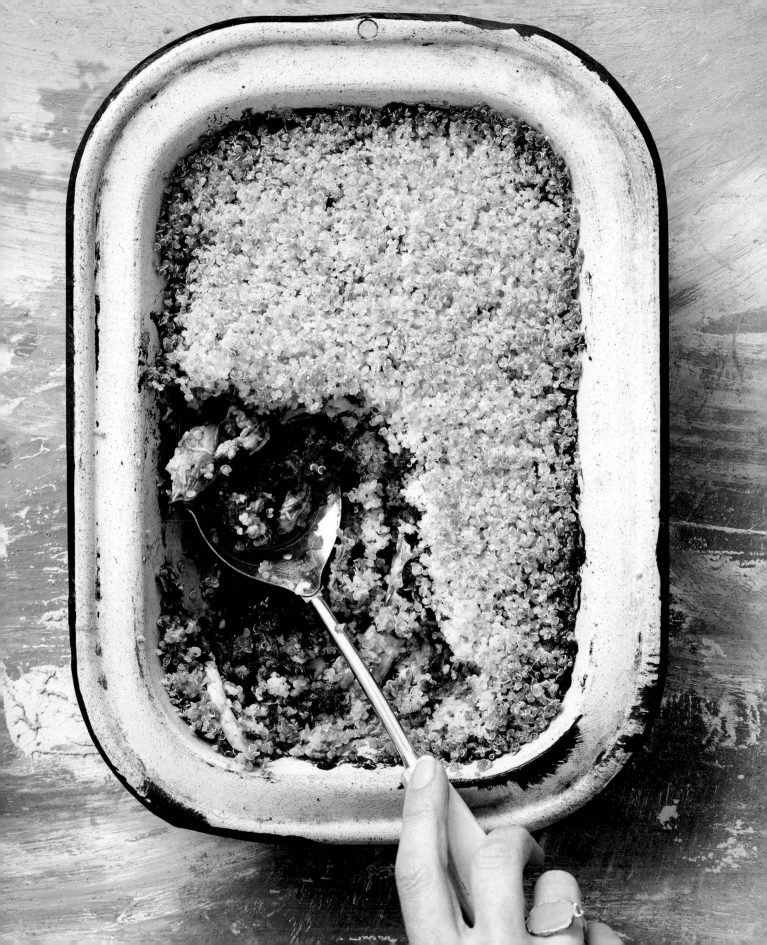

FOUR HEALING THINGS TO DO WITH A CUP OF HOMEMADE STOCK

I pride myself on finding better and simpler ways to maketh some bone broth/stock into a quick, gut-lining meal. (See page 42 for beef, chicken and fish stock recipes.)

You can use any stock for these recipes, but beef and chicken are best.

EGG-DROP SOUP

Whisk 1 egg and pour slowly into a small saucepan of simmering stock, stirring with a spoon. Cook for half a minute and serve with a sprinkle of chopped flat-leaf parsley, if you like.

LEFTOVERS KIMCHI SOUP

Combine equal quantities of stock (preferably chicken, page 42), Shredded Chicken (page 214), water and "But the Kitchen Sink" Kimchi (page 337) in a saucepan. Bring to the boil and simmer for 5 minutes, tossing in some green onions and frozen peas toward the end.

EASIEST-EVER KOREAN BREAKFAST CUSTARD

Whisk 2 eggs with ¼ teaspoon of sea salt and ½ cup of stock in a ramekin or mug until foamy. Place the ramekin in a saucepan of simmering water (the water should come halfway up the sides of the ramekin). Cover the saucepan and gently simmer for 10–15 minutes until the eggs are set but still a bit wobbly. Serve with My Indian Kimchi (page 338), sliced green onions and Seaweed Dukkah (page 45).

MY GUT-HEALING BREW

(see page 87)

Face + head beyond the fold

GREEN GUMBO

LEFTOVER SOUP + LEFTOVER HAM

SERVES 2

Use any greens you like: kale, chard, mustard greens, cavolo nero, parsley, etc.

6 cups chopped leafy greens

2 portions of Slow-Cooked Green Peas and Ham (the soup variation; page 217)

2 teaspoons apple cider vinegar

2 portions of Ham Hock Chunks (page 217)

Celery Leaf Salt (see below), to serve (optional)

Bring a saucepan of salted water to a boil over medium heat. Add the greens and blanch, uncovered, for about 5 minutes, or until quite soft. Drain most of the water out. Add the soup portions and vinegar and simmer for another 5 minutes. Sprinkle over the ham and serve with Celery Leaf Salt, if you like.

CELERY LEAF SALT
LEFTOVER CELERY LEAVES

MAKES ½–1 CUP

Granddad Tim put celery salt on everything. Along with white pepper. I think I've inherited his taste for it. Or perhaps it's the taste of smugness from knowing I've found another way to use stuff that's mostly thrown out. Lovely on eggs and salads and on top of soups.

1 bunch celery, leaves only

sea salt flakes (not ground salt or crystals—Maldon sea flakes are good)

Preheat the oven to 350°F. Place the dry celery leaves on a baking sheet in a single layer. Bake in the oven for 5–8 minutes until dried out and crunchy, but not browned. Remove from the oven, cool and either crumble in your hands into small flakes or process briefly in a food processor. Place in a jar and add salt in a 1:1 ratio if you like lots of salt, or 2:1 ratio if you want a stronger celery flavor. Shake to combine.

3½ SERVINGS VEG + FRUIT PER SERVING

A SMALL CHAPTER
OF SHOW-STOPPING
TREATS

Frankly, I've scaled everything back for this chapter. Originally, my plan was to shrink the whole chapter. Literally. But it was going to make it hard for you to read. And my publisher Ingrid gave me her "Are you serious, Sarah?!" look. So I just concentrated on making sure
the amount
of sugar
sweetener
used
was
small.
Ditto portion sizes. You won't notice, of course. But I wanted to MAXIMIZE my minimizing point. Now. Please enjoy.

LAMINGTON
ICE CREAMS

The lamington is a classic Australian dessert made from sponge cake squares, which are dipped in melted chocolate and wrapped in coconut. This frozen one takes things up a notch.

14 ounce can coconut cream, shaken lightly before opening

⅓ cup cashew butter

1 teaspoon pure vanilla extract (or make your own; see page 45)

1 tablespoon brown rice syrup

7 ounces dark (85–90% cocoa) chocolate, chopped into small pieces

1½ cups desiccated or shredded coconut

⅓ cup Raspberry Chia Jam (page 57)

Line an 8 × 8-inch square baking pan with parchment paper. Pour the coconut cream into the prepared pan and place in the freezer for 2–3 hours until frozen.

Remove the coconut cream slab and break into shards using a potato masher or the end of a rolling pin. Pulse the shards in a food processor until they resemble a fine powder. Add the cashew butter, vanilla extract and brown rice syrup and process until smooth and fluffy like ice cream. Pour the mixture back into the pan and smooth the top with a spatula or palette knife. Freeze for 1–2 hours, until the mixture is firm to the touch but not rock solid.

Melt the chocolate in a bowl in the microwave (or in a heatproof bowl over a saucepan of boiling water, making sure the bottom of the bowl doesn't touch the water). Put the coconut into another bowl.

Remove the ice cream from the freezer and slice into 36 small squares. (You may want to trim the outer edges for a neater result.) Spread 18 squares with a thin layer of jam. Place the remaining squares on top to make "sandwiches."

Using two forks, or a toothpick, gently dip the squares into the melted chocolate, coating all sides, then dip in the coconut until covered, placing them on a lined pan as you go. Store in the freezer in a sealed container for up to 3 months.

If you're serving these straight from the freezer, let them sit out for 2–3 minutes to thaw slightly and they'll be crunchy on the outside and soft and smooth on the inside.

¼ TEASPOON ADDED SUGAR PER SERVING

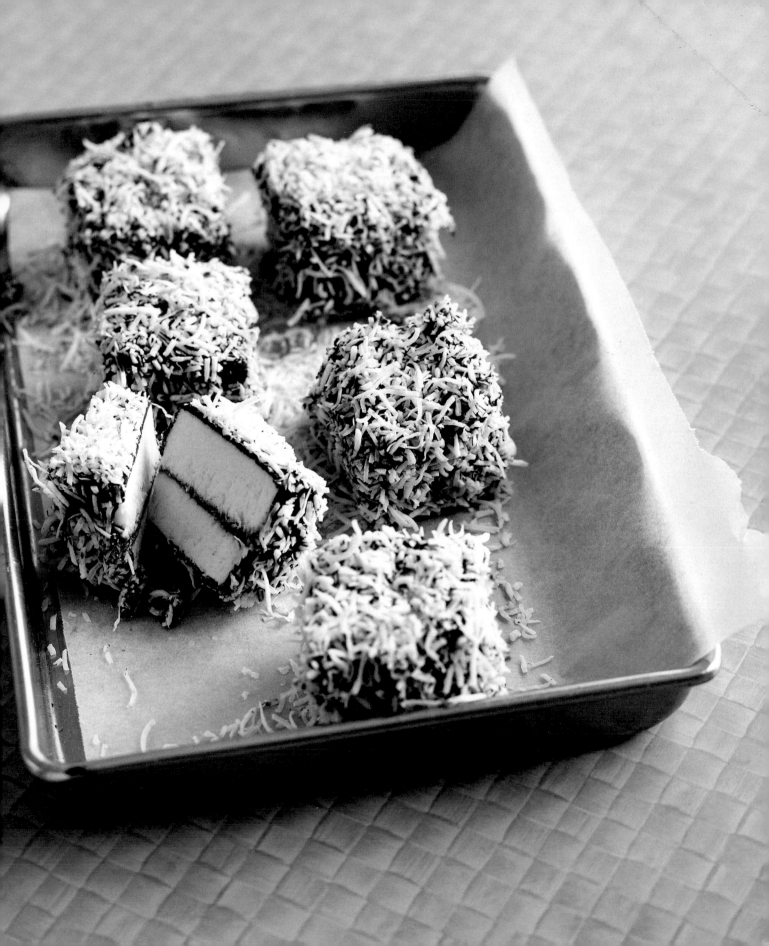

CHOC-BEET
ALLSPICE TRUFFLES

½ cup Cooked 'n' Frozen Beets (page 23) or 1 large beet, trimmed, peeled, chopped and steamed

½ cup heavy cream

1 teaspoon ground allspice (or a big pinch of ground cumin for something quite wild)

1¾ ounces dark (85–90% cocoa) chocolate, roughly chopped

raw cacao powder, for rolling

Purée the beets, then simmer in a small saucepan for 5 minutes, stirring frequently, to remove the excess liquid. In another saucepan, heat the cream and spice until it's simmering. Add the beet purée and chocolate, stirring until the chocolate is melted. Leave in the fridge for a few hours.

Once cold, roll teaspoonfuls of the truffle mix into balls with your hands (refrigerate for an extra 10 minutes if your balls are a little too moist) and then roll in the cacao powder to coat. Store in the fridge for 3–4 days or freeze for up to 3 months.

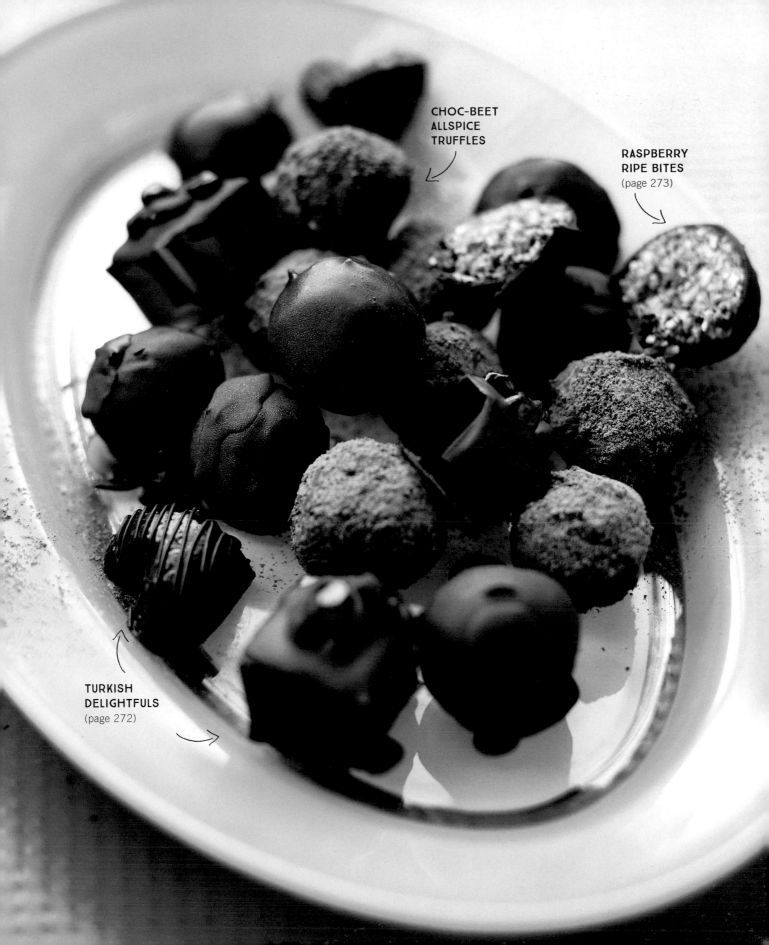

CHOC-BEET
ALLSPICE
TRUFFLES

RASPBERRY
RIPE BITES
(page 273)

TURKISH
DELIGHTFULS
(page 272)

TURKISH DELIGHTFULS

If you can't find a pomegranate, use 1 cup of raspberries or an extra ½ cup of water and 1 tablespoon of beetroot powder.

Two notes on pomegranate
Pomegranate is probably best viewed as a treat food. Its season is short, though you can freeze the seeds. Also, it's not a low-fructose fruit (although the amount you eat means it's not something to be too concerned about).

¼ cup gelatin powder (see page 348)

1 pomegranate (reserve 1 tablespoon seeds for decorating; smash the rest a little to release the juice)

2 tablespoons lemon juice

2 tablespoons brown rice syrup or 4 drops liquid stevia

1–2 teaspoons rose water

You might need up to 1 tablespoon— it depends on the strength of your rose water.

3 cubes frozen Basic Raw Chocolate (page 56) or ¼ cup chopped dark (85–90% cocoa) chocolate (optional)

chopped pistachios, to decorate

"Bloom" the gelatin by stirring it into ⅓ cup of cold water and letting it sit for 5 minutes. Meanwhile, combine the pomegranate pulp and lemon juice in a small saucepan with 1½ cups of water and bring to a boil. Remove from the heat and strain out the pomegranate seeds. Return the pan to the heat and add the brown rice syrup or stevia and the gelatin and stir to dissolve. Remove from the heat and stir in the rose water. Allow to cool slightly, then pour into silicone molds or a glass or plastic dish and set in the fridge for at least 2 hours.

Remove the jelly from the molds (or cut into squares if using a dish). Melt the chocolate in a cup in the microwave (slowly on a low heat, checking frequently). Dunk the jelly shapes into the chocolate or drizzle the chocolate over them. Decorate with the reserved pomegranate seeds and chopped pistachios, using an extra drizzle of chocolate to keep them in place. These will keep in a sealed container in the fridge for up to 1 week.

½ TEASPOON ADDED SUGAR PER SERVING

RASPBERRY RIPE BITES

1¼ cups shredded coconut

1 tablespoon brown rice syrup

1 tablespoon coconut oil, melted

1½ tablespoons coconut milk

1 teaspoon pure vanilla extract (or make your own; page 45), optional

½ cup raspberries or cherries (fresh or frozen)

1 cup Basic Raw Chocolate (page 56) or 1 cup chopped dark (85–90% cocoa) chocolate

Line a baking sheet with parchment paper. Place all of the ingredients (except the chocolate) in a food processor. Pulse until the mixture comes together but still has texture. Roll tablespoons of the mixture into balls, place on the baking sheet and freeze for at least 1 hour.

Meanwhile, make your own raw chocolate, or melt store-bought chocolate in a microwave on low (or in a heatproof bowl over a saucepan of boiling water, making sure the bottom of the bowl doesn't touch the water).

Remove the coconut balls from the freezer and roll them in the melted chocolate so they are completely coated (stabbing the balls with a skewer and dunking works well). Return the balls to the lined sheet and allow to set in the fridge for 30 minutes before serving. These will keep in the fridge for up to 1 week or in the freezer for up to 3 months.

½ TEASPOON ADDED SUGAR PER SERVING

TAM TIMS

These are the bastardized version of the Australian candy favorite (which I renamed to avoid getting sued). Do as the Aussies do: bite off the ends of one and use it like a straw to drink your tea.

1 cup gluten-free plain flour, plus extra for dusting

2 teaspoons granulated stevia

⅓ cup raw cacao powder

⅓ cup cold unsalted butter, diced

¼ cup milk (any kind, though full-fat dairy is best)

GANACHE

2 tablespoons unsalted butter, at room temperature

2 tablespoons brown rice syrup

2 tablespoons raw cacao powder

CHOCOLATE COATING

3½ ounces dark (85–90% cocoa) chocolate, chopped into small, even-sized pieces

Preheat the oven to 350°F and line a baking sheet with parchment paper.

Place the flour, stevia, cacao powder, butter and milk in a food processor bowl and process to make a firm dough. Transfer the dough to a lightly floured work surface and knead until smooth. Roll the dough out between two sheets of parchment paper to make a rectangle (about ¼ inch thick). Cut into 16 smaller rectangles. Transfer to the baking sheet and bake in the oven for 10 minutes.

For a firmer frosting, set the ganache mixture in the fridge for 15 minutes.

Meanwhile, to make the ganache, place all the ingredients in a small bowl and beat until fluffy.

Remove the cookies from the oven and allow to cool. Once cooled, spread a thin layer of ganache over 8 of the cookies and top each one with another cookie, sandwiching them together. Place in the fridge while you make the chocolate coating.

Melt the chocolate slowly in a microwave (or in a heatproof bowl over a saucepan of boiling water, making sure the bottom of the bowl doesn't touch the water). Dip each cookie sandwich in the melted chocolate and place on the parchment paper. Return to the fridge to set before serving. Store in a sealed container in the fridge for up to 1 week or in the freezer for up to 3 months.

1 TEASPOON ADDED SUGAR PER SERVING

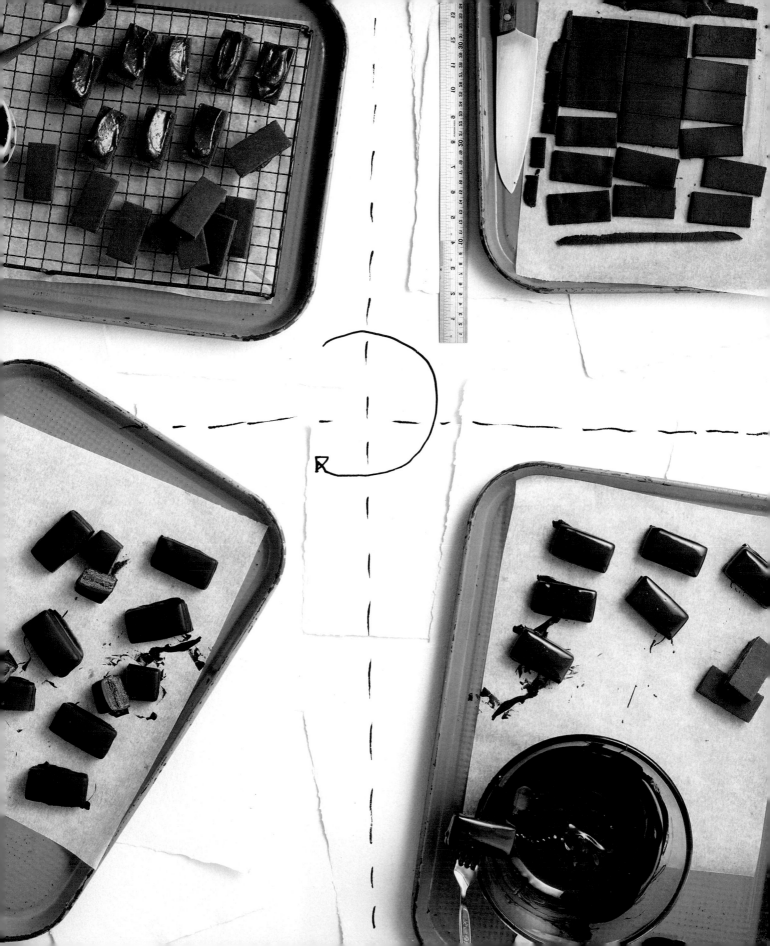

THREE COOKIE DOUGH SLICES

Happily use the BAKED <u>or</u> RAW bases interchangeably, if you like.

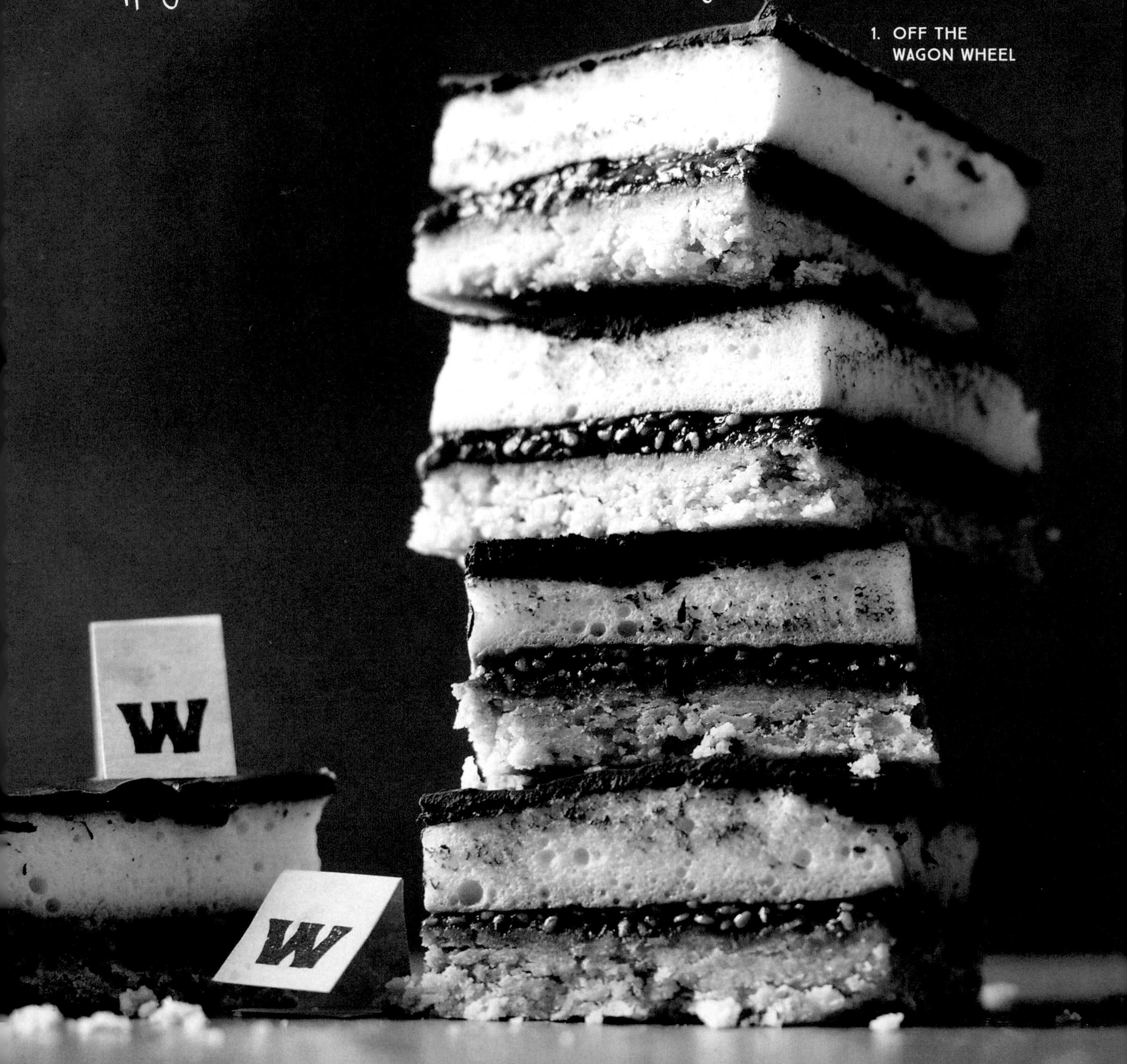

1. OFF THE
   WAGON WHEEL

W

W

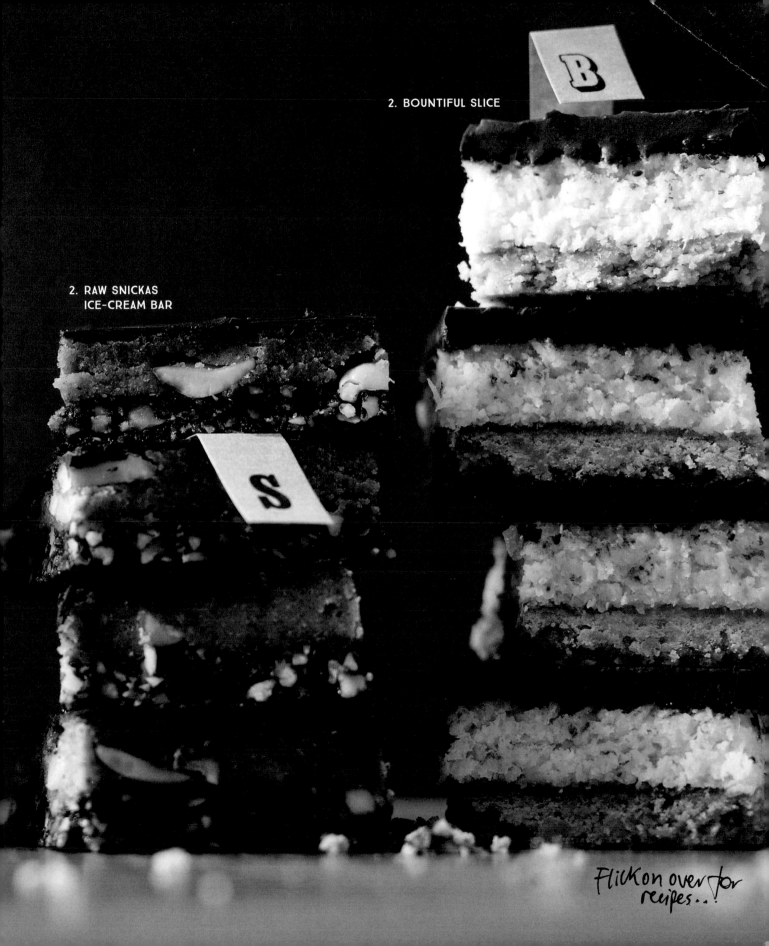

2. BOUNTIFUL SLICE

B

2. RAW SNICKAS
ICE-CREAM BAR

S

Flick on over for recipes...!

1. OFF THE WAGON WHEEL

MAKES 28 SMALL SQUARES

1 cup Raspberry Chia Jam
(page 57)

BAKED COOKIE DOUGH BASE

⅔ cup unsalted butter

2 tablespoons brown rice syrup

¾ cup buckwheat flour

¾ cup gluten-free plain flour

½ cup desiccated coconut

pinch of sea salt

MARSHMALLOW FILLING

1½ tablespoons gelatin powder

¼ cup brown rice syrup

1 teaspoon pure vanilla extract
(or make your own; see page 45)

¼ teaspoon sea salt

CHOC COATING

3½ ounces dark (85–90%
cocoa) chocolate or Basic Raw
Chocolate (page 56)

Yes!!

Preheat the oven to 350°F. Grease and line a 9 × 9-inch square baking pan with parchment paper.

To make the Baked Cookie Dough Base, melt the butter and brown rice syrup in a small saucepan (or in a mixing bowl in the microwave). Combine with the remaining ingredients and mix well. Press the mixture into the prepared pan and bake for 15–20 minutes until light golden. Remove from the oven and allow to cool.

When cool, spread the jam over the base and refrigerate.

Meanwhile, to make the marshmallow filling, "bloom" the gelatin by stirring it into ⅓ cup of water until it dissolves. Allow to sit for 5 minutes—it will become firm like a rubber ball. Meanwhile, combine the brown rice syrup, vanilla and salt in a saucepan with 1 cup of water and bring to a boil. Reduce the heat and simmer, stirring constantly, for 8 minutes. Turn off the heat, add the gelatin blob to the mixture and stir to dissolve. Using an immersion blender, mix until it forms a thick cream (or transfer to a high-powered blender to cut time).

Flick to page 348 to nerd up on gelatin.

Pour the marshmallow over the cooled jam layer. Now rub your hands in coconut oil and use your fingers to smooth the surface. Refrigerate for at least 1 hour, or until set.

Melt the chocolate slowly in a microwave (or in a heatproof bowl over a saucepan of boiling water, making sure the bottom of the bowl doesn't touch the water) and pour over the marshmallow layer, spreading it evenly. Return the tray to the fridge for at least 1 hour or until the chocolate is set. Cut into squares to serve. Store in the fridge in a sealed container for up to 5 days.

¾ TEASPOON ADDED SUGAR PER SERVING

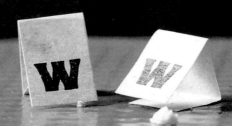

2. RAW SNICKAS ICE-CREAM BAR

Pecans have a good flavor, but almonds, pistachios or hazelnuts are great too.

MAKES 28 SMALL SQUARES

RAW COOKIE DOUGH BASE

2 cups nuts (preferably activated; see page 28)

¼ cup raw cacao powder

¼ cup brown rice syrup

2 tablespoons coconut oil, melted

pinch of sea salt

"NOUGAT"

¾ cup coconut cream

⅓ cup brown rice syrup

good pinch of sea salt

½ cup coconut flour, plus extra if needed

⅔ cup natural peanut butter

¼ cup raw unsalted peanuts

CHOCOLATE TOPPING

3½ ounces dark (85–90% cocoa) chocolate, diced

Line a 9 × 9-inch square baking pan with parchment paper.

To make the Raw Cookie Dough Base, process the nuts in a food processor to a fine crumb. Add the remaining ingredients and process until just combined. Add more coconut oil (if needed) to achieve a dough-like consistency. Alternatively, keep processing until the nuts give up their oil. Press the mixture evenly into the base of the prepared pan. Place in the freezer to set.

Meanwhile, to make the "nougat," place all of the ingredients except the peanuts in a bowl and mix until smooth. (Add extra coconut flour if the mixture is too runny. It should be the consistency of cookie dough.) Fold in the peanuts. Spread the mixture over the chilled cookie dough base and put it back in the freezer.

Melt the chocolate slowly in a microwave (or in a heatproof bowl over a saucepan of boiling water, making sure the bottom of the bowl doesn't touch the water), stirring until melted. Pour the chocolate over the chilled nougat and return to the freezer until ready to serve. Store in a sealed container in the freezer for up to 3 months.

MAKE IT PEANUT-FREE:
Swap the peanut butter and peanuts for cashew butter and cashews.

3. BOUNTIFUL SLICE

MAKES 28 SMALL SQUARES

The taste of paradise . . . with the nutritional profile to match.

1 portion of Baked Cookie Dough Base (opposite)

You can also use the Raw Cookie Dough Base from the Snickas recipe if you prefer. Both work.

1 cup coconut milk

⅓ cup brown rice syrup

¼ cup coconut oil

2 cups desiccated coconut

pinch of sea salt

CHOC COATING

1 batch (1⅓ cups) of Basic Raw Chocolate (page 56)

Make the Baked Cookie Dough Base (opposite) and allow to cool.

Heat the coconut milk, brown rice syrup and coconut oil in a saucepan over low heat. Stir until well combined. Remove from the heat and stir in the desiccated coconut and salt. Spoon over the cookie dough base and press evenly so that it is about ½ inch thick. Freeze until the coconut filling is set (about 1 hour).

Melt the chocolate slowly in a microwave (or in a heatproof bowl over a saucepan of boiling water, making sure the bottom of the bowl doesn't touch the water). Spread the melted chocolate over the coconut layer and return to the fridge for at least 1 hour before cutting into squares. Store in a sealed container in the fridge for up to 1 week or in the freezer for up to 3 months.

MAKE IT A RASPBERRY RIPE SLICE:
Add ½ cup of raspberries to the coconut filling.

CHOCOLATE PEANUT BUTTER CRACKLES

Seven ingredients, one pot, 4½ minutes, some time in the fridge, and you're done.

¾ cup coconut oil

2 tablespoons brown rice syrup

¼ cup raw cacao powder

½ cup crunchy natural peanut butter

½ cup desiccated coconut

½ cup Activated Groaties (page 27)

1½ cups puffed quinoa or puffed rice

Remember you can use the store-bought variety if you like.

Line two muffin pans with 18 paper liners.

Gently heat the coconut oil in a saucepan over medium-low heat. Remove from the heat and stir in the brown rice syrup. Add the cacao powder and peanut butter and stir to combine. Add the coconut, groaties and puffed quinoa or rice and mix well. Spoon the mixture into the prepared pans. Refrigerate for 2 hours to completely set, then serve. Store leftovers in a sealed container in the fridge for up to 2 weeks.

¼ TEASPOON ADDED SUGAR PER SERVING

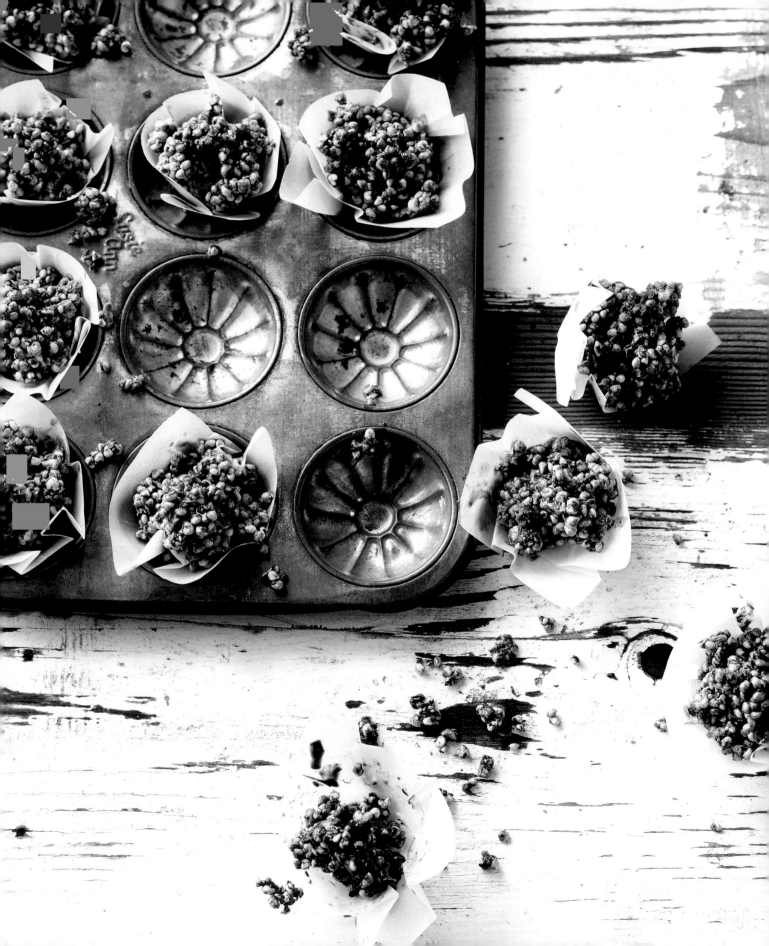

MISO AND WALNUT SLOW BROS

SERVES 16

A slow-cooker brownie . . . yeah! This masterpiece is seriously disaster-proof. And no matter how hard you try to mess it up, it will still come out with a lovely glazed top, crunchy outer bits and a gooey volcano-like center. Serve with yogurt or cream. If your slow cooker is larger than a 4½-quart version, you'll need to double the batch quantity.

coconut oil, butter or ghee, for greasing

1½ cups almond meal

½ cup raw cacao powder

1 teaspoon gluten-free baking powder

½ teaspoon sea salt

½ cup unsalted butter or coconut oil, melted

⅓ cup brown rice syrup

2 tablespoons red miso paste

3 eggs

½ cup chopped walnuts

3 ounces dark (85–90% cocoa) chocolate, chopped into small, even chunks

full-fat organic plain yogurt or cream, to serve

Grease the slow-cooker insert and line it with parchment paper so it reaches halfway up the side.

In a large bowl, combine the almond meal, cacao powder, baking powder and salt.

In a separate bowl, whisk together the melted butter or oil, brown rice syrup and miso paste. Add the eggs and continue whisking until the mixture is well combined.

The center will always be moister than the perimeter of the brownie; don't burn the outside waiting for the center to firm up.

Pour the butter-and-syrup mixture into the dry ingredients and mix thoroughly. Stir through the walnuts and the chocolate chunks. Pour the batter into the lined slow-cooker insert. Cover and cook on low for 2½ hours or 1½ hours on high, or until the outside of the mixture is firm and the center is no longer liquid. Remove the lid and continue cooking for a further 30 minutes, or until the center cooks through.

Once cooked, switch off the slow cooker and leave the cooked mixture to rest for 10–15 minutes. Carefully remove from the slow cooker by grabbing the edges of the parchment paper and gently lifting out. Allow to cool completely before slicing. Store the brownies on the parchment paper in a sealed container for 3–4 days or freeze for up to 4 months.

MAKE IT PEANUT BUTTER SLOW BRO FUDGE:
Follow the recipe above, replacing the walnuts with 3 heaping tablespoons of softened crunchy natural peanut butter. Cook for 3 hours on low or 1½ hours on high.

1½ TEASPOONS ADDED SUGAR PER SERVING

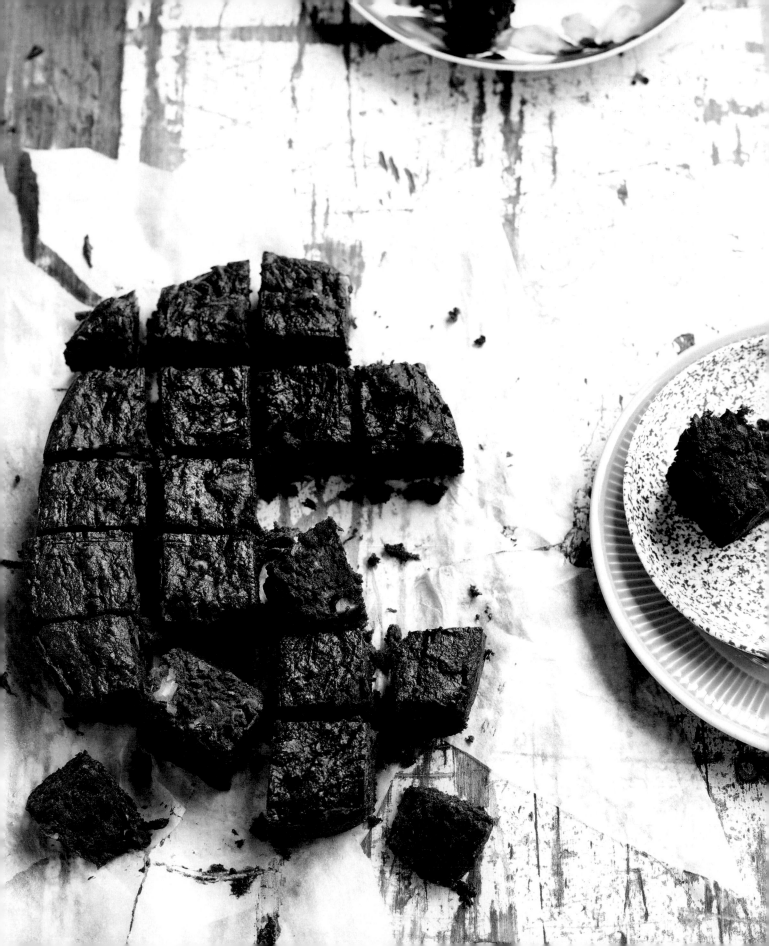

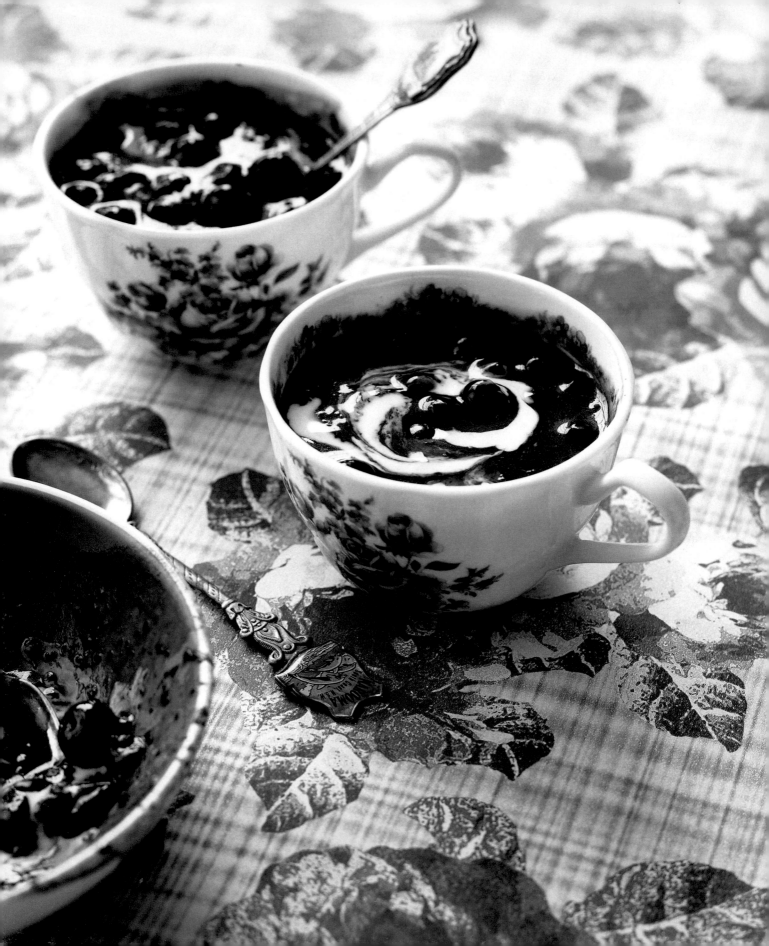

BUTTERED BLUEBERRY AND BLOOD ORANGE SOUP

SERVES 6

So severely simple I feel embarrassed calling it a recipe.

1 tablespoon unsalted butter

1½-inch knob of ginger, minced

3 cups blueberries (fresh or frozen)

juice of 2 small blood oranges
or mandarins (or 1 large orange)

zest of 1 orange or mandarin

1 tablespoon brown rice syrup

Whipped Coconut Frosting (page 56)
or whipped cream, to serve (optional)

pinch of ground nutmeg
or cinnamon, to serve (optional)

Heat the butter in a skillet over medium heat and sauté the ginger for
2–3 minutes. Add the berries, juice, zest and brown rice syrup and sauté
for 5 minutes.

Serve in small bowls (or teacups) with a swirl of cream and a sprinkle
of nutmeg or cinnamon, if you like. Eat with a spoon!

 ½ TEASPOON ADDED SUGAR PER SERVING

 1 SERVING VEG + FRUIT PER SERVING

FRIDAY NIGHT CHOCKITO ON A STICK

MAKES 15–30

When I was a kid, Dad would come home with a Friday Night Surprise each week. Mostly it was the one Chokito bar—a caramel fudge, rice crispy, chocolate log thing—divided between all five of us kids (as we were back then). Perhaps you've not encountered a Chokito. That's because it periodically gets discontinued. I think the Big Food Giant responsible for this might like to reformulate its next incarnation without sugar. Here's a recipe for them now. On a stick.

CARAMEL FILLING

⅓ cup coconut oil, slightly softened

2 tablespoons hulled tahini

2 tablespoons brown rice syrup

½ cup almond meal

½ cup Activated Groaties (page 27) or crushed peanuts

30 lollipop sticks (or use bamboo skewers cut in half)

3½ ounces dark (85–90% cocoa) chocolate

To make the caramel filling, place the coconut oil, tahini and brown rice syrup in a bowl and mix until smooth. Stir in the almond meal. Refrigerate the mixture for 1 hour to firm.

or just do stickless truffles instead

Roll teaspoons of the mixture into balls and coat each one in groaties or peanuts. Insert a lollipop stick or skewer into the center of each ball and place upside down on a baking sheet or plate lined with parchment paper. Pop in the freezer for at least 10 minutes.

Melt the chocolate in a heatproof bowl over a saucepan of boiling water, making sure the bottom of the bowl doesn't touch the water. Dip the balls in the chocolate and coat well. Refrigerate for at least 1 hour, or until the chocolate is set. These will keep in the fridge in a sealed container for up to 2 weeks, or in the freezer for 3–4 months.

¼ TEASPOON ADDED SUGAR PER SERVING

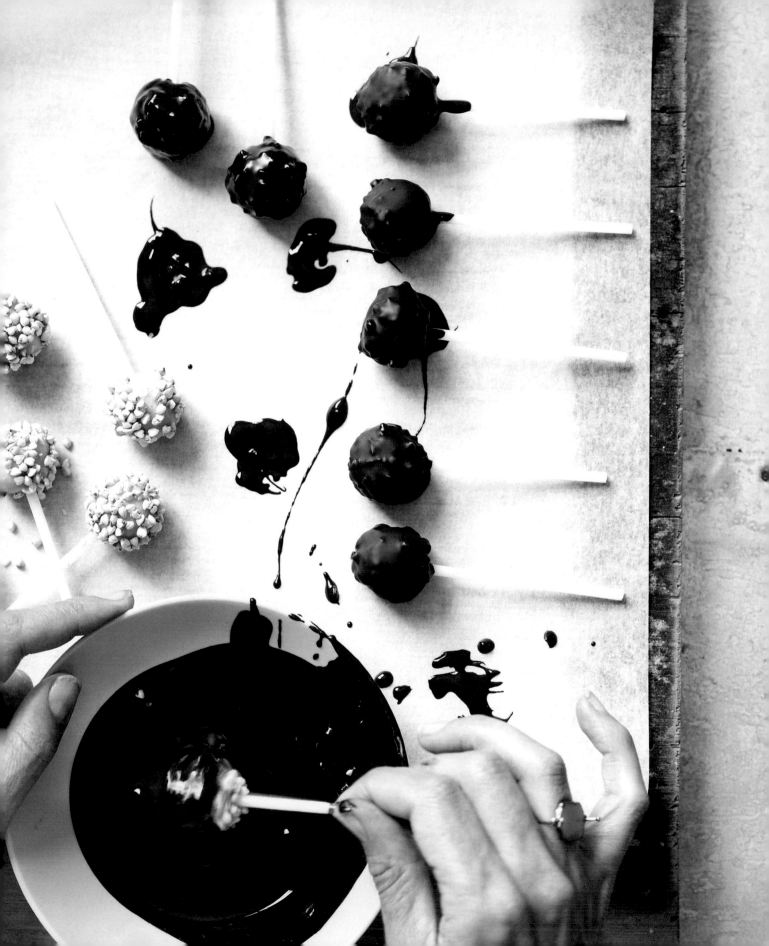

FOUR VERY LUSH MUG CAKES

Treats for one made in the microwave in two.

1. GINGERBREAD MUGGIN

¼ cup almond meal
or gluten-free self-rising flour

2 tablespoons desiccated coconut

¼ teaspoon baking powder

¼ teaspoon ground ginger

½ teaspoon Pumpkin Spice Mix
(page 45) or ground cinnamon

1 tablespoon crushed pecans,
plus extra to serve

½ teaspoon brown rice syrup

1 cube frozen Sweet Potato Purée
(page 23) or ¼ cup grated sweet potato

¼ cup milk (any kind)

full-fat organic plain yogurt, to serve

Place all of the ingredients in a
microwave-safe porcelain mug and
mix with a spoon. Microwave on
high for 2 minutes. Serve with yogurt
and pecans.

½ TEASPOON ADDED SUGAR PER SERVING

 ½ SERVING VEG + FRUIT PER SERVING

2. CHOC-GINGER AND PEAR MUGGIN

¼ cup almond meal
or gluten-free plain flour

2 tablespoons desiccated coconut

¼ teaspoon baking powder

1 teaspoon raw cacao powder

½ teaspoon ground ginger

¼ pear, cored and chopped

¼ cup milk (any kind)

1 cube frozen Basic Raw Chocolate
(page 56)

pear wedges, to serve

Place all of the ingredients, except
the cube of frozen chocolate, in
a microwave-safe porcelain mug
and mix with a spoon. Place the
chocolate cube in the center of the
mixture and push down. Microwave
on high for 2 minutes. Serve with
pear wedges.

4. LEMON SYRUP AND POPPY SEED MUGGIN

¼ cup almond meal or gluten-free plain flour

2 tablespoons desiccated coconut

¼ teaspoon baking powder

zest of ½ lemon

1 tablespoon lemon juice

1 teaspoon poppy seeds,
plus extra to serve

½ teaspoon brown rice syrup

¼ cup milk (any kind)

Homemade Cream Cheese (page 46),
to serve

Place all of the ingredients in a
microwave-safe porcelain mug and mix
with a spoon. Microwave on high for
2 minutes. Serve with a dollop of cream
cheese and a sprinkle of poppy seeds.

½ TEASPOON ADDED SUGAR PER SERVING

3. STRAWBERRY CHEESECAKE MUGGIN

¼ cup almond meal
or gluten-free plain flour

2 tablespoons desiccated coconut

¼ teaspoon baking powder

1 tablespoon pistachios, chopped,
plus extra to serve

1 tablespoon Strawberry Chia Jam
(page 57) or 2–3 strawberries,
chopped, plus extra to serve

¼ cup milk (any kind)

1 tablespoon full-fat ricotta, plus
extra to serve (or use Homemade
Cream Cheese; page 46)

Place all of the ingredients in
a microwave-safe porcelain
mug and mix with a spoon.
Microwave on high for 2 minutes.
Serve with a dollop of ricotta and
the extra pistachios and jam or
strawberries.

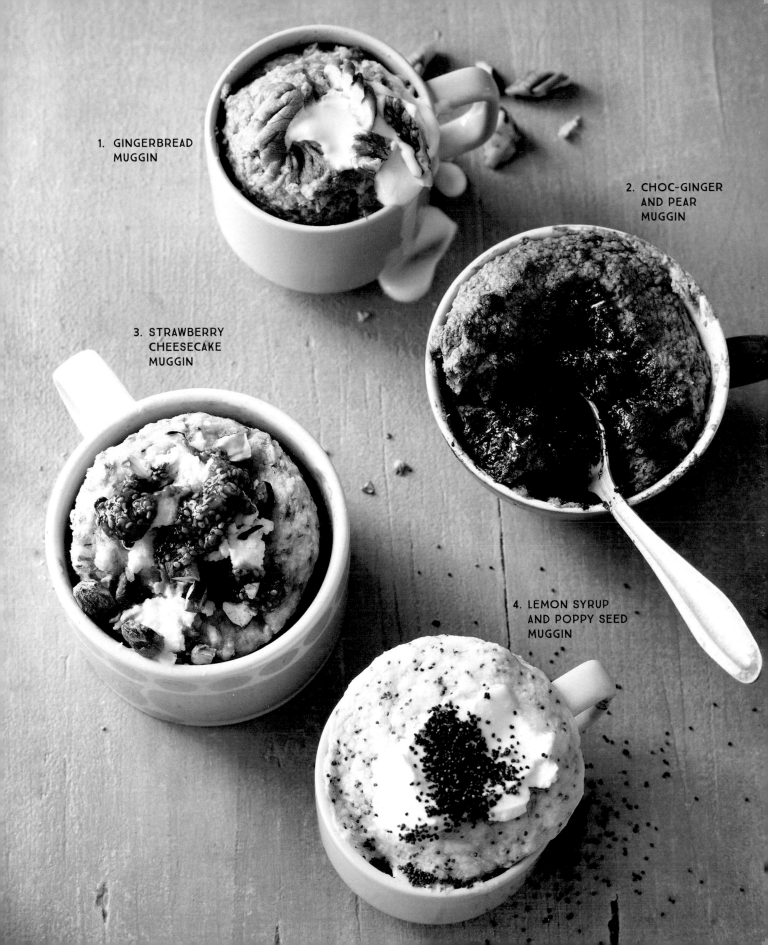

1. GINGERBREAD
MUGGIN

2. CHOC-GINGER
AND PEAR
MUGGIN

3. STRAWBERRY
CHEESECAKE
MUGGIN

4. LEMON SYRUP
AND POPPY SEED
MUGGIN

PULL-APART CATERPILLAR BIRTHDAY CAKE

SERVES 13 ⎯⎯⎯

A cupcake pull-apart cake is the best way to manage portion control with kids.

Double the recipe if you've been roped into making a cake for the whole class and make him a fat, hungry caterpillar with two cupcakes per "segment."

14-ounce can black beans, rinsed and drained

1 cup Sweet Potato Purée (page 23)

4½ ounces coconut oil

⅓ cup brown rice syrup

1½ teaspoons ground cinnamon

1½ teaspoons baking powder

1 teaspoon baking soda

5 eggs

½ cup raw cacao powder

ICING

1½ tablespoons frozen raspberries, thawed and mushed through a sieve to extract the juice

several pinches of pure vanilla powder (optional)

1½ cups Cream Cheese Frosting (page 56) or Supercharged Coconut Frosting (page 56)

1 cup baby spinach leaves, puréed with 3 teaspoons water and pressed through a sieve

a few blueberries and tiny Swiss chard leaves, for garnish

Preheat the oven to 325°F. Line one or two muffin pans with 13 paper liners.

Place the beans, sweet potato, coconut oil, brown rice syrup, cinnamon, baking powder, baking soda and 1 of the eggs in a food processor. Process until smooth. Add the remaining eggs and the cacao powder and process until combined. Divide the mixture between the cups, overfilling one of the paper liners (with an extra 1–2 tablespoons of mixture) to make the head. Bake for 25 minutes, leaving the larger cupcake for another 3 minutes. Leave in the cups for 5 minutes, then transfer to a wire rack to cool.

Assemble the caterpillar on a baking sheet or serving tray lined with parchment paper (or other paper).

To make the icing for the head, mix the raspberry juice with 1 teaspoon of the frosting in a cup. Mix in a pinch of vanilla powder (if using) and spread evenly over the largest cupcake.

To make the icing for the body, add the spinach juice to the remaining frosting (reserve a tiny amount of cream-colored frosting for the eyes, if you like), a little at a time. Add a few pinches of vanilla powder and mix until thick. Spread over the remaining cupcakes and decorate as desired. I use half a blueberry to make each pupil, a blueberry sliver for the mouth and tiny chard leaves for the antennae.

1 TEASPOON ADDED SUGAR PER SERVING

To reduce the sugar load, I suggest making the frosting with no added sweetener

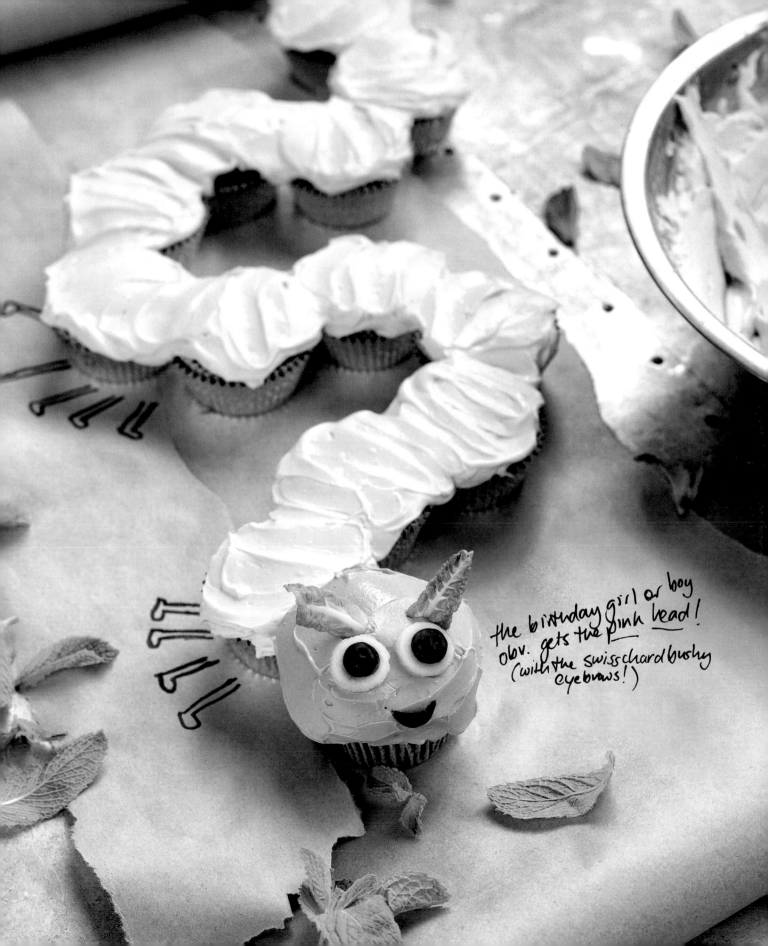

the birthday girl or boy
obv. gets the pink head!
(with the swisschard bushy
eyebrows!)

PARTY POLENTA CAKES WITH POPPING TOPPING

MAKES 12

6 ounces unsalted butter, cubed and at room temperature, plus extra for greasing

½ cup brown rice syrup

3 eggs

8 ounces almond meal

3½ ounces coarse polenta

1 teaspoon baking powder

1 teaspoon pure vanilla extract (or make your own; see page 45)

½ teaspoon ground turmeric

zest of 2 oranges

juice of ½ orange

1 cup Cream Cheese Frosting (page 56)

TOPPING

⅓ cup popcorn kernels

1 tablespoon unsalted butter

1 tablespoon brown rice syrup

big pinch of sea salt

Preheat the oven to 350°F and grease a 12-cup muffin pan with butter or line with paper liners.

Beat the butter until pale. Add the brown rice syrup and beat until light and creamy. Beat in the eggs one at a time. Fold in the almond meal, polenta, baking powder, vanilla, turmeric and the orange zest and juice and mix until just combined. Spoon the mixture into the pan and bake for 45 minutes or until just golden and the sides are coming away from the cups (or liners). Set aside to cool.

Meanwhile, for the topping, place the popcorn kernels in a large bowl with the butter. Cover with a plate and heat in the microwave on high for 2½–3 minutes until the popping eases off. While the popcorn is still hot, drizzle it with the brown rice syrup and sprinkle with salt. Toss to combine.

Smooth the frosting over the cooled cakes and top with the popcorn. Store in a sealed container in the fridge for 3–4 days.

2 TEASPOONS ADDED SUGAR PER SERVING

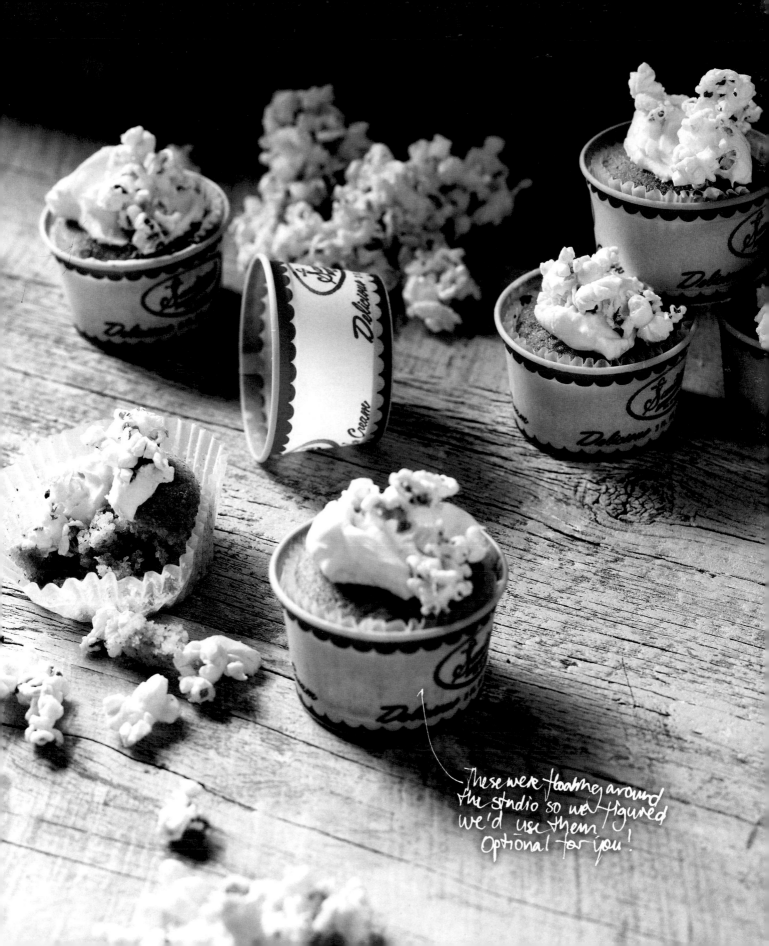

These were floating around the studio so we figured we'd use them. Optional for you!

CHEESECAKE-STUFFED PEACHES WITH BASIL

SERVES 12

6 peaches, halved and stones removed

¼ cup unsalted butter, melted

2 teaspoons ground cinnamon

1 cup Homemade Cream Cheese (page 46)

2 tablespoons brown rice syrup

1 egg

1½ teaspoons pure vanilla extract (or make your own; see page 45)

basil leaves, to serve

Preheat the oven to 350°F and line a baking sheet with parchment paper.

Trim a very thin slice from the round side of each peach half (so the halves don't topple in transit). Coat each peach half in melted butter and place, cut side up, on the lined baking sheet. Sprinkle with cinnamon.

Beat the cream cheese in a bowl with an immersion blender until smooth. Add the brown rice syrup, egg and vanilla and mix together until creamy. Spoon the mixture into the peach centers. Bake for 35 minutes, until everything is crispy and golden.

Serve with a sprinkle of basil leaves.

½ TEASPOON ADDED SUGAR PER SERVING

½ SERVING VEG + FRUIT PER SERVING

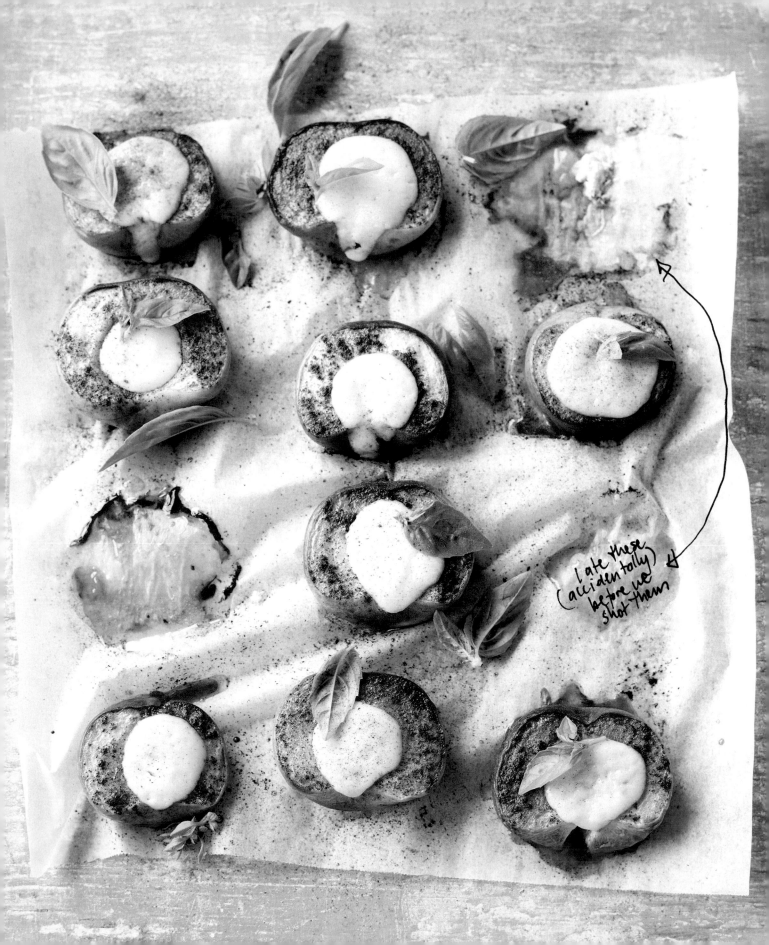

I ate these
(accidentally)
before we
shot them

GOLDEN
HAPPY TIMES

The original commercial version of this ice cream is an Australian national treasure. We make them healthy enough to actually feed to kids (though note that they do contain nuts).

14-ounce can coconut cream

⅓ cup almond butter
or cashew butter

1 tablespoon pure vanilla extract
(or make your own; see page 45)

¼ teaspoon sea salt

1½ tablespoons brown rice syrup

1 teaspoon each coconut oil
and brown rice syrup, melted

½ cup Activated Groaties (page 27)

½ cup Basic Raw Chocolate (page 56)

In a small saucepan, combine ½ cup of the coconut cream with the nut butter, vanilla, salt and brown rice syrup and whisk continuously over very low heat until a thick caramel forms (about 10 minutes). Remove from the heat and stir in the rest of the coconut cream until the mixture is creamy. Pour into ice pop molds, add the sticks, and freeze for 4 hours or until set.

Preheat the oven to 350°F and line a baking sheet with parchment paper.

Since you have the oven on, you might like to make a big batch of these and keep as toppers for yogurt, oatmeal, cakes or smoothies. Store in a sealed container for up to 2 months.

Mix the melted coconut oil and brown rice syrup with the groaties and spread them out on the baking sheet. Bake in the oven for 10 minutes, or until browned. Use your fingers to break up any clusters and set aside.

When the ice creams are set, melt the chocolate in a cup in the microwave (do it gradually on low). Remove the ice creams from their molds by running the molds under warm water. Dip each ice cream into the melted chocolate (you might like to do a few coats) and then sprinkle the groaties over the top. You will need to work quickly, as the chocolate will set fast. Place the ice creams on a lined baking sheet and freeze for another 5 minutes before serving. Store these in a sealed container in the freezer for 3–4 months.

¾ TEASPOON ADDED SUGAR PER SERVING

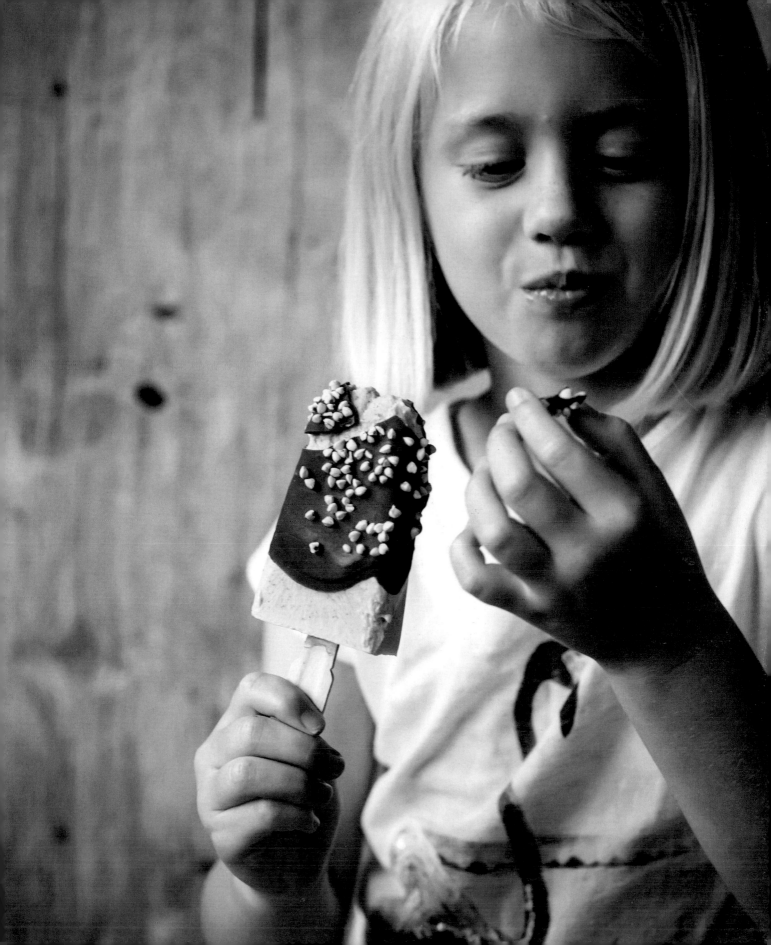

SUNFLOWER STRAWBERRY THUMBLES

MAKES ABOUT 16

In Australia, these are usually called thimbles, after the sewing thingamajig you're supposed to use to make the little jam indents. No one I know owns a thimble. Thumbs can be used instead.

1½ cups sunflower seeds

½ cup buckwheat flour

1½ tablespoons arrowroot

1 teaspoon baking powder

pinch of sea salt

¼ cup butter or coconut oil, melted

2 tablespoons brown rice syrup

1 egg, separated

1 teaspoon pure vanilla extract (or make your own; page 45)

2 tablespoons Strawberry Chia Jam (page 57)

Preheat the oven to 350°F and line a baking sheet with parchment paper.

Spread the sunflower seeds on the baking sheet and roast in the oven for 10 minutes, tossing them around after 5 minutes, until lightly browned. Put three-quarters of the sunflower seeds into a high-speed blender or food processor and pulse until a coarse meal forms. Transfer to a large mixing bowl and stir in the buckwheat flour, arrowroot, baking powder and salt.

In a small bowl, combine the butter, brown rice syrup, egg yolk and vanilla and whisk with a fork. Fold into the dry ingredients and stir until a dough forms.

Whisk the egg white in a small, clean bowl until foamy. Coarsely chop the remaining sunflower seeds and place in another small bowl.

Roll dessert spoons of the dough into balls. Roll each ball in the foamy egg white and then coat it in the sunflower seeds. Arrange on the baking sheet and push down with your thumb (or use a thimble!) to create a well in the center. Repeat with the remaining dough. Fill each well with ½ teaspoon of jam. Bake for 10–15 minutes, until lightly golden. Transfer to a wire rack and leave to cool; they will firm up once they cool. Store these in an airtight container in the fridge for 4–5 days or freeze for up to 1 month.

Handy for lunchboxes if you pop in a couple of frozen ones.

¼ TEASPOON ADDED SUGAR PER SERVING

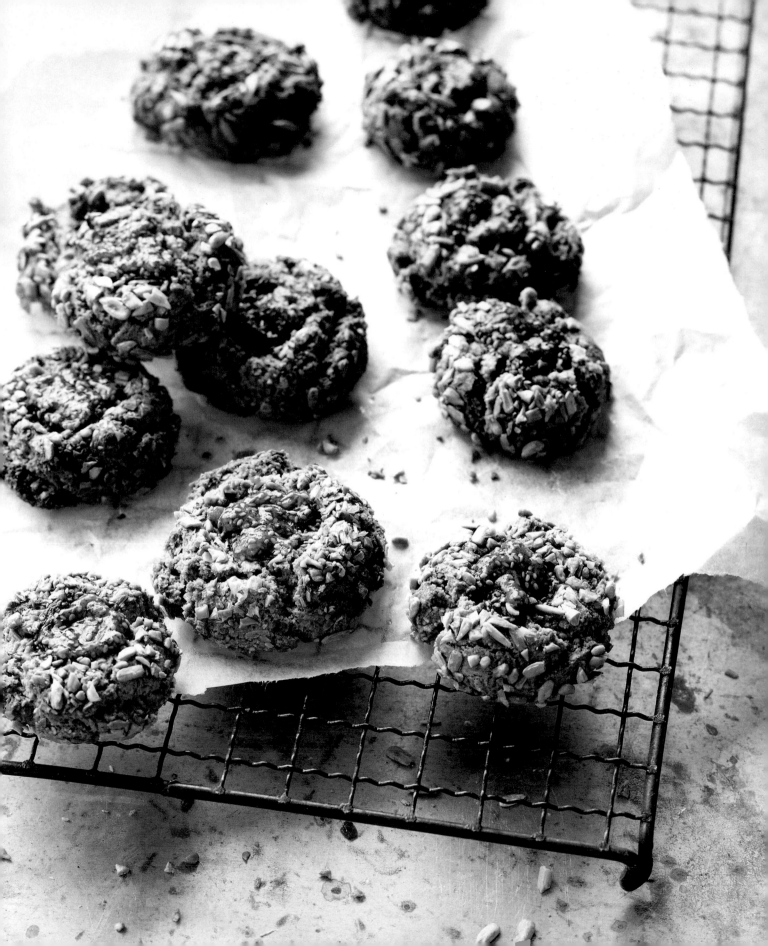

A
CELEBRATION
MENU

kids' birthdays

CHRISTMAS

Easter

special afternoon teas

weddings...

all of which are
STILL rather healthy

dinner parties

(and LOOK MORE FANCY
than they really are!)

(but don't look too earnest
either!!!)

TOTALLY GAUDY CHRISTMAS TREE CHEESE BALL

18 ounces cream cheese, preferably homemade (see page 46), at room temperature

9 ounces cheddar, finely grated (or use 4½ ounces cheddar and 4½ ounces feta or gorgonzola)

1 tablespoon Dijon mustard

3 green onions, thinly sliced

sea salt and freshly ground black pepper

½ cup finely chopped flat-leaf parsley

TO GARNISH

Bacon Bits (page 44)

almond flakes

pomegranate seeds

Blend the cream cheese, cheddar and mustard in a bowl with an immersion blender. Stir through the green onions and season with salt and pepper. Cover and refrigerate for at least 2 hours or overnight (heaps better) to firm.

Get organized! You can make your tree ball to this stage and freeze for up to 2 months.

Before serving, form into a ball and then into a tree shape. Roll the tree-shaped cheese mixture in the parsley, reshaping it with your hands as necessary. Decorate with bacon bits, almond flakes and pomegranate seeds.

Serve with crackers or crudités.

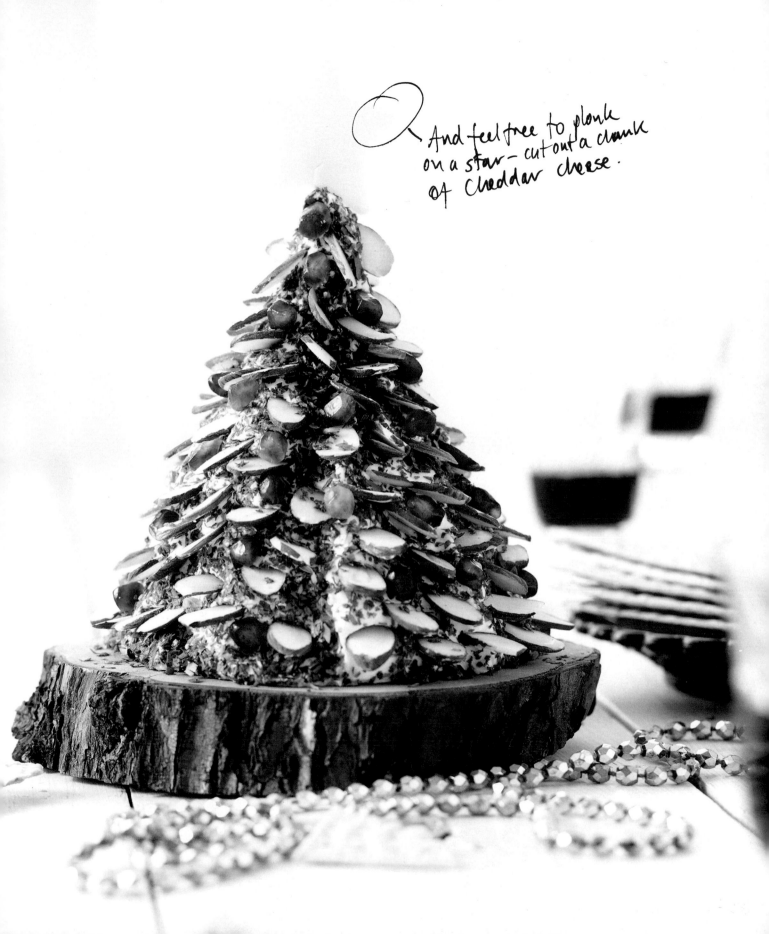

And feel free to plonk on a star—cut out a chunk of Cheddar cheese.

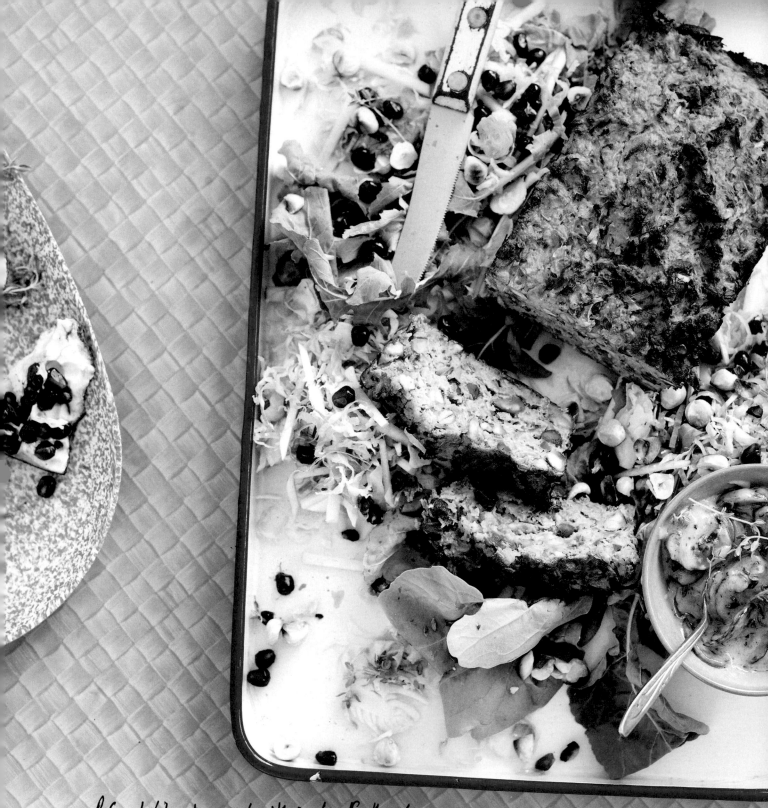

P.S. I like to make this loaf the day
after making a big roast (the Jerk Pork)
I cook extra veg + reserve some of the
juices + add to the mushroom sauce. →

BAKED STUFFING LOAF

WITH MUSHROOM SAUCE AND SHAVED SPROUTS AND PECORINO SALAD

SERVES 6–8

Yep, a vegetarian baked dinner in a loaf with added bits
to make it a dish worthy of a celebration.

*A combo of cauliflower, sweet
potato and celery is great; or
a combo of parsnip, squash
and carrot also works well.*

5 cups chopped raw veggies

1 onion, chopped

4 cloves garlic, skin on

3 eggs

1 teaspoon chopped rosemary

1 tablespoon chopped thyme
plus extra sprigs to garnish (optional)

good pinch of sea salt

2 tablespoons flour (any kind)

2 tablespoons coconut oil, melted

1 cup chopped pistachios

MUSHROOM SAUCE

3 knobs of butter

pinch each of sea salt and
freshly ground black pepper

5 ounces button mushrooms, sliced

½ cup cream

Preheat the oven to 400°F and line a baking sheet and a 9 × 5-inch loaf pan
with parchment paper.

*To make it with leftover
veggies, use 4 cups of
Roasted Roots (page 23),
skip the roasting step
and follow the rest of
the recipe (oh, and use
1 tablespoon of melted
coconut oil instead of 2).*

Place the vegetables and garlic on the baking sheet and roast for 30 minutes.
Transfer to a food processor (squeeze the garlic out of its skin first) and pulse
until the vegetables resemble bread crumbs. Add the eggs, herbs and salt and
blend until combined, leaving some chunks. Stir in the flour, coconut oil and
pistachios.

Pour the mixture into the lined loaf pan and bake for 40–50 minutes, until a
skewer inserted into the center of the loaf comes out clean. (Remove from the
oven after 25 minutes and press the extra thyme sprigs into the top of the loaf,
if you like.) Set aside to cool a little.

To make the mushroom sauce, place the butter, salt, pepper and mushrooms in
a skillet over low heat. Cook the mushrooms for 10 minutes, until softened, then
stir in cream. Reduce the sauce until the desired consistency is reached.

Lift the loaf from the pan and slice into thick slices. Serve with the Shaved
Sprouts and Pecorino Salad (see below) and the mushroom sauce.

SHAVED SPROUTS AND PECORINO SALAD

SERVES 6–8 AS A SIDE

1 green apple, cut into matchsticks

14 ounces brussels sprouts, shaved
or grated (about 4 cups)

½ cup Powerhouse Dressing (page 53)

2 big handfuls of arugula or watercress leaves

1 cup grated pecorino or Parmesan

chopped hazelnuts and pomegranate seeds,
to garnish (optional)

Toss the apple, sprouts and dressing in a large bowl and leave to sit for
20 minutes. Serve with the leaves and grated cheese, sprinkled with the
hazelnuts and pomegranate seeds, if using.

3 SERVINGS VEG + FRUIT PER SERVING

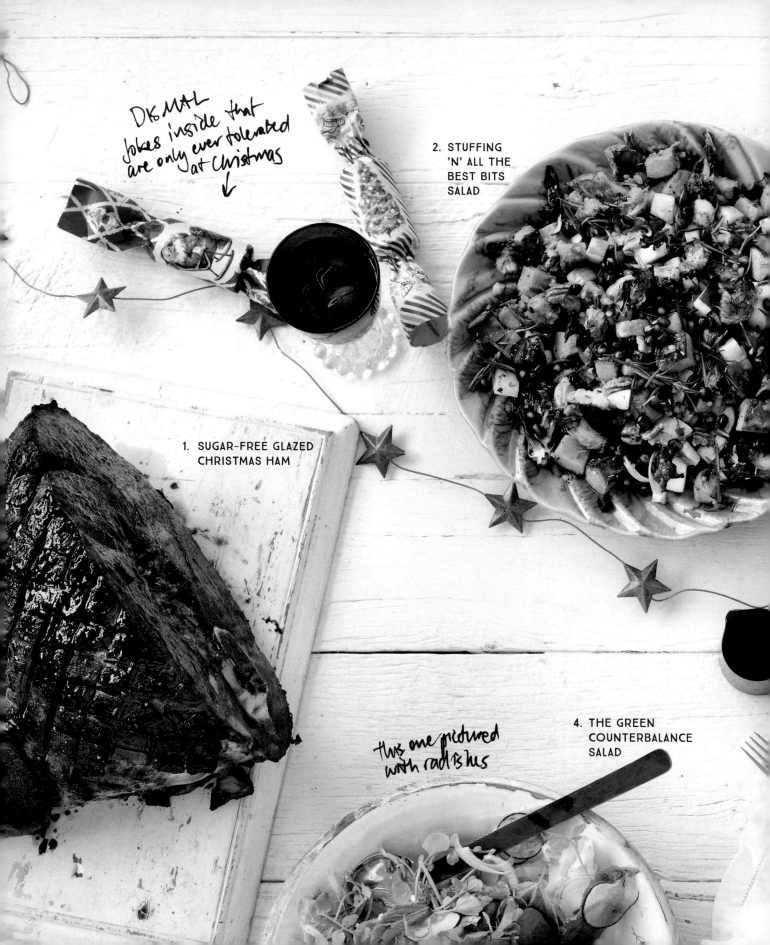

DISMAL jokes inside that are only ever tolerated at Christmas ↓

2. STUFFING 'N' ALL THE BEST BITS SALAD

1. SUGAR-FREE GLAZED CHRISTMAS HAM

this one pictured with radishes

4. THE GREEN COUNTERBALANCE SALAD

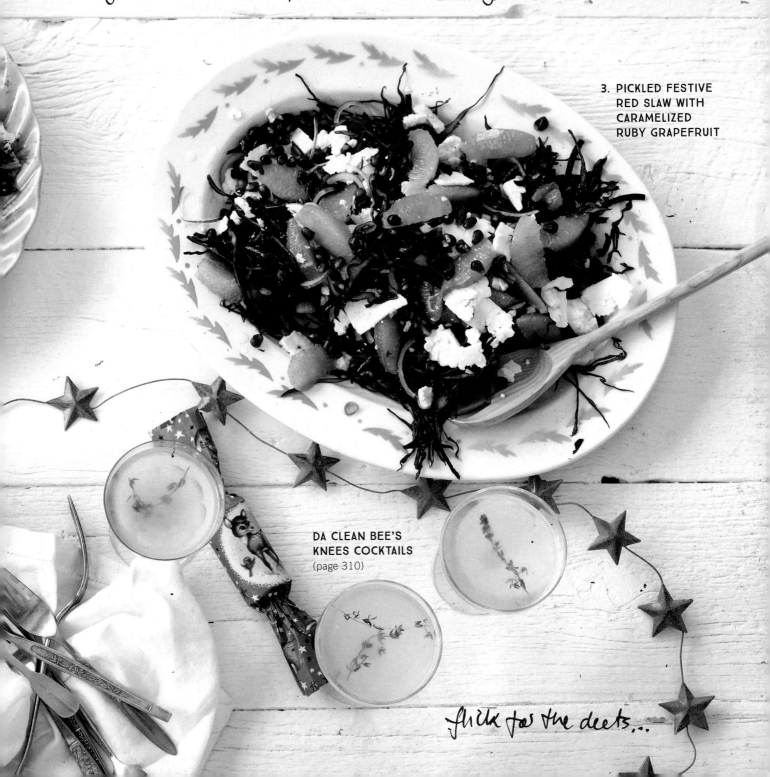

A HEALTHY CHRISTMAS DAY SPREAD

Designed to save time, pans, effort + family conflict!

3. PICKLED FESTIVE RED SLAW WITH CARAMELIZED RUBY GRAPEFRUIT

DA CLEAN BEE'S KNEES COCKTAILS
(page 310)

flick for the deets...

1. SUGAR-FREE GLAZED CHRISTMAS HAM

SERVES 8, PLUS LOTS OF LEFTOVERS

Pork neck is an economical cut and pork leg (leg of ham) is, too, surprisingly. Because so few people buy them fresh (everyone buys them pre-smoked as ham), you can get them for a good price.

4 pounds pork neck
or 4½ pounds leg of ham

½ cup brown rice syrup

¼ cup olive oil

1 tablespoon paprika

2 teaspoons ground cloves

1 teaspoon ground cinnamon

1 teaspoon each sea salt and freshly ground black pepper

zest of 1 orange

2 tablespoons orange juice

Christmas Eve: Line a baking dish with parchment paper. Wash the meat under cold running water and pat dry with paper towels.

Place the brown rice syrup and olive oil in a jug with ¼ cup of water. Stir in the spices, salt, pepper and orange zest and juice. Pour over the pork, using your hands to rub the marinade well into the meat. Place in the prepared baking dish. Cover and marinate in the fridge for at least 8 hours or overnight.

Christmas Day: Preheat the oven to 400°F. Remove the ham from the fridge and allow it to stand for 10 minutes. Add 1 cup of water to the base of the dish and pop the lot in the oven. Bake for 30 minutes, then turn the baking dish around and bake for another 30 minutes, adding another ½ cup of water if necessary. Bake for another 30 minutes, turning the dish around after 15 minutes. Serve warm with the salads on these pages.

2. STUFFING 'N' ALL THE BEST BITS SALAD

SERVES 8

18 ounces brussels sprouts

1¾ pounds butternut squash

Cut 'em all into 1-inch chunks.

2 large parsnips

3 sprigs rosemary or thyme, leaves picked and roughly chopped, plus extra to garnish

7 ounces pancetta, cut into ⅜-inch cubes

½ cup olive oil or coconut oil

sea salt and freshly ground black pepper

2 cups Cooked Buckwheat (page 27)

1 cup pecans, roughly chopped

1 Pink Lady apple, cut into ⅜-inch cubes

dash of apple cider vinegar

pomegranate seeds, to garnish

Christmas Eve: Preheat the oven to 400°F. Spread the vegetables, herbs and pancetta on one or two baking sheets. Coat with oil and season to taste with salt and pepper. Roast for 45 minutes, turning halfway.

Spread the buckwheat and pecans on another baking sheet and place in the oven. Roast everything (including the veggies) for another 10 minutes, or until the pecans are golden. Remove from the oven and allow to cool. Once cooled, transfer each sheet of goodies to separate containers and keep them somewhere cool (the basement, perhaps . . . no need to take up fridge space).

Root vegetables improve with cooling—both in texture and flavor—and also provide great resistant starch . . . which will help with post-Christmas digestion.

Christmas Day: In a large serving bowl, toss the vegetables with the roasted buckwheat and pecans. Add the cubed apple and drizzle with a dash of apple cider vinegar. Garnish with pomegranate seeds and the extra rosemary or thyme.

some of this drains away

1½ TEASPOONS ADDED SUGAR PER SERVING

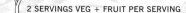 2 SERVINGS VEG + FRUIT PER SERVING

3. PICKLED FESTIVE RED SLAW WITH CARAMELIZED RUBY GRAPEFRUIT

SERVES 8

½ red cabbage, shredded

2 beets, trimmed, scrubbed and grated

2 purple (or orange) carrots, grated

1 red onion, thinly sliced

½ cup Powerhouse Dressing (page 53)

sea salt and freshly ground black pepper

2 ruby grapefruit or 3 blood oranges or 2 oranges, segmented

a few dobs of butter

½ cup crumbled feta, to serve

Christmas Eve/morning: Toss the red cabbage, beets, carrot and onions in a bowl with the dressing. Season with salt and pepper. Cover and leave in the fridge overnight (or for a few hours if you want to prepare it on the day).

Christmas Day: Place the grapefruit or orange segments on a tray lined with parchment paper. Dot with butter and a sprinkle of salt. Place under the broiler (or in a hot oven—with the ham!) and cook for 5–8 minutes. Allow to cool.

To serve, add the caramelized grapefruit or orange to the slaw and sprinkle with the crumbled feta.

4. THE GREEN COUNTERBALANCE SALAD

SERVES 6–8

1 large bunch watercress, leaves picked (or arugula leaves and/or Belgian endive leaves, halved)

2 small fennel bulbs, stalks removed, cored, halved and thinly sliced (reserve the fronds)

2 handfuls of mint leaves

½ red onion, halved and thinly sliced

1 green apple, halved and thinly sliced or 6 radishes, thinly sliced

⅓ cup Powerhouse Dressing (page 53)

Place the leaves, fennel, mint, onion and apple or radish in a large bowl (or on a platter). Pour the dressing over the salad and mix. Toss the fennel fronds on top.

MAKE IT BULKIER:

Add 2 cups of Cooked Quinoa (page 26) or a 14-ounce can of brown lentils, rinsed and drained, along with 1 cup of frozen peas, cooked in hot water for 2 minutes, and ½ cup of toasted pepitas.

something bitter + green to get gastric juices fired up

1 SERVING VEG + FRUIT PER SERVING

1 SERVING VEG + FRUIT PER SERVING

THREE CLEAN DIGESTIVE COCKTAILS

I called on my friends the Trolley'd boys—two guys who serve cocktails from an old airline trolley at events—to help fine-tune these boozy treats. All three cocktails serve as refreshing aperitifs, with gut-boosting properties.

1. THE BRIGHT SIDE

MAKES 8

1½-inch knob of turmeric, peeled and sliced

1 teaspoon fennel seeds

2 tablespoons brown rice syrup

1 cup boiled water

5½ ounces grapefruit juice

8 ounces vodka

fennel flowers, to serve

Muddle the turmeric in a bowl (smash around a little with a spoon to release the juices). Add the fennel seeds, brown rice syrup and boiled water and allow to brew for 20 minutes. Strain and cool.

Make two cocktails at a time by shaking one-quarter of the fennel and turmeric liquid with one-quarter of the remaining ingredients. Strain into chilled cocktail glasses and garnish with fennel flowers.

2. THE CULTURED MULE

MAKES 8

12 ounces vodka

⅓ cup lime juice

2 tablespoons brown rice syrup (mixed with 1–2 teaspoons hot water)

22 ounces plain Kombucha (page 344) or use store-bought kombucha

ice and lime wedges, to serve

Combine all of the ingredients in a large jug. Pour into tall glasses over ice and lime wedges.

3. DA CLEAN BEE'S KNEES

MAKES 8

1 cup boiled water

2 tablespoons brown rice syrup

12 sprigs thyme, plus extra to serve

12 ounces vodka or gin

4 ounces lemon juice

4 ounces apple cider vinegar

You may want to add more syrup if you like

Combine the boiled water, brown rice syrup and thyme in a jug and allow to brew for 20 minutes. Strain and cool.

Make two cocktails at a time by shaking one-quarter of the thyme liquid with one-quarter of each of the remaining ingredients. Strain into chilled cocktail glasses and garnish with a sprig of thyme.

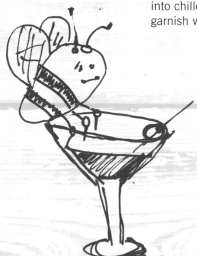

¾ TEASPOON ADDED SUGAR PER SERVING   ¾ TEASPOON ADDED SUGAR PER SERVING   ¾ TEASPOON ADDED SUGAR PER SERVING

"MAPLE SYRUP" PORK BELLY WITH PECANS

SERVES 6–8

Pork belly is a very fatty, rich piece of meat, but beautifully succulent.
Be sure to eat it with plenty of greenery.

2 pounds pork belly, cut into 6–8 thick slices

⅓ cup brown rice syrup

2 cinnamon sticks

1 large red chili, finely chopped

8 cloves

3 cloves garlic, minced

⅓ cup soy sauce or tamari

½ cup Homemade Chicken Stock (page 42)

zest of ½ orange, flesh cut into segments (seeds removed)

2 tablespoons apple cider vinegar

TO SERVE

6 cups steamed greens (broccolini, zucchini and kale make a good combo)

½ cup pecans, lightly toasted

If the top of your pork hasn't browned in the slow cooker, place on a foil-lined baking sheet and pop under a hot broiler for 5 minutes to crisp.

In the morning: Place the pork slices in the slow-cooker insert, fatty side up (try to wedge them all in so they fit in one layer). Pour the brown rice syrup over the pork, then add the remaining ingredients. Cover and cook on low for 6–7 hours or high for 4 hours.

Just before serving: Remove the pork and keep warm. Skim off as much fat from the top of the cooking liquid as you can, place in a jar and refrigerate (lard is great for cooking). Strain the sauce through a fine sieve and return it to the slow-cooker insert. Cook on high with the lid off to thicken while you steam your greens.

Serve the pork with the steamed greens. Sprinkle with the pecans and pour the sauce over all.

!) as I say, this is a rich dish

2 TEASPOONS ADDED SUGAR PER SERVING

CACAO CAYENNE PECANS

These make a great grown-up Christmas gift. A dad who came to one of my events with his daughter took me aside and told me I should do more "chocolate stuff for men." Hopefully this fits the bill and his daughter finds this recipe.

butter, for greasing

3 egg whites

pinch of sea salt

⅓ cup brown rice syrup

⅓ cup raw cacao powder

½ teaspoon ground ginger

¼ teaspoon cayenne pepper (add more if you like a bit of heat)

1 teaspoon ground cinnamon

4 cups pecans (preferably activated; see page 28)

Preheat the oven to 175°F and grease a stainless-steel baking sheet with butter.

Beat the egg whites and salt in a clean bowl. Gradually add the brown rice syrup, then stir in the cacao powder and spices and mix well. Fold in the pecans until well coated. Spread the pecans on the baking sheet and place in the oven for 1½ hours, or until the coating hardens. Once cool, store in airtight jars for up to 1 month.

USE THE LEFTOVER EGG YOLKS:
Make an omelette or frittata.
Or freeze them (see page 25).

1 TEASPOON ADDED SUGAR PER SERVING

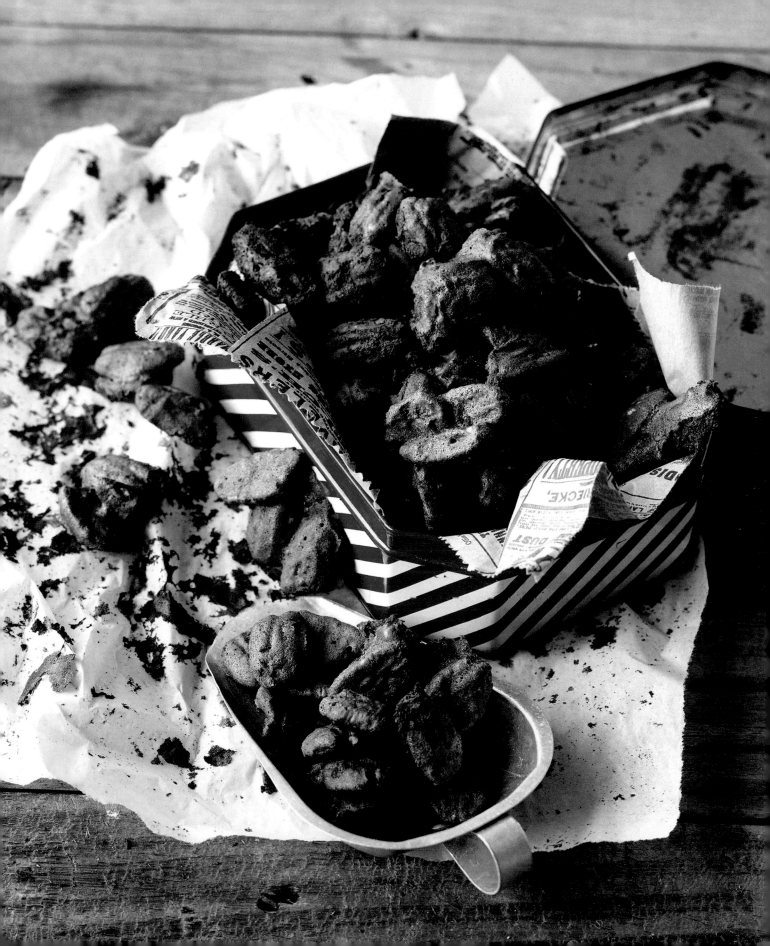

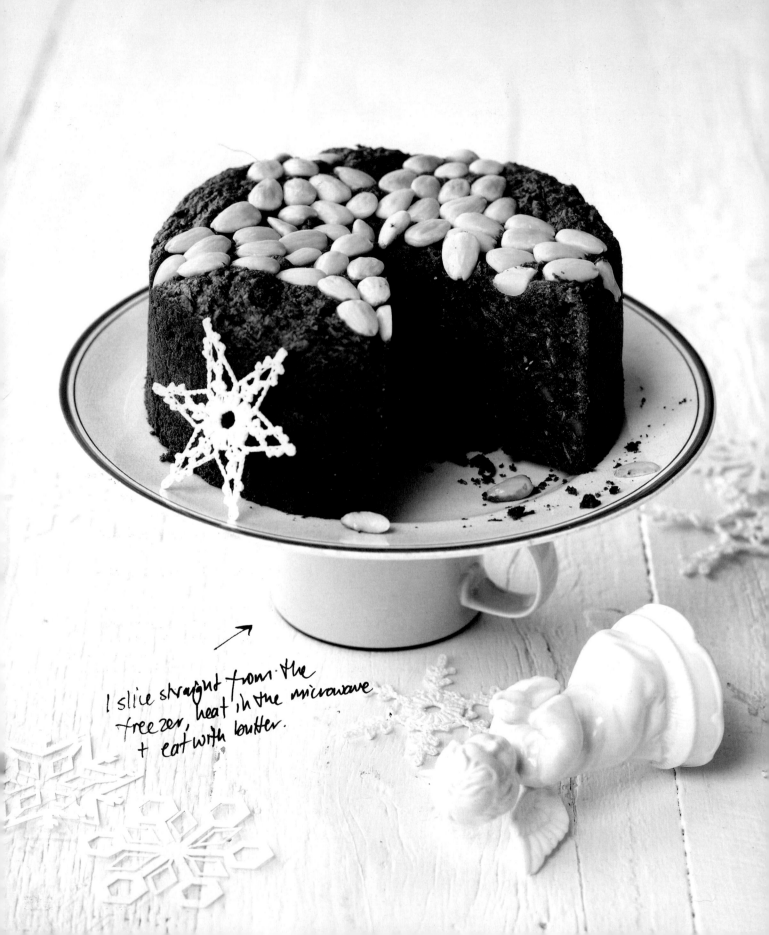

I slice straight from the
freezer, heat in the microwave
+ eat with butter.

MY TOTALLY MESSED-WITH CHRISTMAS CAKE

SERVES 16 ——————————————————————————————

I've taken out the dried and glacéed fruit and the gluten but kept the brandy and almonds, then added dark chocolate, coconut, walnuts and, yeah, beets.

A storage warning
The reason traditional fruit-filled Christmas cakes last for so long is that they're full of sugar and alcohol. Both work as preservatives and in some cases they can keep the cake moist and mold-free for several months. This cake ain't like that. Store it in an airtight container and it should keep for up to a week. Or freeze it for up to 2 months.

2 cups gluten-free self-rising flour

1 cup shredded coconut

1 cup almond meal

¼ cup raw cacao powder

1 tablespoon gluten-free baking powder

2 teaspoons ground cinnamon

2 teaspoons ground ginger

2 teaspoons ground cardamom

½ teaspoon ground cloves

1 tablespoon orange zest

1 cup walnuts, chopped

3½ ounces dark (85–90% cocoa) chocolate, coarsely chopped

1¾ sticks butter, cubed

½ cup brown rice syrup

4 eggs

2 tablespoons brandy

2 cups grated beets (about 2–3 beets)

½ cup blanched almonds (optional)

Preheat the oven to 325°F and grease an 8-inch-diameter springform cake pan.

In a large bowl combine the flour, coconut, almond meal, cacao powder, baking powder, spices and zest. Stir in the walnuts and chocolate.

Melt the butter and brown rice syrup in a small saucepan over medium heat (or in the microwave). Cool slightly.

Break the eggs into a separate bowl and whisk. Stir in the brandy, then whisk in the melted butter and brown rice syrup.

Pour the wet ingredients into the dry ingredients. Add the beets and stir well. Transfer the mixture to the prepared pan and smooth the top. Decorate with blanched almonds (if using). Cover the pan with foil and bake for 1 hour 15 minutes. Remove the foil and cook for another 15–25 minutes until a skewer inserted into the center comes out clean. Allow the cake to cool for 20 minutes before removing from the pan.

This cake can be served warm or cold.

1½ TEASPOONS ADDED SUGAR PER SERVING

ISRAELI WHOLE-BAKED CAULIFLOWER

I loved the idea of serving a whole cauli on the table for dinner ('cos I love cauli *that* much) so I did just that, but gave it an Israeli twist. It makes a great dinner-party conversation starter.

1 cup full-fat organic plain yogurt (preferably Greek-style)

3 teaspoons Ras el Hanout Mix (page 45) or 1 teaspoon each sweet paprika, ground cumin and ground coriander

2 teaspoons sumac (optional)

2 teaspoons ground turmeric

1 tablespoon chopped thyme or 1 teaspoon dried thyme

2 cloves garlic, minced

¾-inch knob of ginger, minced

1 teaspoon sea salt

zest and juice of 1 lemon

1 head cauliflower, leaves and stalk trimmed

1 tablespoon coconut oil

Green Minx Dressing (page 54), Leftovers Pesto (page 55) or TMT Dressing (page 53), to serve

If your cauli is quite large, feel free to precook it: simmer it in a stockpot with enough water to cover for 20 minutes. Then bake for 40 minutes only.

In a large mixing bowl, combine the yogurt, spices, thyme, garlic, ginger, salt, zest, and half of the juice. Place the cauliflower headfirst into the yogurt mixture, moving it around until the entire top is coated. Using your hands, make sure the mixture gets under the florets on the base of the cauliflower. Cover and place in the fridge to marinate for at least 1 hour, preferably overnight.

Preheat the oven to 350°F and line a baking sheet with parchment paper.

Remove the cauliflower from the bowl, reserving the leftover marinade for serving. Place the cauli on the baking sheet and drizzle it with the coconut oil. Bake for 1½ hours on the middle shelf of the oven or until the cauli is soft.

Remove from the oven and slice into 6 wedges (do it at the table for effect). Mix the leftover marinade with the remaining lemon juice to make the dressing. Serve the cauli with the marinade dressing and a robust salad—try The Green Counterbalance Salad (page 309) or A Salad of Crushed Olives (page 170).

1 SERVING VEG + FRUIT PER SERVING

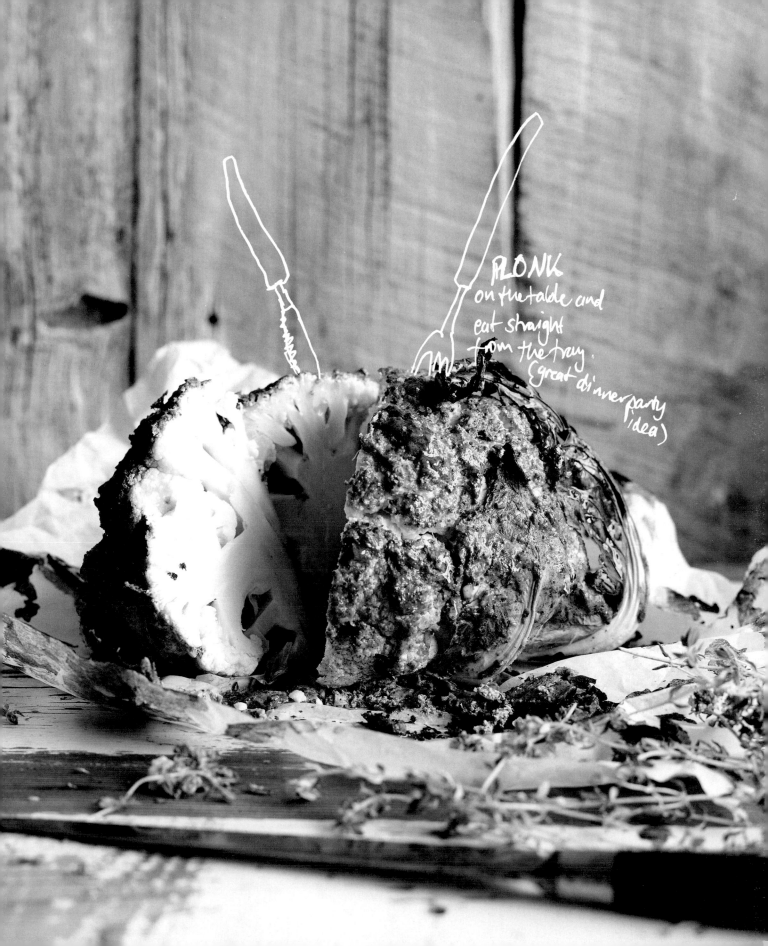

PLONK
on the table and
eat straight
from the tray.
(great dinner party
idea)

CARDAMOM AND SEA SALT GANACHE TART

SERVES 16

9 ounces coconut cream

2 tablespoons cardamom pods, lightly crushed with a flat blade until the outer husks crack

½ teaspoon pure vanilla powder or 1 teaspoon pure vanilla extract (or make your own; see page 45)

3½ ounces dark (85–90% cocoa) chocolate, chopped

pinch of sea salt, plus coarse sea salt, to garnish

berries, edible petals and Activated Groaties (page 27), to garnish (optional)

CRUST

⅓ cup coconut oil

¼ cup brown rice syrup

2 cups shredded coconut

1 tablespoon raw cacao powder

Preheat the oven to 350°F.

To make the crust, melt the coconut oil and brown rice syrup in a saucepan. Remove from the heat, add the shredded coconut and cacao powder and mix well. Press the mixture into the bottom and up the sides of a quiche or tart pan—no need to grease it—so that the mixture's approximately ¼ inch thick all over. Bake the crust for 15–20 minutes. Remove from the oven and set aside to cool and firm up.

Meanwhile, heat the coconut cream, cardamom pods and vanilla in a saucepan to a simmer, then turn off the heat and cover with a lid. Allow to steep for 10 minutes.

Strain the coconut cream mixture into a bowl, reserving ¼ cup in the pan for emergency use later, if needed. Discard the cardamom pods (or save to spice up chai tea). Add the chocolate and salt to the bowl, whisking it through until silky and melted. If the fats separate and your ganache develops a chocolatey cottage-cheese appearance, just add the reserved coconut cream, whisking swiftly to bring it all back together.

Once silky, pour into the tart shell and refrigerate until the ganache sets (at least 2 hours). Garnish with a pinch of coarse sea salt and berries, petals and Activated Groaties, if desired.

1 TEASPOON ADDED SUGAR PER SERVING

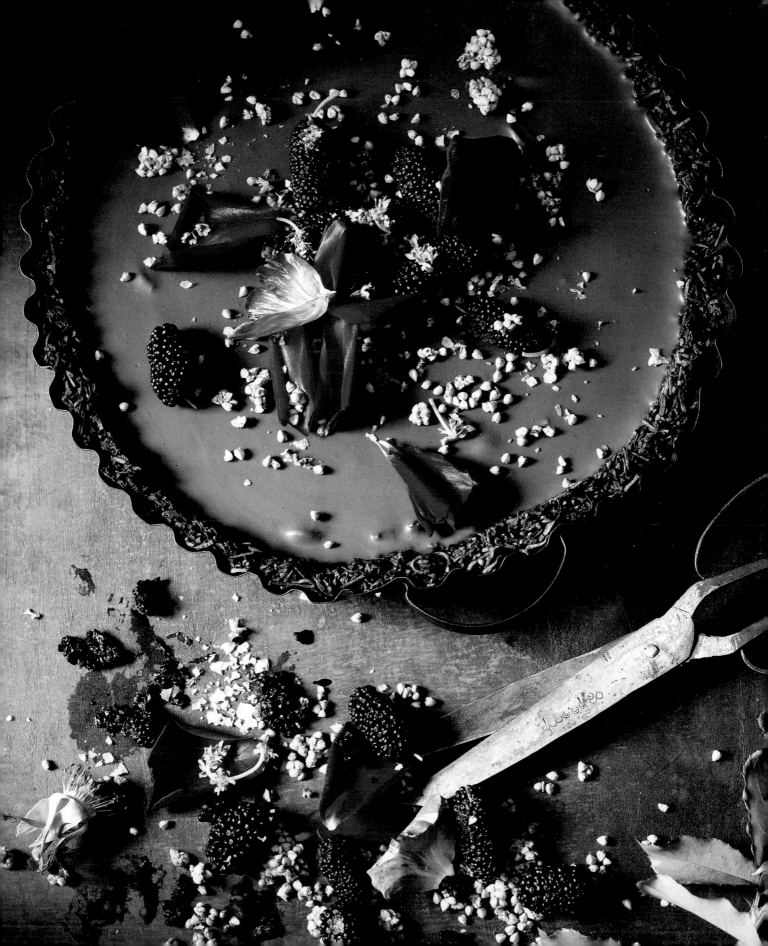

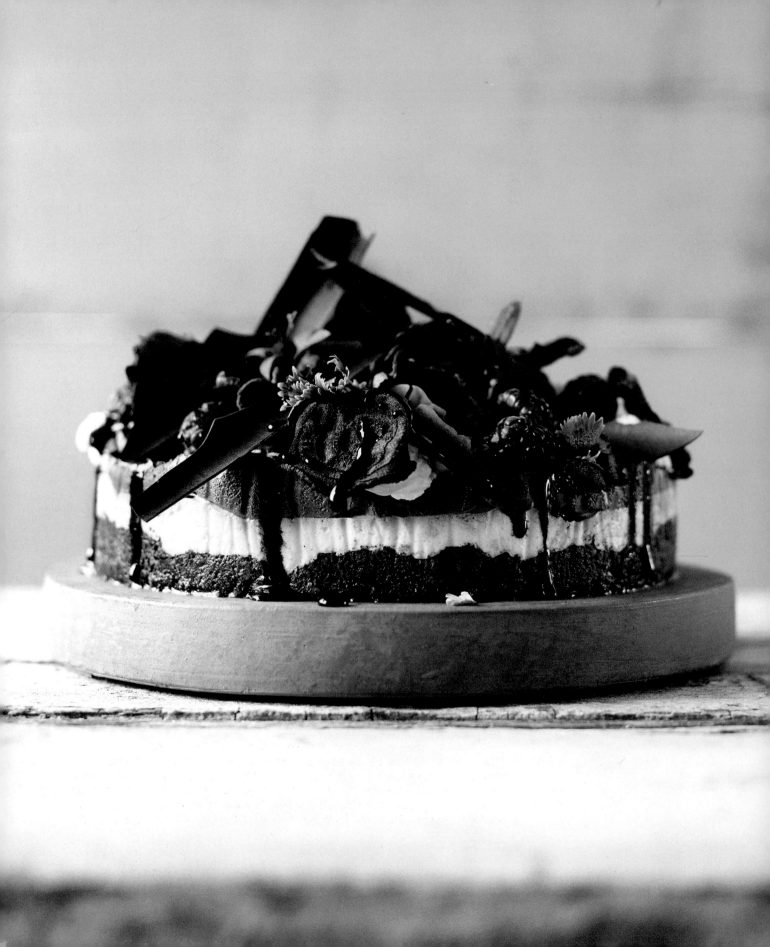

BEET RED VELVET CHEESECAKE

IN WHICH I "PIMP" TWO FAVORITE TREATS

SERVES 12

I put out a "What would you like to see in my next cookbook?" call to action on the web. I was overwhelmed with requests to "pimp" the Crunchynut Cheesecake from my first book as well as the Beetroot Red Velvet Cupcakes from iquitsugar.com. So I figured I'd do the whole crazy thing in the one springform cake pan!

The recipe might look tricky . . . but there is an extraordinary amount of flow to it.

CANDIED BEET

1 beet, trimmed and peeled

2 tablespoons brown rice syrup

½ teaspoon pure vanilla powder

BASE

1 cup nuts (preferably activated; see page 28; skinless hazelnuts are best, but you can use pistachios too)

1 cup desiccated coconut

½ cup almond meal

½ cup raw cacao powder

1¼ sticks unsalted butter, softened

CHEESECAKE FILLING

27 ounces Homemade Cream Cheese (page 46; or use store-bought), at room temperature, plus extra to garnish

2 tablespoons full-fat organic plain yogurt or sour cream

¼ cup coconut cream

¼ cup brown rice syrup

1 egg

pinch of pure vanilla powder

¼ cup raw cacao powder

GARNISH

1¾ ounces dark (85–90% cocoa) chocolate, chopped

edible flowers and raspberries, to garnish

Preheat the oven to 250°F and line a baking sheet with parchment paper.

To make the candied beet, slice the beet thinly (about ⅛ inch) using a sharp knife or mandoline. In a small saucepan, heat the brown rice syrup and vanilla with ½ cup of water, stirring until the syrup dissolves. Bring to a boil. Add the beet slices and top with more water so that the beet is just covered. Return to a boil and simmer for 20 minutes, or until the beet slices are tender and translucent. Remove the beet, reserving the leftover liquid for making the cheesecake filling. Lay the beet slices on the prepared sheet and bake for 1 hour, or until crispy. Remove from the oven and allow to cool.

To make the base, increase the oven temperature to 350°F and line a 9-inch-diameter springform cake pan with parchment paper. Grind the nuts in a food processor until semi-fine. Transfer to a mixing bowl with the coconut, almond meal, cacao powder and butter and rub with your fingers to make a dough. (The more you rub, the more you'll release the oils in the nuts and achieve the right consistency.) Add more butter if required. Press the mixture evenly into the bottom of the pan so

1½ TEASPOONS ADDED SUGAR PER SERVING

continued over...

BEET RED VELVET
CHEESECAKE

[. . . CONT'D]

the crust is about ½ inch thick. Bake for 10 minutes. Remove and allow to cool completely.

To make the cheesecake filling, combine the cream cheese, yogurt or sour cream, coconut cream, brown rice syrup, egg and vanilla in a large bowl. Don't overmix, and try to keep the aeration to a minimum while stirring (too much air will make the filling puff up and then collapse during cooking). Transfer half of the mixture to another bowl and stir in 2–3 tablespoons of the reserved beet liquid and the cacao powder. Spoon the vanilla layer onto the cooled bottom, then layer the beet-and-cacao mix on top. Return to the oven for 20–30 minutes, until the mixture pulls away from the side a little and the center is custard-like (don't overcook). Place in the fridge for at least 2 hours to firm.

To make chocolate shards for the garnish, melt the chocolate slowly in a microwave (or in a heatproof bowl over a saucepan of boiling water, making sure the bottom of the bowl doesn't touch the water). Pour onto a sheet of parchment paper and spread evenly with a palette knife. Cover with a second sheet of parchment paper and smooth out any bubbles. Gently roll up to form a 1½-inch tube. Place in the fridge for 30 minutes to set. Unroll carefully to reveal instant shards.

Adorn the cold cheesecake with the candied beet chips, edible flowers, chocolate shards and raspberries, using the extra cream cheese to keep things in place.

THAI LATTES

MAKES 6

1½ tablespoons gelatin powder (see page 348)

3 teaspoons lemongrass-and-ginger tea leaves (or use 3 teabags)

½ small red chili, chopped, or 2 kaffir lime leaves, chopped (optional)

2 tablespoons brown rice syrup

1 cup Supercharged Coconut Frosting (page 56)

¼ cup roasted peanuts and/or coconut flakes, toasted

shredded kaffir lime leaves or lime zest, to serve

"Bloom" the gelatin by stirring it into ⅓ cup of cold water until dissolved. Let it sit for 5 minutes until it becomes rubbery.

Meanwhile, place the tea (in a tea ball if using leaf tea), chili or kaffir lime leaves (if using) and brown rice syrup in a saucepan with 2 cups of boiling water. Leave to steep, then remove the tea and chili or kaffir lime leaves and strain. Use a whisk or an immersion blender to blend the gelatin into the mixture until smooth.

Pour into teacups or glasses and chill in the fridge for 4 hours to set.

To serve, top with the coconut frosting, sprinkle with peanuts and/or coconut and garnish with shredded kaffir lime leaves or lime zest.

1½ TEASPOONS ADDED SUGAR PER SERVING

MY SPECTACULAR
POPSTICK CAKE

For many, the end of a dinner party is the real test of their no-sugar resolve. So, here you go: dessert, chocolate and vodka all combined into one fun, distracting package. I used an old polystyrene ball chopped in half to poke the sticks into. You could use some of your kid's play dough or I guess an orange, halved, would do it. But that would seem a waste of an orange. Source flowers from your garden/neighborhood to add extra flourish and dig up some sparklers from that drawer where such things get lost.

POMEGRANATE AND COCONUT
VODKA POPSTICKS

MAKES 6

COCONUT LAYER

3½ tablespoons gelatin powder
(see page 348)

9-ounce can coconut cream

½ teaspoon granulated stevia,
or to taste

VODKA LAYER

3½ tablespoons gelatin powder

¾ cup boiling water

½ teaspoon granulated stevia,
or to taste

¾ cup vodka

1–2 teaspoons rose water,
to taste (you may need to use
more, depending on the strength)

seeds of 1 pomegranate

To make the coconut layer, "bloom" the gelatin by stirring it into ⅓ cup of cold water until dissolved. Let it sit for 5 minutes until it becomes rubbery.

Put the coconut cream and stevia in a saucepan and heat until almost boiling. Remove from the heat and add the bloomed gelatin, breaking up the blobby bits and using an immersion blender to purée. When cooled a little, pour into ice pop molds to one-third full and freeze for 1 hour.

To make the vodka layer, make up another batch of jelly, blooming the gelatin as above. Combine the boiling water with the stevia. Allow to cool a little, then stir in the vodka and rose water. Sprinkle pomegranate seeds over the set coconut layer and pour the vodka mixture over the top. Insert the ice pop sticks and return to the freezer to set. Serve with a few more pomegranate seeds sprinkled on top, if you like.

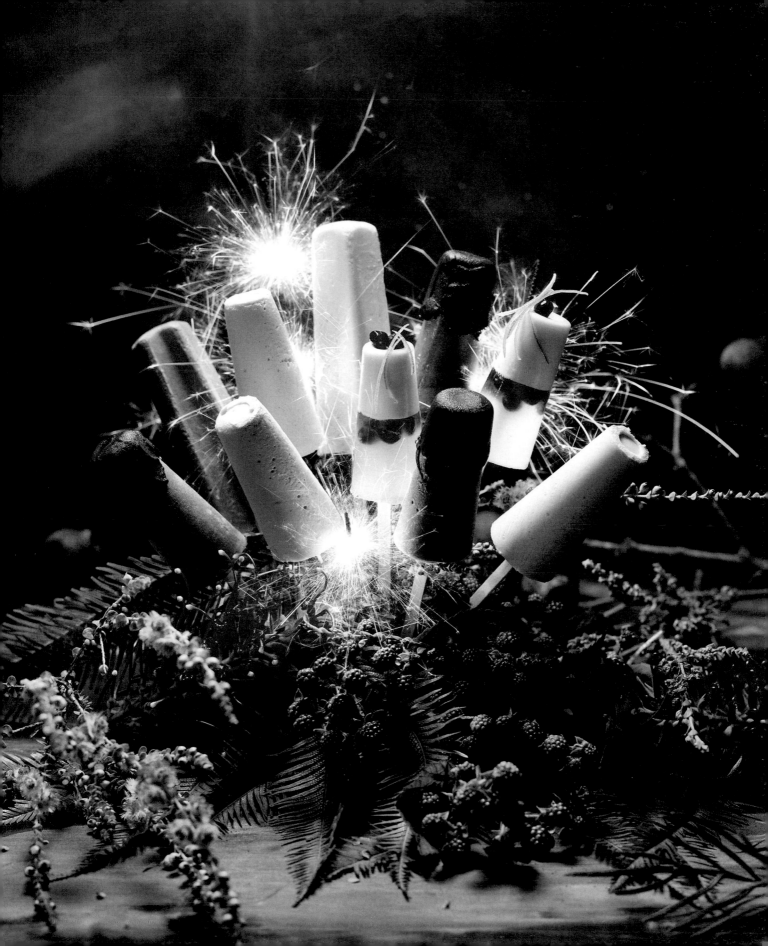

MARGARITA POPSTICKS

MAKES 6

juice of 5 limes,
plus 1 lime, peeled
and cubed

*Made specifically for
my friend Zoe, who's
partial to some salt
and lime on a rim.*

1½ cups coconut milk

1 large avocado

¼ cup tequila, or to taste

1¼ tablespoons brown rice syrup
or 5 drops liquid stevia

1½ teaspoons sea salt

Place everything except the lime
chunks in a blender and blend until
smooth. Pour the margarita mixture
into six ice pop molds. Add chunks
of lime and insert ice pop sticks.
Freeze for at least 1 hour until
slushy, and then stir to distribute
the lime chunks evenly. Freeze for
another 3 hours.

CHOCOLATE AND RED WINE CREAMSTICKS

MAKES 6

¾ cup leftover red wine

1 cinnamon stick or 1 teaspoon
ground cinnamon

1 teaspoon ground allspice

1 teaspoon cloves

1 cup coconut cream

½ avocado

1 tablespoon brown rice syrup
or 4 drops liquid stevia

2 tablespoons raw cacao powder

1¾ ounces dark (85–90% cocoa)
chocolate, or 3 cubes frozen Basic Raw
Chocolate (page 56)

Heat the wine and spices in a saucepan over
medium heat. Simmer for 10 minutes (it will
reduce quite a bit). Cool slightly, then strain and
pour into a blender. Add the coconut cream,
avocado, brown rice syrup or stevia and cacao
powder. Blend until smooth. Pour into ice pop
molds and insert the sticks. Freeze for at least
4 hours.

Melt the chocolate in a cup in the microwave
(do it gradually on low), or in a heatproof bowl
over a saucepan of boiling water, making sure the
bottom of the bowl doesn't touch the water. Dip
the top of each creamstick into the chocolate and
return to the freezer (use your mold to keep them
propped vertically) until ready to serve.

½ TEASPOON ADDED SUGAR PER SERVING

½ TEASPOON ADDED SUGAR PER SERVING

PUMPKIN SPICE-A-CHINO

1½ tablespoons gelatin powder (see page 348)

2 x 14-ounce cans coconut cream

1 cup Squash Purée (page 23)

2 tablespoons brown rice syrup

2 teaspoons Pumpkin Spice Mix (page 45)

ground cinnamon or grated dark (85–90% cocoa) chocolate, to serve

CHINO FOAM

⅔ cup coconut cream (reserved from above)

1 tablespoon gelatin powder

2 teaspoons brown rice syrup

"Bloom" the gelatin by stirring it into ⅓ cup of cold water until dissolved. Let it sit for 5 minutes until it becomes rubbery.

Place 2 cups of the coconut cream in a saucepan with the Squash Purée and brown rice syrup. (Refrigerate the remaining coconut cream for the Chino Foam.) Heat gently, then remove and stir in the gelatin and Pumpkin Spice Mix. Using an immersion blender, blend the mixture until smooth. Pour into cups or glasses and refrigerate for 4 hours, or until set.

About 10 minutes before the mixture is set, make the Chino Foam. Remove the reserved coconut cream from the fridge and blend with an immersion blender. Slowly pour in the gelatin in a thin stream, followed by the brown rice syrup. Continue mixing until the mixture is fluffy (2–3 minutes).

To serve, top with Chino Foam and sprinkle with cinnamon or chocolate.

MAKE IT AN AUSTRALIANA MANGO FLAT WHITE:

Follow the recipe above, replacing the Squash Purée with 1 cup of chopped mango and omitting the Pumpkin Spice Mix. Top with Chino Foam and serve with a pinch of lime zest and frozen mango cubes, if you have some.

1½ TEASPOONS ADDED SUGAR PER SERVING

HOT CROSS MUFFINS

I've spent four Easters perfecting a HXB that contains no gluten,
no dried fruit and no gooby additives that no one has in their pantry . . .
but that still tastes like the things Australian supermarkets start selling
shortly after Christmas. Here she is . . .

3½ tablespoons coconut oil or butter, melted, plus extra for greasing

1½ cups almond meal

¼ cup arrowroot

1½ teaspoons baking powder

1 teaspoon ground cinnamon

1 teaspoon ground ginger

1 teaspoon ground nutmeg

1 teaspoon Pumpkin Spice Mix (page 45) or ¾ teaspoon ground cinnamon and ¼ teaspoon ground nutmeg

¼ teaspoon ground cloves

pinch of sea salt

¼ cup chopped pecans

1¾ ounces dark (85–90% cocoa) chocolate, roughly chopped

zest of 1 orange

1 teaspoon pure vanilla extract (or make your own; page 45)

1 tablespoon brown rice syrup

3 eggs, lightly beaten

¼ cup gluten-free plain flour (regular plain and spelt are fine too)

butter, to serve

Preheat the oven to 350°F and grease an 8-cup muffin pan.

Place the almond meal, arrowroot, baking powder, spices, salt, pecans, chocolate and orange zest in a mixing bowl and stir until combined.

In a separate bowl, lightly whisk the melted butter or coconut oil, vanilla, brown rice syrup and eggs. Pour the wet ingredients into the dry ingredients and mix until smooth. Spoon the mixture evenly into the muffin cups.

Whisk the flour with 2–3 tablespoons of water to make a thick paste. Spoon the mixture into a piping bag (or a plastic zipper bag with one corner snipped), and squeeze onto each muffin to make a cross. Bake for 15 minutes, or until brown on the top. Cool for a minute or so, then slice open and serve with a dollop of butter.

½ TEASPOON ADDED SUGAR PER SERVING

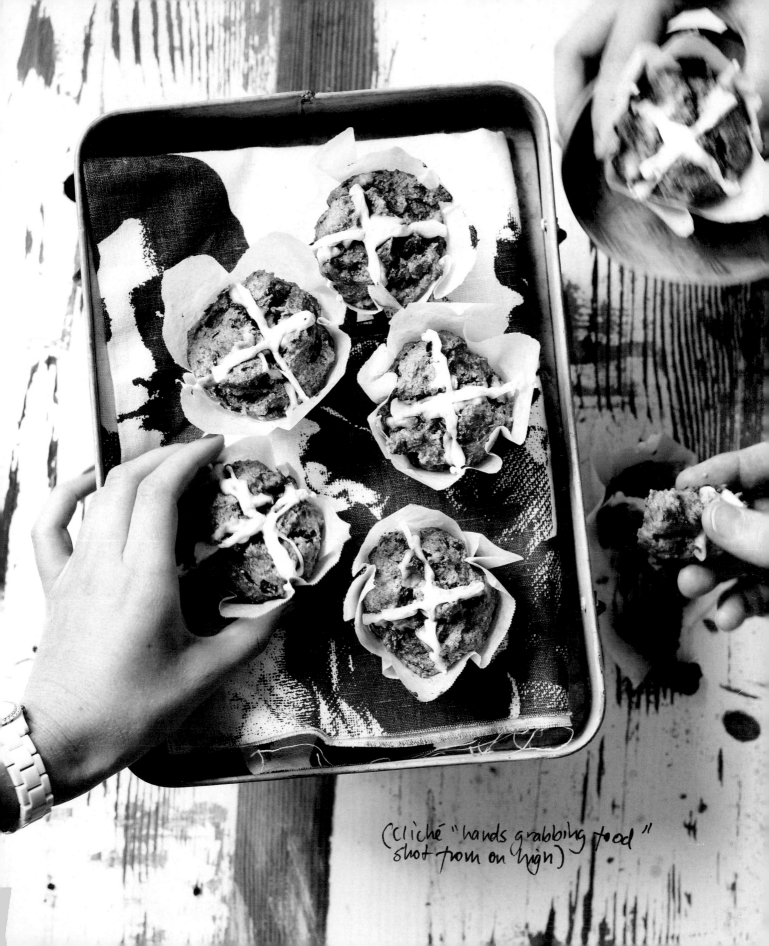

(cliché "hands grabbing food" shot from on high)

GREEN SMOOTHIE CAKE WITH LEMON CHEESE WHIP

butter or coconut oil, for greasing

1 bunch spinach (about 10½ ounces), roots trimmed, leaves and stems roughly chopped

zest and juice of 1 lemon

3 eggs

½ cup brown rice syrup

2 teaspoons pure vanilla extract (or make your own; page 45)

1½ cups brown rice flour mixed with 2½ teaspoons baking powder

⅓ cup extra-virgin olive oil

1¾ cups almond meal

1 zucchini, finely grated and squeezed in a clean dishtowel to remove moisture

1½ cups Cream Cheese Frosting (page 56)

Preheat the oven to 350°F. Grease and line an 8-inch square or round cake pan with nonstick parchment paper.

Place the spinach in a food processor and process until very finely chopped. Add the lemon juice and process to form a paste.

Beat the eggs and brown rice syrup in a large bowl until thick and glossy—this will take about 4–5 minutes using an electric mixer. (A ribbon should fall from the beaters when lifted.) Beat in the vanilla and lemon zest. Using a large metal spoon, gradually fold in the flour alternately with the oil. Fold in the almond meal and mix until smooth, then stir through the spinach and zucchini. Spoon the mixture into the prepared pan and smooth the surface. Bake for 45–50 minutes, or until a skewer inserted into the center comes out clean. Leave in the pan to cool completely.

When cool, use a small spatula to ice the cake with the frosting. Cut into slices to serve.

This cake is best served fresh but can be stored in an airtight container in the fridge for 3 days. Or you can slice and freeze it for up to 1 month.

1½ TEASPOONS ADDED SUGAR PER SERVING

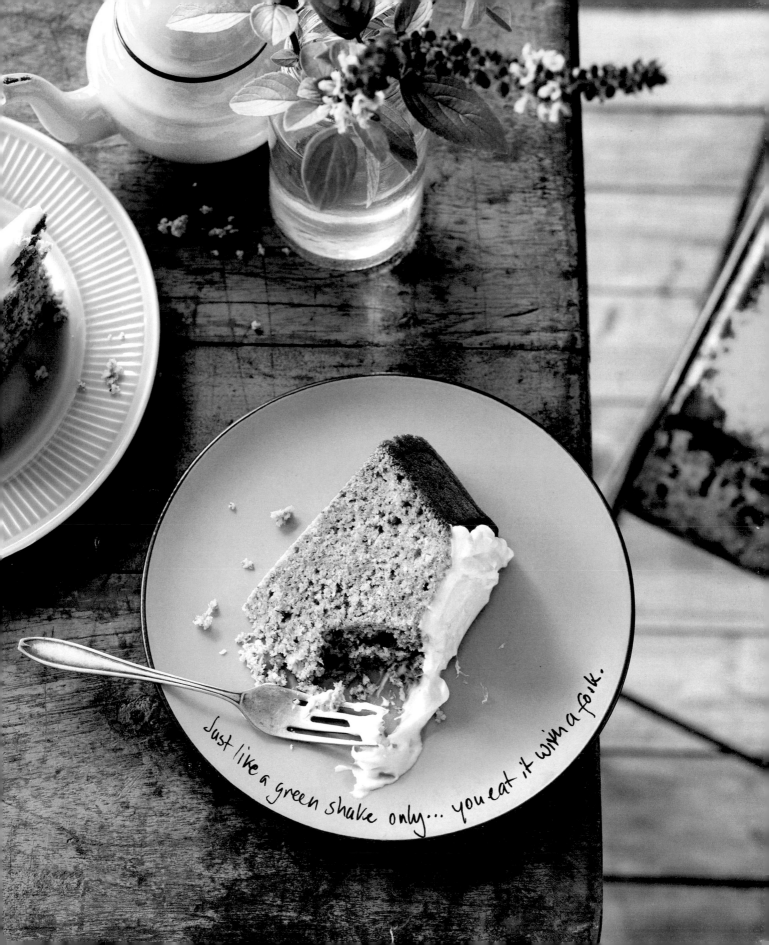

Just like a green shake only... you eat it with a fork.

FERMENTS AND OTHER
GUT-HEALING
FUNCTIONAL FOODS

witchy FERMENTED, sprouted
and BACTERIA-blooming
stuff

for STUPENDOUSLY
healthy, happy, balanced
interior health. ☺

FERMENTED VEGETABLES.

New to the concept? Jaded by the multi-step hoopla? I've given the fad a simplicious makeover and streamlined things for us all.

WHY FERMENT?

It saves food

Lacto-fermentation has been around for eons as a way to preserve food when it's in seasonal abundance. Unlike pickling (which uses heat, vinegar and sugar), lacto-fermentation uses salt (and sometimes whey) to encourage the veggie's natural "good" (*lactobacillus*) bacteria to flourish, producing lactic acid that staves off dodgy bacteria. Pickling, on the other hand, pretty much kills off everything.

It's a condiment flavor bomb

Ferments are a condiment on their own and ferment juices add kick to sauces, deglazes, dressings and leftovers.

It unlocks extra nutrition

Lactic acid activates enzymes in the vegetable that aid digestion, and unlocks a bunch of vitamins, including vitamin C and vitamin A as well as the much-revered vitamin K[2]— a known cancer fighter.

It builds gut health

It promotes the growth of healthy flora in the intestine.

It cuts sugar content

The sugar in the veggie is what ferments; the same process sees red wine end up almost fructose-free.

And reduces sugar cravings

This is the other BIG reason to ferment— it helps you quit the white stuff. Scientists have found that gut bacteria actually secrete special proteins that are similar to hunger-regulating hormones, affecting both our food cravings and mood. In other words, the little buggers try to get us to eat foods that *they* thrive on. So if you eat lots of sugar, you feed the bacteria that love it, locking yourself into the craving cycle. Eating fermented food, however, amps up the healthy bacteria, overpowering the sugar-lovin' microbes and weakening the craving signals.

WHAT DO YOU NEED?

You could follow all the complex methods . . . or you can do as I do and cut steps and ingredients and then to the chase. You just need:

- super-fresh and organic vegetables that are currently abundant

- a few glass jars (about 1 quart is ideal) with tight-fitting lids

- a fair dose of salt and/or whey (see page 46 for how to make your own whey), both of which work as fermenting starters

- some spices to help act as fungicides (fenugreek, fennel, coriander, mustard, caraway or chili seeds, or just peppercorns)

- something to act as a weight (see "Always submerge your ferments," right)

Which salt?

Himalayan rock salt is best. It's a very dry salt and contains no harmful molds (which can be found in some sea salt). Don't use bog-standard table salt— for anything!—as the iodine will kill the ferment.

WHAT TO KEEP IN MIND

Follow these tips to make your ferments fabulous.

Always submerge your ferments

Your vegs will ferment instead of rot *only* if they're fully covered in liquid—either brine or salt-released veggie juices. If you ever come up short, add some brine.

The best way to keep the vegetables from floating above the liquid is to cut a cabbage-leaf circle slightly larger than the mouth of the jar and fit it over the vegetables. Or use a small glass jar that fits snugly into the mouth of your jar, filled with water. Or a clean stone!

Temperature matters

Around 61–72°F is ideal and will ensure a nicely paced ferment. In colder climates, stick your ferment on top of the fridge and perhaps use a little whey. In warmer places, you'll just have to put up with a faster ferment that's not quite as tangy.

Always add spices and herbs

Chili, garlic, peppercorns, caraway, fenugreek, fennel, coriander and mustard seeds are chucked in for a reason—they act as mold inhibitors.

Keep the lid loose

This stops the jar from exploding. You might like to place a bowl underneath in case it does bubble over. I do.

Don't fret about mold

You might see a white furry film develop on the surface. It won't hurt you. Skim it off as soon as you see it.

CHOPPED SALAD PICKLE

MAKES A 1-QUART JAR

This is the simplest ferment doing the rounds. And so pretty to boot.

1 teaspoon spices or herbs (chili flakes, black or white peppercorns, bay leaf, dill seeds, fennel seeds, coriander seeds)

3 cups chopped vegetables (cauliflower, zucchini, beans, beet, carrot, radishes, bell peppers, turnip, broccoli, red onion, green onions)

2 cups water mixed with 1 tablespoon Himalayan pink salt

I use my pickle as I would gherkins—diced and added to mayo to make a tartar sauce, or to a salsa for an extra boost.

Place the spices or herbs in the base of your jar. Arrange the chopped veggies in lovely layers, leaving 1½ inches of room at the top. Pour in enough brine to cover, leaving 1¼ inches clear of the rim. Place a cabbage leaf or weight on top to submerge the veggies. Seal loosely (or cover with a cloth) and keep at room temperature for 2–7 days (the colder it is, the longer it will take). You'll need to try it after the second day. Once it tastes tart and the liquid is a bit fizzy, seal and transfer to the fridge, where it will keep for several months.

If you use bell peppers in your pickle, use 1 tablespoon of salt for every cup of water.

MAKE IT A CHARD STEM PICKLE:

Use 3 cups of chard or beet leaf stems sliced into ¾-inch pieces, 1 small sprig of dill or thyme and ½ teaspoon each of chili flakes, fennel seeds and coriander seeds and follow the recipe above.

Just a note: These stems can go mushy easily, so don't use whey. Also, try to make it during cooler periods and use 3 tablespoons of salt.

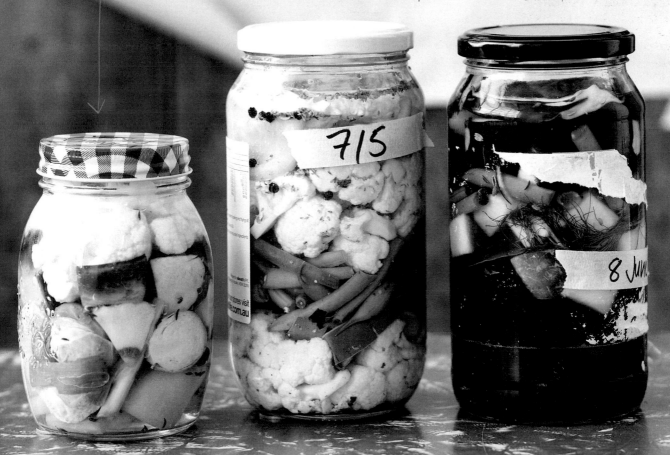

'BUCHA MUSTARD

MAKES 1 JAR

As little as 1 teaspoon of mustard seeds will provide a potent injection of antioxidants and anti-inflammatory helpers selenium and magnesium. So goes the research. Ferment the little things with life-giving kombucha and the ante is upped that little bit more.

½ cup whole mustard seeds (brown or yellow)

Plain Kombucha (page 344) or use store-bought

Fill a glass jar (preferably broad mouthed) with mustard seeds to about one-third full. Add enough kombucha to cover the seeds. Place the lid on loosely (or cover with a dishtowel) to allow air to release, and leave on the kitchen counter for 5–10 days (fewer days in summer). Check the seeds each day and add extra kombucha to ensure the seeds stay covered in a little liquid and remain moist. The seeds will swell and come to fill the jar—pretty fun to watch! Once they stop absorbing liquid, and you see bubbles forming, blend into a paste using an immersion blender (if you've used a broad-mouthed jar, you can do this in the jar).

MAKE IT GARLICKY:
Add a clove or two before pouring on the kombucha.

MAKE IT COOLING FOR PITTA TYPES:
Add some coriander seeds before pouring on the kombucha.

Brown or yellow mustard?
In Ayurvedic parlance, mustard seeds increase Pitta (fire) while minimizing Vata (air) and Kapha (earth and water). Brown mustard seeds are hotter and more pungent and potent. They are balancing for Kapha and Vata. Yellow seeds impart a milder Dijon flavor and are better for Pitta types (also see the "Make it cooling" variation).

Food Nerd Tip: Coconut oil turns from solid to liquid at 72°F. I use a jar of it to gauge my perfect ferment conditions!

SIMPLICIOUS SAUERKRAUT

MAKES 3–4 CUPS

In my previous books, I've shared a recipe that involves shredding and hammering and pushing and fussing a big ball of cabbage into submission. Since then I've gotten creative with my 'kraut. I'm rather happy with the far more elegant result.

Red cabbage makes a slightly sweeter and crunchier 'kraut.

1 small (or ½ large) white or red cabbage, cored, cut into wedges and rinsed

1 tablespoon caraway seeds

2 tablespoons Himalayan pink salt

Shred the cabbage in a food processor using the grater option (or use a hand grater . . . tedious!). Toss with the caraway seeds and salt in a big bowl and let it sit for 30 minutes. Spoon into a large jar (or several), pressing down as you go so the juices come to the top of the cabbage. Fill each jar, leaving 1¼ inches of room at the top. Place a weight on top (to help the juices rise), then seal loosely and keep at room temperature for 1–3 days. Transfer to the fridge, where it will keep for several months.

MAKE IT YOUR OWN FLAVOR:
Substitute the caraway seeds for mustard seeds, cumin seeds or white peppercorns.

MAKE IT A PINK SAUERKRAUT:
Replace half of the cabbage with 1–2 beets, scrubbed, and follow the recipe as above. (Oh, and use a red cabbage.)

Salt versus whey
Salt encourages the growth of local bacteria found on the vegetable itself, which is always best. It also slows and tempers the ferment process. Plus salt hardens the pectins in vegetables, giving them added crunch and a bitier flavor.

Whey produces a more rounded flavor in ferments than salt, but can also lead to slightly mushy vegetables, in part because it speeds up the ferment process.

I tend to use whey in winter, and in sauces, mayo and pesto. I use salt when the temperature is around 73°F or higher.

"BUT THE KITCHEN SINK" KIMCHI

MAKES ABOUT 8 CUPS

This is one of my favorite ferments. Mostly 'cos you can make huge quantities with minimal effort and then use it with gay abandon to boost casseroles and stews and toasties (see page 84). Feel free to choose your own veggies (though cabbage is a staple). Beans and okra also work well.

12 radishes or 1 small daikon

2 carrots (orange, yellow or purple)

1 green apple

1 onion or ½ bunch green onions, chopped

1 napa cabbage, coarsely chopped (or ½ red cabbage, shredded)

1 bunch bok choy or ½ bunch kale, stems removed (or ½ bunch dandelion greens), coarsely chopped

Or you can use brussels sprouts, quartered

2-inch knob of ginger or turmeric, minced

5 cloves garlic, minced

1–2 large red chilies, finely chopped or 1½ teaspoons chili flakes

2 tablespoons fish sauce or dulse flakes (or a couple of canned anchovies, chopped)

2 tablespoons Himalayan pink salt

Shred the radishes or daikon, carrots, apple and onion using a blender with a grater option (or use a grater) and place in a large glass or ceramic bowl. Add the remaining ingredients and, using your bare hands, massage and squeeze the mixture to release the juices. Cover with a dishtowel and let it sit overnight.

The next day scoop into a large jar (or two smaller ones), leaving 2 inches clear at the top. Try not to leave much more than this—more air means more chance of the ferment going moldy. And make sure the ingredients are completely submerged in liquid (if not, add a little water). Place a weight on top to submerge the veggies, put the lid on loosely and leave on the counter (ideally at 68–72°F) for 2–3 days, until it starts to fizz a little. Screw the lid on tight and store in the fridge for up to 3 months.

MY INDIAN KIMCHI

MAKES 4–6 CUPS

There are four reasons I wrap my turmeric-stained arms around this sweet-but-tangy mix-up of the Korean classic. Daikon boosts the digestive enzymes we need to break down fats, complex carbohydrates and proteins. It's also been shown to counteract the carcinogens in processed and fried foods, which is why it is traditionally served with tempura in Japan. Even better, when eaten with foods high in beta-carotene (um, like carrots!!) daikon improves the body's ability to absorb vitamin D. And, even betterer . . . When's the best time to make this little combo I've put together, you may ask? Funnily enough, at the end of summer, when carrots and daikon are at their peak . . . and just as we're heading into the darker months. Which is when our vitamin D levels drop. Oh, it's all such a beautiful thing!

FIVE WAYS TO USE KIMCHI:

1. Toss it through a Crisp Bibimbap Skillet Pancake (page 250).
2. Make a Kimcheese Toastie (page 84).
3. Make Kimchi Instant Noodles (page 116).
4. Add kick to an Abundance Bowl (pages 126–37).
5. Make Leftovers Kimchi Soup (page 264).

1¾–2 pounds carrots, peeled

1 daikon, peeled

2–3-inch knob of turmeric, peeled

2 large red chilies, finely chopped (or 3 teaspoons chili flakes)

2 teaspoons fenugreek seeds

2 teaspoons mustard seeds

2 tablespoons Himalayan pink salt (in summer) or 1 tablespoon salt and ¼ cup Homemade Whey (page 46; in winter)

I use salt to make kimchi because to get the best "fizzy" vibe, the ferment needs to be slowed down a little. Of course, if your house is cooler than, say, 68°F, feel free to prod things and use a bit of whey and less salt.

Grate the carrots, daikon and turmeric (use the grater attachment on your blender or food processor) and place in a glass or ceramic bowl. Add the rest of the ingredients. Mix and let sit for 20 minutes to allow the salt (and whey, if using) to release the juices. If it's not looking juicy enough, use a mallet or pestle to "massage" the veggies to release the juices.

Spoon into a large jar with a lid. Press down on the veggies so the juices rise up to cover them. Put a weight on top to submerge the veggies and put the lid on loosely. Allow to sit at room temperature for 3–5 days (1–2 weeks if you don't use whey) before sealing tightly and moving to the fridge, where it will last for up to 3 months.

½ SERVING VEG + FRUIT PER SERVING

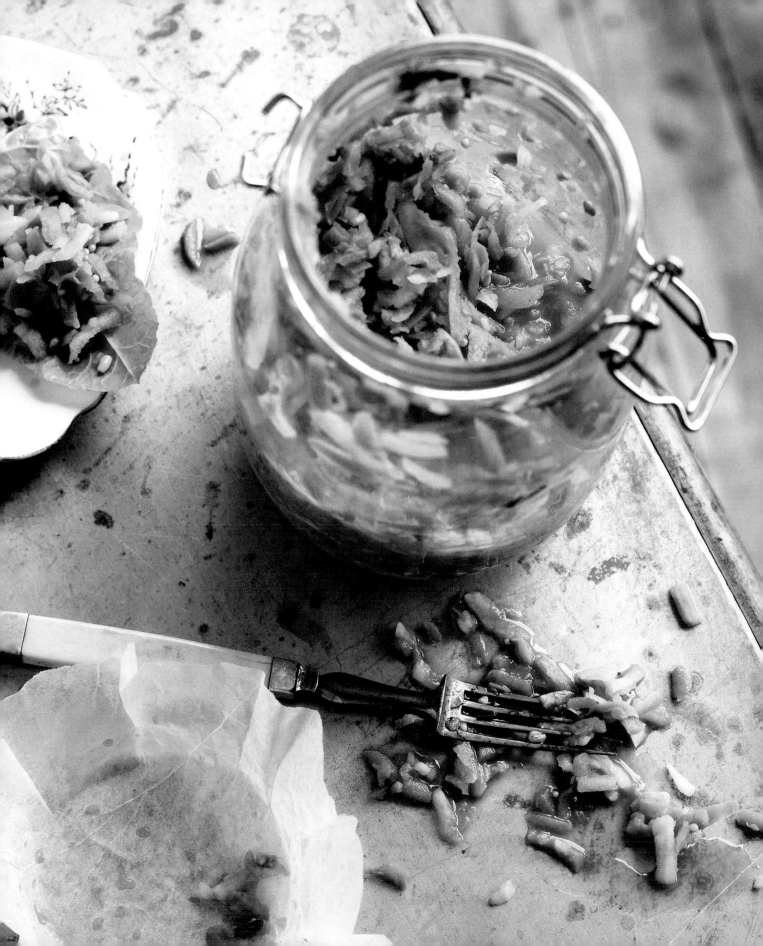

FIVE WAYS TO GET
A GOOD DOSE OF
TURMERIC PASTE:

1. Warming Golden Milk
   (page 81).

2. Golden Milkshake
   (page 81).

3. TMT Dressing (page 53).

4. My Gut-Healing Brew
   (page 87).

5. Thai Coconutty Cabbage
   (page 182).

FERMENTED TURMERIC PASTE

MAKES 1 CUP

Turmeric is an Ayurvedic staple, long known to have anti-inflammatory, antibacterial and antifungal properties. Its active ingredient, curcumin, is also a rich source of antioxidants and is said to have anti-platelet properties that help protect against strokes and heart attacks. However, curcumin is not easily absorbed by the body *unless* you eat it with fat (it's fat soluble) or black pepper (the piperine in pepper ramps up the absorption by 2,000%) or you ferment it. Herewith two recipes that ensure you get the full benefits from this amazing little root.

7 ounces fresh turmeric, peeled and roughly chopped

½ teaspoon organic freshly ground black pepper or cumin

¼–½ teaspoon sea salt

¼ cup Homemade Whey (page 46), plus extra to cover

Cumin also increases curcumin's bioavailability.

Be prepared to stain your blender doing this.

Blend the turmeric to a smooth paste in a high-powered blender (or use a mortar and pestle). Stir in the pepper or cumin, salt and whey. Press into a jar and top with a little more whey so the turmeric is completely submerged. Cover with a lid and place in a cool, dark place for about 5 days or so, adding extra whey if required. Seal and store in the fridge for up to 6 months.

If you prefer (I do), you can use the leftover fermented turmeric from my Lemon and Turmeric Tonic-Ade (page 347) to make your paste. Whatever works for you.

MAKE IT EASY TURMERIC PASTE:

If you can't find fresh turmeric, make this.

¼ cup ground turmeric

¾ teaspoon finely ground black pepper

Place the turmeric and pepper in a saucepan with ½ cup of water and bring to a boil over medium heat. Reduce the heat and simmer, stirring vigorously, until the mixture forms a thick paste (about 5–7 minutes). Allow to cool, then transfer to a sealable jar. This will keep in the fridge for 2 weeks.

GOOD FOR YOUR GUTS GARLIC

MAKES 4 CUPS

Garlic has amazing properties and is particularly good for fighting off infections in the digestive tract and lungs, but it can be rough on your guts when eaten raw. Relate much? Fermenting famously fixes most things, including this issue. Plus, if you hate peeling garlic, then doing up a bunch of heads in one fell swoop makes a lot of sense. Note my nifty peeling trick, below.

6–8 heads garlic

1 teaspoon Himalayan pink salt

1 tablespoon Homemade Whey (page 46) or 1 teaspoon salt

1 teaspoon dried oregano or basil (optional)

1 bay leaf (optional)

Preheat the oven to 200°F. Place the garlic heads on a baking sheet and bake for 1 hour, or until the cloves begin to pop out of their skins. (Some ovens may take longer, but don't be tempted to crank the temp!) Cool a little, then simply pop the cloves from their skins, being sure to leave the ends intact.

Place in a 1-quart preserving jar with the rest of the ingredients and top with water, leaving 1¼ inches clear at the top. Seal loosely and leave on the counter for 3–5 days (a little longer if you don't use whey). Then seal tightly and place in the fridge for 6 months. Best left for a couple of weeks before eating.

Be gentle with garlic
Avoid damaging the flesh of the garlic clove, especially the root end (don't cut it off). Any cuts will cause it to ferment unevenly and make the clove turn blue . . . which is nothing to be worried about; it's merely an amino acid reacting with the acid. All good. Just not pretty.

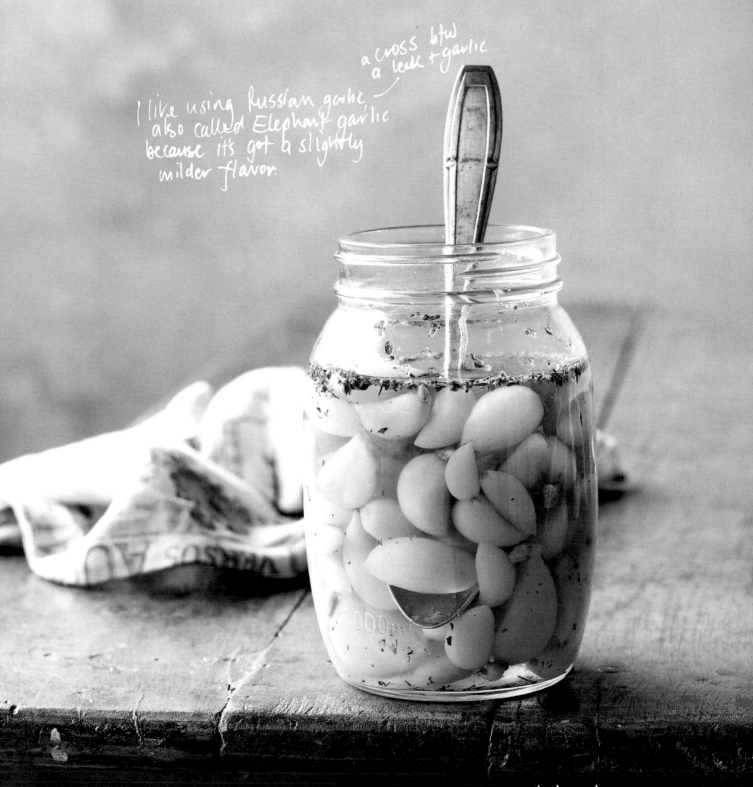

a cross btw
a leek + garlic

I like using Russian garlic,
also called Elephant garlic
because it's got a slightly
milder flavor.

P.S. As you eat your ferment, transfer
the remainder to a 'smaller' jar to
reduce oxygen + thus spoilage.

KOMBUCHA

A fizzy-drink addict? Loved a sugar-laced iced tea in your past life? Let me introduce you to The 'Bucha. You might have seen kombucha-crazed kids parodied about town and rolled your eyes with the masses. Fair enough. It's kind of boundary-pushing stuff. But I'll try to ground it for us.

Kombucha is a slightly fizzy, fermented "iced tea" made by adding a disgusting-looking creature called a SCOBY (short for "symbiotic culture of bacteria and yeast") or "mother" to a batch of brewed tea. This spongy, mushroomy thing activates and propels the drink (by eating sugar—yes, sugar!!) to become an "alive" gut-healing beverage. With bubbles. And tang. Oh goodness, I know . . . Please don't leave me yet.

The stuff is brimful of probiotics and is a standout for digestive health. I go on about it over at sarahwilson.com if you'd like to learn more. For now, know this much: countless studies have shown it can assist in the treatment of arthritis, depression, heartburn and candida. It's also great for liver detoxification, plus it improves pancreatic function and increases energy.

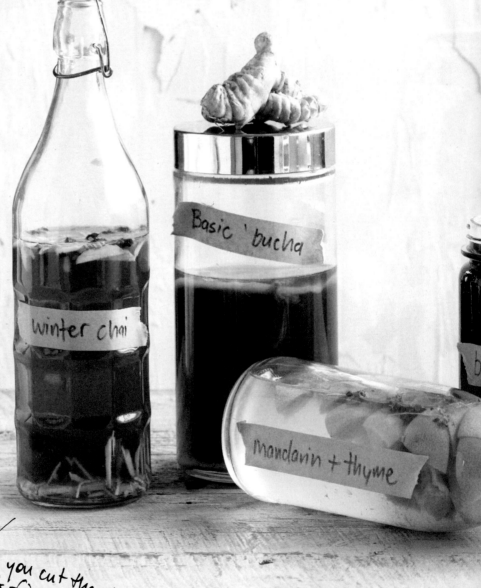

The sugar content of most fermented drinks here is about ½ tsp sugar for 100 ml of goodness.

Basic 'bucha

winter chai

mandarin + thyme

make sure you cut the ginger + other bits fine enough so they'll come back out.

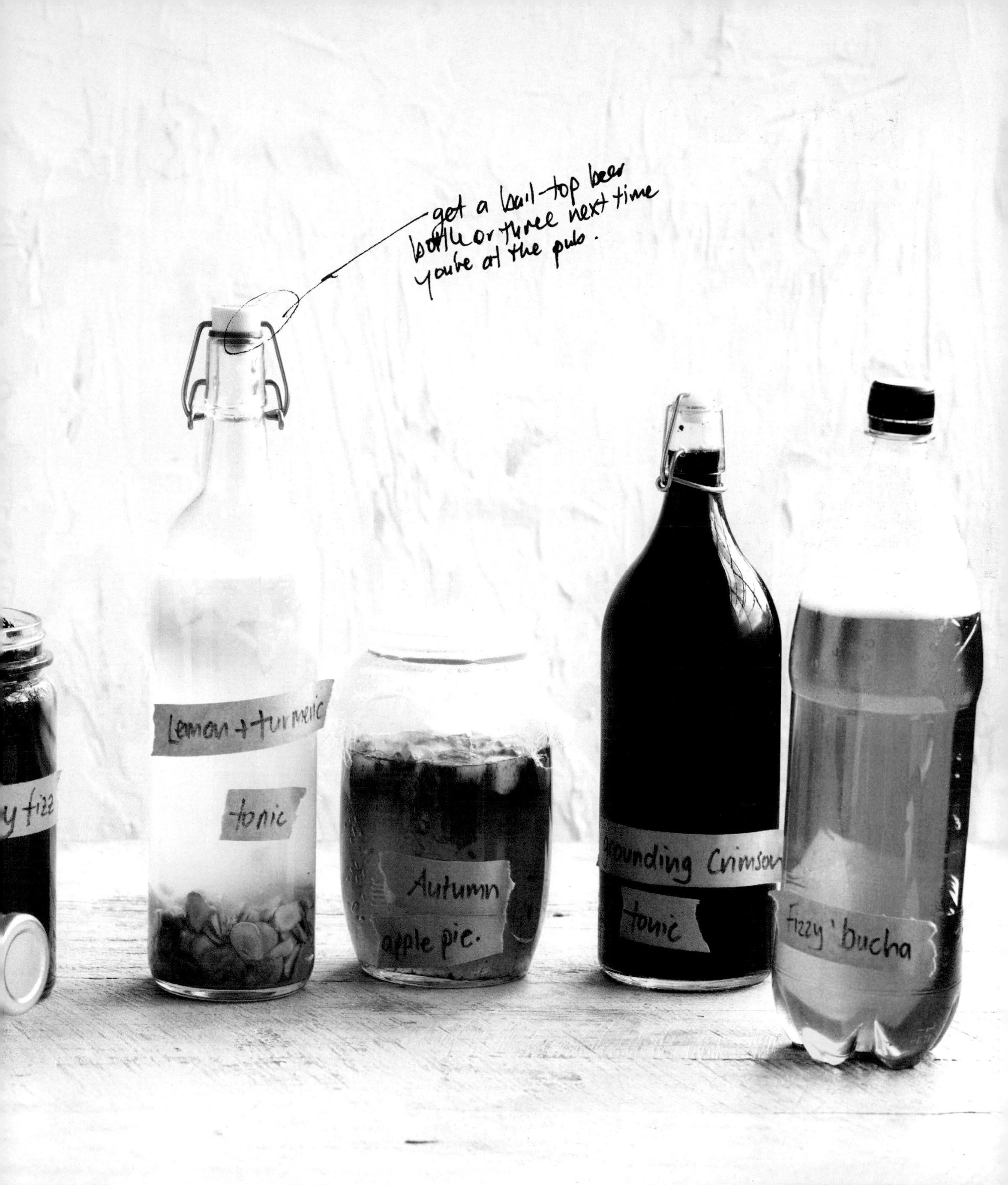

get a bail-top beer bottle or three next time you're at the pub.

y fizz

Lemon + turmeric

tonic

Autumn apple pie.

grounding Crimson

tonic

Fizzy 'bucha

Do you have to use sugar?

No. I'd read that honey doesn't work when making kombucha—the theory being that the honey's natural antibacterial agents kill the SCOBY. So I was a little concerned about using brown rice syrup instead of sugar. (Brown rice syrup is a fermented product and I pictured the different bacteria squabbling for attention in the bowl, eventually annihilating each other.) I chatted to various experts and Googled the bejesus out of the topic—no one had tried it. So I did. The result? Brown rice syrup maketh for a wonderful kombucha. You just have to leave it to ferment a day or two longer than its sugary cousin, and I think it does produce a slightly tarter brew. Which I kinda love.

Where does one obtain this SCOBY fellow?

This is the fun bit . . . You have to become part of a very cool witchy 'bucha community to get hold of one. SCOBYs can't be manufactured as such but are spawned from a "mother" when one makes a batch of brew. Regular kombucha makers are always happy to give away a baby SCOBY.

How do I drink the stuff?

Straight from the fridge. About 3½ ounces (one-third of a glass) a couple of times a day. First thing in the morning before breakfast is fab (I have some before heading off for exercise and it's beautifully energizing); so is after dinner as something of a digestive chaser. I like to team it with a dash of soda water for extra fizz.

Check out sarahwilson.com for details on finding one online.

PLAIN KOMBUCHA

MAKES ABOUT 3½ CUPS

a long-looking recipe. Don't be daunted!

¼ cup brown rice syrup, or sugar if you prefer

2 organic black tea bags (many say non-organic tea just doesn't work as well)

½ cup kombucha (from a previous batch or store-bought)

1 SCOBY

Sterilize a broad-mouthed glass or ceramic bowl or jug with boiling water. (It needs a wide opening to allow plenty of contact with oxygen.)

Combine the brown rice syrup or sugar in a saucepan with 1 quart of water and bring to a boil. Remove from the heat, add the tea bags, cover and allow to steep for 15 minutes. Remove the tea bags and pour the liquid into the sterilized container. Leave it to cool to around body temperature. Or cooler.

This is an important bit, okay? Hot tea will kill your mother!

Add the kombucha and then gently place the SCOBY on top (it may sink, but this is okay, says my friend Kate). Cover with a clean dishtowel or muslin and leave to sit for 7–10 days (a week will be plenty in warm weather and/or if you use sugar). The temperature needs to be around 75–86°F.

If it's cool where you live, stick the bowl on top of the fridge.

At the end of 7–10 days, a "baby" SCOBY will have formed on top of the "mother." Remove both SCOBYs, placing them in a glass container. Pour a little of the kombucha liquid onto the SCOBYs, then pour the rest into a 1-quart bail-top bottle (one with a hinged lid and rubber stopper), or a plastic soft-drink bottle, and refrigerate, ensuring you leave a ¾–1¼-inch space at the top.

You could use one to start a new batch and give the other to a friend.

MAKE IT FIZZIER:

Get a little more fizz going by adding a dash of extra brown rice syrup or a little chopped fruit and securing the lid. Leave the bottle out at room temperature for an additional 2–4 days. The live yeast and bacteria will continue to consume the residual sugar from both the first fermentation, plus the extra dash you've just added. In the absence of oxygen (now that the whole thing is lidded), carbon dioxide is produced (and trapped), thus building up the fizz. (If you like a 'bucha with fizz, you may wish to use sugar instead of brown rice syrup in the fermenting stage. It fizzes faster.)

WINTER CHAI KOMBUCHA

3 cups Plain Kombucha
(see opposite)

5 cloves or cardamom pods

1 cinnamon stick, broken up

1¼-inch knob of ginger or turmeric,
cut into matchsticks

1 star anise

Place all the ingredients in a large jar with a tight seal or a 1-quart bail-top bottle and let it sit at room temperature for 3–4 days. You can choose to strain the spices after 2 days and rebottle, though I don't as I prefer the mixture to become stronger with time.

**USE THE LEFTOVER
GINGER OR TURMERIC:**
Add it to smoothies.

AUTUMN APPLE PIE KOMBUCHA

3 cups Plain Kombucha
(see opposite)

½ apple, cored and chopped

½–1 teaspoon Pumpkin Spice Mix
(page 45)

Place all the ingredients in a large jar with a tight seal or a 1-quart bail-top bottle and let it sit at room temperature for 3–4 days. Strain the apple out after 2 days and rebottle, if you wish, or leave it in so that the flavors become stronger with time.

MAKE IT SQUASH PIE KOMBUCHA:
Add ¼ cup of Squash Purée (page 23) instead of the apple. Toss in a bit of grated ginger, too.

SPRING STRAWBERRY AND VANILLA KOMBUCHA

3 cups Plain Kombucha
(see opposite)

6–8 strawberries
(fresh or frozen)

Or use 2 leftover vanilla pods when you've used the seeds for something else.

1 vanilla pod, split, or ¼ teaspoon pure vanilla extract (or make your own; page 45)

Place all the ingredients in a large jar with a tight seal or a 1-quart bail-top bottle and let it sit at room temperature for 3–4 days. You can choose to strain the strawberries and vanilla pod out after 2 days and rebottle, if you like.

**USE THE LEFTOVER
FERMENTED STRAWBERRIES:**
Have them with yogurt for dessert or breakfast.

Discomfort or pain associated with intestinal gas may subside soon after eating 4–6 strawberries. I'm not exactly sure why this works, but it seems to give quick relief for some people.

SUMMER PEACH AND BASIL COLADA

3 cups Plain Kombucha
(see opposite)

1 large ripe peach, stone removed and chopped

5 basil leaves

Place all the ingredients in a large jar with a tight seal or a 1-quart bail-top bottle and let it sit at room temperature for 3–4 days. Strain out the peach and basil after 2 days and rebottle if you like, or if you prefer a stronger flavor, leave them in.

when done, use the fermented peach pieces in a smoothie or atop yogurt for dessert.

GUT-HAPPY TONICS

Fiddly, witchy kombucha making ain't for everyone. Forthwith, a bunch of super-simple probiotic drinks that cut out as much palaver as possible.

A few things to know about these tonic-y things

* Always make two batches back to back, re-using the remaining fruit and roots, adding another tablespoon of salt and leaving to ferment for the same period.
* Once you've done two batches, keep the fruits 'n' roots and eat them—they're lovely and activated!
* If it's winter, or if you're not keen on using so much salt, add 1–2 tablespoons of Homemade Whey (page 46) or some sauerkraut juice (see page 337) or some leftover tonic from a previous batch and halve the salt.
* To increase carbonation, decant the tonic into a wine bottle and cork it, or into a recycled plastic soft-drink bottle and cap tightly. Leave at room temperature until you can see a rim of bubbles at the top of the wine bottle or until the plastic bottle bulges from CO_2 pressure buildup.

HARDCORE FLU TONIC

MAKES 1 JAR

This stuff is seriously potent and will fix the worst kind of man flu (and lesser variants). I gargle 1–2 tablespoons straight and then swallow several times a day. Again, I've kept the amounts loose. We'll work to proportions on this one. (P.S.: Don't fret; you really can't get it wrong.)

EQUAL PARTS FRESH:

garlic, peeled

onion, peeled

chili (hot jalapeño is best)

ginger, unpeeled

turmeric, unpeeled

horseradish, peeled (optional)

PLUS:

apple cider vinegar

Place all of the ingredients except the vinegar in your blender and blend. Add a dash of apple cider vinegar (enough to form a pourable slurry). Transfer to a jar large enough to three-quarters fill. Add a little more apple cider vinegar to your blender and swirl to capture any remaining slurry. Pour into the jar, leaving a 1¼-inch space at the top. Seal and shake. Leave on the counter for 2–4 weeks, shaking daily (you might need to release the lid occasionally to prevent an explosion!). Strain into a bail-top bottle. Store in the fridge for 6 months (maybe even longer).

USE THE LEFTOVER FERMENTED VEGGIES AND SPICES:
These add umami flavor to a stew, soup or stir-fry.

GROUNDING CRIMSON TONIC

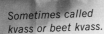
Sometimes called kvass or beet kvass.

MAKES ABOUT 1 QUART

¾ cup coarsely chopped beets

¼ cup chopped turmeric

1 tablespoon salt

Place all the ingredients in a 1-quart jar with a lid. Top with water, stopping ¾ inch from the rim. Screw on the lid and leave on your kitchen counter, shaking a few times a day, for 2–6 days, depending on the season (winter requires longer fermentation). Keep an eye on the bubbles. Once they start to appear, open the jar to release some of the CO_2 and have a taste. Strain, leaving the beets and turmeric in the jar along with enough liquid to cover them. Pour the rest of the tonic into a bail-top bottle and store in the fridge for up to 1 week.

USE THE LEFTOVER BEETS:
Add it to Abundance Bowls (pages 126–37) or mix it with yogurt, with a sprinkle of apple cider vinegar or ground cumin as a side at dinner.

USE THE LEFTOVER TURMERIC:
Purée and keep in a jar in the fridge for up to 2 months and use in place of minced turmeric.

LEMON AND TURMERIC TONIC-ADE

MAKES ABOUT 1 QUART

½ cup sliced turmeric or ginger, unpeeled

½ cup sliced lemon or lime, unpeeled

1 tablespoon brown rice syrup or sugar

1 tablespoon salt

Place all the ingredients in a 1-quart jar with a tight-fitting lid. Top with water, stopping ¾ inch from the rim. Screw on the lid and leave on your kitchen counter for 2–6 days, shaking a few times a day. How long you leave it will depend on the season (winter requires longer fermentation). Keep an eye on the bubbles. Once they start to appear, open the top to release some of the CO_2 and have a taste. (I brew mine a little longer than most—I like a tarty, less sugary flavor.) Strain into a 1-quart bail-top bottle and store in the fridge for up to 1 week.

USE THE LEFTOVER LEMON OR LIME:
Keep it in a clean jar in the fridge for 2 months and use with Sweet Persian Tagine (page 224) or in any recipe calling for lemon or lime zest.

APPLE AND BLACKBERRY CARDAMOM FIZZ

MAKES ABOUT 1 QUART

½ cup sliced apple, unpeeled

½ cup pitted cherries or blackberries

1 tablespoon brown rice syrup or sugar

½ teaspoon ground cardamom

½ teaspoon ground cinnamon

Place all the ingredients in a 1-quart jar with a lid. Top with water, stopping ¾ inch from the rim. Screw on the lid and leave on your kitchen counter, shaking a few times a day, for 2–6 days, depending on the season (winter requires longer fermentation). Keep an eye on the bubbles. Once they start to appear, open the jar to release some of the CO_2 and have a taste. Strain into a bail-top bottle and store in the fridge for up to 1 week.

MAKE IT A MANDARIN AND THYME FIZZ:
Use 1 cup of chopped mandarin oranges (seeds removed, peel left on) and a few sprigs of thyme.

GUT-GIVING GUMMIES

Gelatin, a collagen powder made from the bones, hides and connective tissues of animals, is the gift our tired guts have been waiting for. This might be enough for you to give gelatin a go. If so, skip to my gummy recipes. If not, read on for the finer claims made of the stuff.

How to buy and eat gelatin

* Only get stuff made from pasture-fed cows. This is non-negotiable when you're eating the very gelatinous fiber of their being.
* The best stuff comes as a powder (as opposed to sheets and envelopes). 1 envelope granulated gelatin = 1 tablespoon powdered gelatin = 3 sheets of leaf gelatin.
* Start with ½–1 tablespoon per day and slowly increase to about 2–3 tablespoons a day.
* Since gelatin is a protein, it's important to eat it with fats to stimulate strong digestive juices and allow the body the fuel to use the protein properly.
* Get gelatin made from complete collagen, not collagen hydrolysate, to make these gummies.
* You can purchase bone gelatin via the The Kit (see page 5).

Gummies for insomnia? Eat one gummy before bed.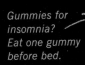

What you need to know about gelatin:

* It helps heal our tired gut linings by boosting acid production and restoring the mucosal lining.
* It reduces heartburn, ulcers and acid reflux by binding gut acids with the foods.
* It balances out meat intake. Muscle meats contain elevated levels of certain amino acids that can be inflammatory over time (you know those headlines about red meat being harmful?). Gelatin contains two anti-inflammatory amino acids, thus balancing, completing and complementing the other meat sources. This is particularly important for autoimmune sufferers.
* It helps your liver do its detox thing. Gelatin provides the amino acid glycine, which assists the liver in ridding toxins from your body.
* It boosts metabolism and can be used for weight loss.
* It's great for injury. It not only reduces inflammation, which can trigger pain receptors and cause stiffness in the joints, but it can also help repair small tears in the cartilage.
* And it helps with insomnia. Research has shown that taking glycine just before bed can actually enhance sleep quality, reduce daytime sleepiness and even improve memory.

Gummies for weight loss?

I don't advocate weight-loss obsessing, but if you're trying to curb late-night eating try this: stop eating at least 3 hours prior to bedtime and consume at least 1 tablespoon of gelatin powder right before bed.

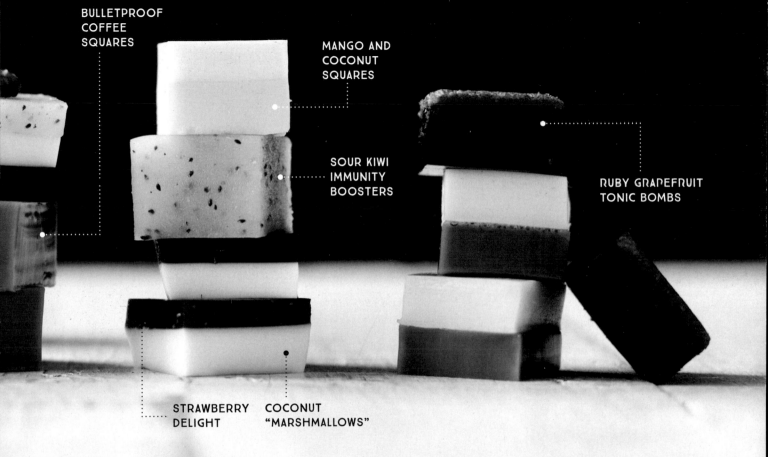

BULLETPROOF COFFEE SQUARES

MANGO AND COCONUT SQUARES

SOUR KIWI IMMUNITY BOOSTERS

RUBY GRAPEFRUIT TONIC BOMBS

STRAWBERRY DELIGHT

COCONUT "MARSHMALLOWS"

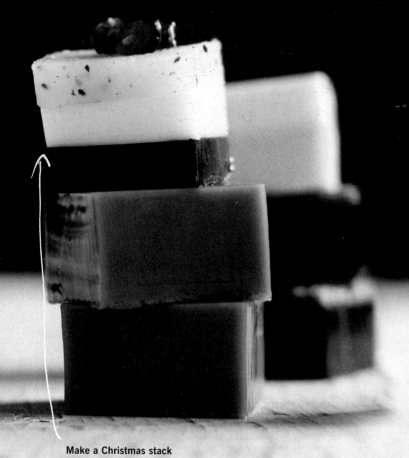

BASIC GELATIN GUMMIES

MAKE ABOUT 15

Use this basic recipe to make
the delights that follow.

3½ tablespoons gelatin powder

1½ cups chopped fruit or 1–1½ cups liquid

½ tablespoon brown rice syrup or 2 drops
liquid stevia (optional)

"Bloom" the gelatin by stirring it into
⅓ cup of cold water until dissolved. Let
it sit for 5 minutes; it will expand and
become "rubbery."

Heat the fruit or liquid and sweetener (and
any spices or essences) in a small saucepan
until it's almost boiling and the fruit has
softened. Turn off the heat and add the
bloomed gelatin (break the large blob into
little blobby bits) and stir until dissolved,
then use an immersion blender to purée.
Pour into molds or a 4 × 6-inch glass
dish (or similarly sized plastic one—I use
a lunchbox). Cool a little then place in the
fridge to set for 1 hour. Cut into rectangular
blocks. Store in the fridge in an airtight
container for up to 1 week.

 LESS THAN ¼ TEASPOON ADDED SUGAR PER SERVING

Make a Christmas stack

Make one portion of Strawberry
Delight (see opposite) and pour into
a slightly deeper dish. Allow to set for
1 hour, then add a layer of Coconut
"Marshmallows" (opposite) and a layer
of Sour Kiwi Immunity Booster (right),
allowing each layer to set. Top with
some pomegranate seeds to make
them special.

SOUR KIWI IMMUNITY BOOSTERS

In my obsessed reading on the
subject, I came across gelatin
devotees who think the acid in
kiwi stops the gelatin from goobing
correctly. I beg to differ. These
things wobbled out a treat.

½ cup lemon juice

4 ripe kiwi fruit, peeled and chopped

1½ tablespoons vitamin C powder (optional;
added after the gelatin has been mixed in
and the liquid has cooled a little)

*Note: You'll need to use sweetener for
this one . . . it's rather tarty. Also, feel
free to use 4 tablespoons of gelatin.*

COCONUT "MARSHMALLOWS"

9-ounce can coconut milk

½ cup cream

½ teaspoon pure vanilla extract
(or make your own; page 45)

pinch of sea salt

BULLETPROOF COFFEE SQUARES

½ cup black coffee

½ cup almond milk

¼ teaspoon pure vanilla extract
(or make your own; page 45)

MAKE IT A BUBBLE TEA:
Add bulletproof coffee squares
to a glass of cold milk.

STRAWBERRY DELIGHT

1 cup strawberries

1 teaspoon rose water

Add the rose water to the gelatin.

MANGO AND COCONUT SQUARES

½ cup chopped mango
(about ½ mango)

½ cup coconut cream or milk

juice of 1 lime

¼ teaspoon pure vanilla extract
(or make your own; page 45)

big pinch of cardamom powder

You're a vegan or veggo?
The best option would be to
use agar, derived from a
seaweed, although it doesn't
create the same "creamy"
texture, nor does it possess the
same gut-giving gifts. It sets
more firmly than gelatin, so
you'll only need 1¼ tablespoons
of agar powder (though this
varies between brands).
Although, bearer of bad news
and all, if you take any kind
of vitamin capsule or eat
commercial gummy bears or
snake lollies, um, you're eating
beef gelatin, albeit inferior stuff.

GREEN JUICE DETOX JELLIES

1½ cups green smoothie
of your choice

2 scoops of green supplement powder
(optional)

If using the green powder, add after
the gelatin has been mixed in, once
the liquid has cooled a little.

PROBIOTIC BERRIES 'N' CREAM CHEWS

½ cup frozen blueberries,
strawberries or raspberries

½ cup coconut cream

3 probiotic capsules (optional)

If using probiotic capsules, add them
after the gelatin has been mixed in,
once the liquid has cooled a little.

RUBY GRAPEFRUIT TONIC BOMBS

1 ruby grapefruit or 2 blood oranges,
peeled, pith and pips removed, chopped

½ cup Grounding Crimson Tonic
(page 347)

Add the tonic after the gelatin has
been mixed in, once the liquid has
cooled a little.

VANILLA PEACH KOMBUCHA GUMS

3 peaches, peeled (if you want,
I don't) and chopped

½ cup kombucha

¼ teaspoon pure vanilla extract
(or make your own; page 45)

Add the kombucha after the gelatin
has been mixed in, once the liquid
has cooled a little.

SPROUTS
IN A JAR

This recipe pares the sprouting caper back to basics—
no fancy sprouting kits required.

The deal with sprouts

Unsprouted beans, grains, nuts and seeds (BGNSs) contain enzyme inhibitors that prevent them from growing until the conditions are just right for germination. These anti-nutrients hinder our own enzymes from digesting them, blocking our ability to absorb their goodness. BGNSs also contain phytic acid (mostly in the bran) to deter bugs from munching them. Problem is that this acid binds to minerals, making them unavailable for absorption in our intestines.

But! Soaking and sprouting deactivates the bothersome acids and inhibitors, making the BGNSs far more digestible and absorbable, saving (indeed, boosting) our bodies' enzymes for other things. They turn the little buggers into living things, making a bunch of vitamins and minerals in the process.

The depletion of our bodies' enzymes is, in fact, the aging process. So . . . eating sprouts slows down the aging process!

2–4 tablespoons raw legumes, seeds and/or nuts of your choice

dash of apple cider vinegar or lemon juice

Place the legumes, seeds or nuts and apple cider vinegar or lemon juice in a large wide-mouthed jar and cover with water. Place a piece of muslin, cheesecloth or nylon cloth over the mouth and secure it with a rubber band. Leave to soak for 12 hours or overnight.

In the morning, drain (pouring the water through the cloth). Rinse and drain again (your cloth is still on!) and then leave the jar inverted at an angle out of direct sunlight—on your dish rack is a great idea. Repeat this rinse and drain business twice a day for the next day or three until your sprouts have tails.

Ensure your beloved sprouts are completely drained after the final rinse and store in an airtight container in the fridge for several days.

Keep your sprouts spritely by rinsing and draining as often as possible.

MAKE IT A MIXED BAG:

Combine a number of legumes in one jar, ensuring you use legumes that take the same amount of time to sprout. Lentils, mung beans and chickpeas are a good combo.

MAKE IT HEALTHIER:

Do the final drain in a sunlit position to allow the chlorophyll and carotenes to develop.

MAKE IT LAST LONGER:

Remove the mold-attracting hulls before the final rinse (dump in a bowl and cover in water so the hulls rise to the surface), and drain. Rinsing them daily once you've refrigerated them will also help them last up to 1 week.

FIVE WAYS TO USE YOUR SPROUTS:

1. Sprinkle on top of or mix into a salad.
2. Blend into a smoothie or shake (mung bean sprouts are great for this).
3. Add to a stir-fry just before serving.
4. Make **Indian Sprouts Raita**: Mix 1 cup of sprouts with 1 cup of full-fat organic plain yogurt, a handful of chopped mint and 1 teaspoon ground cumin. Chill for 1 hour. Done.
5. Add sprouts that are "turning" to soups and stews in the final 5 minutes of cooking.

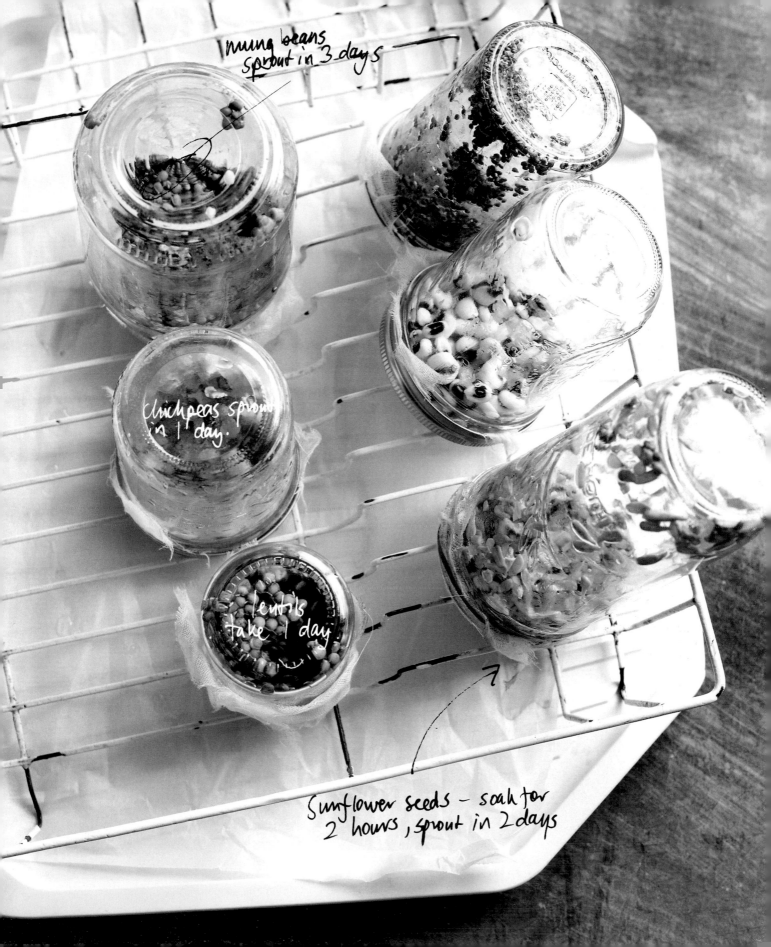

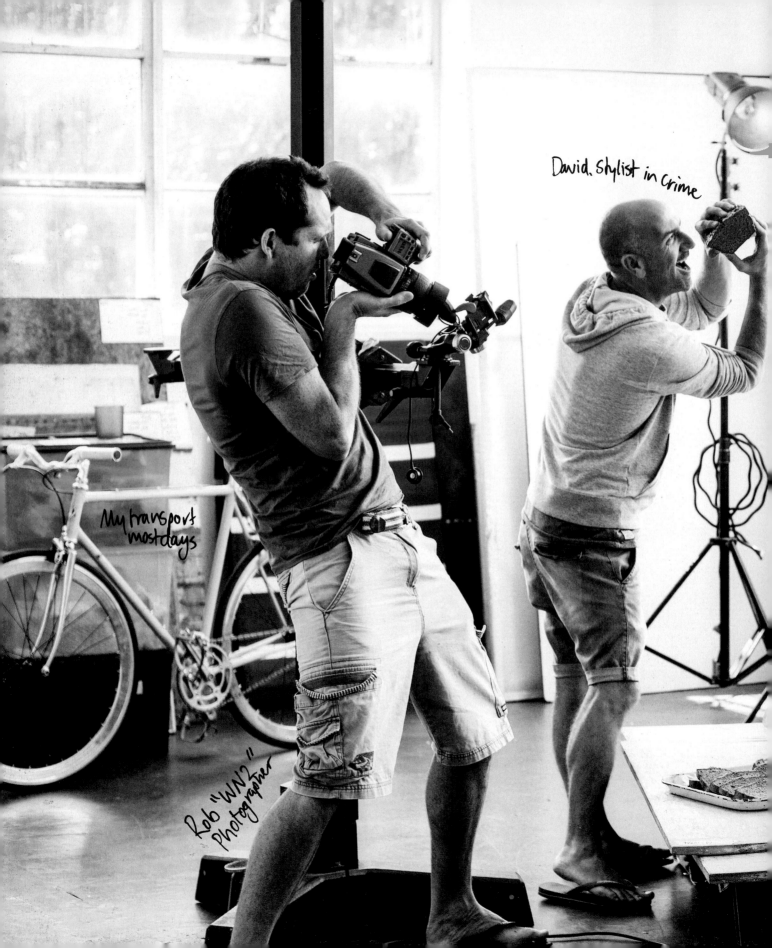

David, Stylist in crime

My transport mostdays

Rob "WN2" Photographer

Q **Gosh, am I eating too much sugar?**

A Not sure. This is how you work it out:

1. Look at the sugar content in the "per serving" column on your label (not the "per 100 g" column).

2. Divide that quantity (it's in grams) by 4 (1 teaspoon is about 4 g of sugar) to get the rough number of teaspoons.

3. For dairy products, remember to subtract the first 4.7 g per 100 g (which is lactose). For example, if the serving size is 50 g, 2.3 g is lactose.

4. Double or triple the serving amount if you tend to eat more, as I do. Be realistic!

Q **What sweetener do you use, then?**

A **Stevia:** a natural sweetener derived from the leaves of the *Stevia rebaudiana* plant. It's 300–450 times sweeter than sugar. I use it in liquid form (you can also get it granulated or powdered).

Brown rice syrup: a natural sweetener made from fermented, cooked rice and a blend of complex carbohydrates, maltose and glucose. It is relatively slow releasing so does not dump on the liver as much as pure glucose.

Q **So I can eat as much of the "safe" sweetener as I want, then?**

A Nope. To live sugar-free successfully I suggest minimizing all sweeteners. The science now shows that even brown rice syrup, stevia and artificial sweeteners can cause blood-sugar spikes and mess with the reward center in our brains—continuing the sugar addiction.

Q **What about artificial sweeteners?**

A Studies have shown that artificial sweeteners are correlated with a host of health complications. The body ingests sugar alcohols like sorbitol and isomalt poorly. Instead they end up in our bloodstream and feed the bacteria in our large intestine. Studies have also shown that artificial sweeteners can cause weight gain, contribute to diabetes, lead to cancer and muck up our gut microbiome.

Q **What about honey; it's natural, surely!?**

A Sugarcane could equally be described as natural. Regardless, our bodies don't really care where the fructose comes from.

Dates: 30% fructose (total sugar content 60%)
Honey and maple syrup: 40% fructose
Agave: 70–90% fructose
Coconut sugar/nectar/syrup: 38–49% fructose

Be aware: I try to reference studies that are as close to "gold standard" as possible. However, nutritional science is rarely "gold," being frequently conducted on rats (not humans), and neither controlled nor randomized.

Hopefully the above rant will set the pesky doubters straight. You're welcome!

AYURVEDA 101

A traditional Indian healing system, Ayurveda is more than 5,000 years old. It gave us yoga and meditation, and Buddhism stemmed from it 3,000 years ago. Ayurveda says we're made up of three doshas (energy types)—Vata, Pitta and Kapha. Each of us is a combination of all three doshas, but we generally have one that dominates. When our dominant dosha is out of balance, we get wobbly and unwell.

Vata types are lanky, flighty and easily excited, and they hate the cold. Their dominant force is wind, so they do not like sitting idle, preferring to seek constant action. When out of balance, Vatas often experience problems with digestion and malabsorption, get anxious and distracted, and suffer insomnia.

For Vatas to stay in balance, they need warm, "sweet," mushy foods to bring them back down to earth—stews, soups, sweet potato and spices such as cinnamon, ginger and cardamom. And to slooooow down.

Vatas love sugar! It provides temporary stimulation, but adds to the flightiness. Not good.

Pitta types have a medium but strong build and possess great concentration, but they can also be angry and judgmental. Their force is fire, so when out of balance, Pittas can get "hot under the collar." They don't tolerate summer well.

For Pittas to stay in balance, they need cooling foods, such as salads. They should avoid chilies and hot spices.

Pittas love a greasy burger. Pitta peeps tend to go for alcohol, meat and fatty, salty, sour or spicy foods, which make them more intensely driven. Not good.

Kapha types have a "thick" frame, oily skin, strong teeth and thick hair. They also have a slow metabolism and pace. Kaphas are earthy types (their force is earth and water) and when out of whack they can become heavy and phlegmatic and require firing up.

For Kaphas to stay in balance, they need stimulating spices, such as pepper, chili and cumin and aerobic exercise.

Kaphas love doughnuts and meat pies. They search out sugary, salty, dairy-based or fatty foods, which reinforce their natural lethargy. Not good.

Whatever your dosha, balancing Vata is key.

This is because when our Vata gets overstimulated, it can throw all our doshas out of whack. And so the recipes in this book mostly work to pacify Vata energy. Thus:

- Warming, slow-cooked foods "sweetened" with cinnamon, ginger and cardamom are great.

- Fewer ingredients are best (simplicious!). Lots of flavors are hard to assimilate. When a recipe requires a big bunch of different ingredients, we cook them for a while as a one-pot meal so they have time to "get to know each other."

- Foods high in nutrients can also be tough to digest, so simple combinations of these are best.

- For more, head to The Kit (see page 5).

FYI: I'm a vata-pitta, with a fair bit of deranged vata going on! :-)

VERY FREQUENTLY ASKED QUESTIONS ALL IN ONE SPOT

NB: I count ½ banana and ½ mango (and other high-fructose, often tropical, fruits) as 1 serving.

Q CAN I DRINK ALCOHOL WHEN I QUIT SUGAR?

A Yup. Sort of.

Wine: Contains minimal fructose. How so? It's the fructose in the grapes that ferments to become alcohol, leaving red wine low in sugar. It can contain very low levels of residual sugar—less than ¼ teaspoon per liter in the case of dry reds. White wine contains more residual sugar and should be avoided.

Sparkling wine (champagne): Bubbles retain quite a lot of the sugar (fructose). Avoid.

Spirits: Dry spirits like gin, vodka and whiskey contain little or no fructose.

Beer: Doesn't contain fructose. The sugar in beer and stout is maltose, which we can metabolize fine.

Dessert wine: A stack of sugar remains unfermented. Don't touch the stuff.

Q CAN I EAT CHOCOLATE?

A Well, yes. But it depends what kind.

Homemade chocolate: If you make it with raw cacao powder, which is less than 1% sugar, and coconut oil (and perhaps a little brown rice syrup) it is fructose-free. Great! This is how I eat my chocolate.

Store-bought plain chocolate: The majority is made with cocoa (the refined version of cacao containing fewer nutrients) that comprises less than 50% of the ingredients (the other 50% is largely sugar). It also often contains bad oils and additives (look for versions that use cacao butter, not vegetable oil). However, there are now varieties with 85% cocoa. This means that a 3½-ounce block will contain ½ ounce or 3½ teaspoons of sugar. And if you eat just a couple of squares (say, ¾ ounce) it equates to about ¾ teaspoon of sugar—not that much.

Q CAN I EAT FRUIT?

A Yes, please do.

Fruit can contain a fair whack of sugar—up to 3 teaspoons apiece. So I advise keeping to 1–2 servings a day, steering your way to low-fructose fruits like kiwi fruit, blueberries, raspberries and honeydew melon, and never eating grapes (unless you can stick to just a few at a time). On my 8-Week Program I advise cutting out fruit from Week 2 to Week 6 so that your body can properly recalibrate and your taste buds can regroup.

Q SHOULD I QUIT CARBS WHEN I QUIT SUGAR?

A I wouldn't. Do one thing at a time.

Quitting sugar is a big undertaking and one that will require your focus and willpower. Once you have mastered quitting sugar and if you feel a desire to do so, try cutting carbs for about 4–6 weeks and see if it suits YOUR body. Don't get caught up in what everyone else is doing. Experiment and learn for yourself—it's the only way to truly know if something works for you.

TEN DAYS OF DINNER FOR FOUR
(REQUIRING ONLY THREE COOK-UPS!)

head to The Kit for the full shopping list. (see page 5)

Here's how to use cook-ups to extend things further. Feel free to draw up your own version on your own fridge planner, inserting other bulk cook-ups and secondary dishes.

P.S. I've designed this to allow for flexibility – you can use leftover cooked veggies and meat, or meat and veggie scraps. As you clear the fridge out, you can make a quick trip to grab a head of broccoli or a bag of beans. It's the ultimate perpetual meal!

SUNDAY: Chicken Pot-au-Feu (page 214). *Reserve the leftover veggies, chicken and stock.*

1

MONDAY: The Fish That Got Away Pie (page 261) made with chicken and veggies from last night. *While the oven is on, feel free to roast some more veggies at the same time (see page 23) to use later in the week.*

just crank the temp to 400°F once your pie is out.

2

TUESDAY: Sweet Potato, Miso and Sage Soup (page 244) with Poached Egg Floaters (page 245) made with Sunday's chicken stock.

3

WEDNESDAY: The Cheapest Stew Ever (page 212) made with brisket in a slow cooker and served as a veggie soup with a few beef cubes on top. *Reserve most of the beef and 2 cups of stock.*

4

THURSDAY: Last Night's Dinner with an Egg Stuck in It (page 256) made with leftover roasted veggies from Monday and some of the brisket from Wednesday. Serve with steamed greens and peas and any leftovers from the previous week.

5

FRIDAY: Fridge-Door Tonnato (page 254) made with the remaining leftover brisket from Wednesday and an egg or two. *Boil up the whole dozen eggs while you're at it.*

6

SATURDAY: Jerk Pork Shoulder Roast (page 222) made in the oven. *Roast some extra roots at the same time (see page 23).*

7

SUNDAY: Baked Stuffing Loaf (page 305) made with last night's roast veg and served with steamed greens or green salad.

8

MONDAY: "Pizza" Bread-and-Butter Crumble (page 262), made with leftover Pulled Pork from Saturday, and greens. Throw in a spare boiled egg or three.

9

TUESDAY: Vegan Whatchagot Quiche (page 260) made with whatever veggies you have left, or Green Scraps Shakshouka (page 248) if you also have some uncooked eggs that need to be used.

Now, repeat . . .

10

A MINDFUL LEFTOVERS INDEX

By leftovers I'm referring not only to the peels, stalks, cores, scraps, bones, skin and pan juices left behind after cooking, but also the veggies at the bottom of the crisper that you bought up and forgot about – or indeed any ingredient that you need to use up to avoid waste.

A

apple
| Blaukraut | 182 |
| Green Apple Pie Smoothie Bowl | 72 |

asparagus ends
Add to your veggie stock bag 43
Leftovers Pesto 55

asparagus
Add to Abundance Bowls 126–37
Spring Socca Pizza 106

avocado
Green Minx Dressing	54
Green Spaghetti and Meatballs	145
Margarita Popsticks	326
Misomite	54
The BLAT	75

B

bacon
Bacon 'n' Egg Oatmeal	66
Bacon Granola	108
Blaukraut	182
The BLAT	75
Zucchini No-Carbonara	188

bacon fat
Use to roast potatoes and root vegetables, to fry eggs, sauté onions or greens, or as a spread.

bacon rind
Add to your stock bag.

banana
Slice, freeze and add to smoothies and smoothie bowls.
Not Quite Banana Bread 69

beans, green
| Bloke Beef 'n' Beer with Mash | 206 |
| Persian Lamb Salad | 221 |

beet leaves
Leftovers Pesto	55
Massaged Beet Greens	23
Green Scraps Shakshouka	248

beets
Beet, Beet Leaf 'n' Apple Borscht	244
Beet That Popstick Salad	191
Pink Sauerkraut	337
Pretty in Pastel Pink Parsnip Pasta	137

| Red Velvet Crunch Bowl | 72 |
| Warming Berry and Beet Smoothie | 80 |

berries
Blueberry Banana Bread	69
Buttered Blueberry and Blood Orange Soup	285
Warming Berry and Beet Smoothie	80

bones, carcasses
Homemade Stock 42–43

bread
Make breadcrumbs: Dry, process and mix into meatballs, or toast crumbs then use as a topping for pasta or gratins, as a coating for pan-fried cutlets or as a thickener for blended soups.

broccoli
Asian Cashew Crisp	184
Broc Bites	92
Crunchy Broccoli Buckwheat Tabbouli	187
Lebanese Roll Pizza	186
The Whole Brassicus Hummus	187
Zesty Caper Crunch	185

broccoli stems/stalks
| Leftovers Pesto | 55 |
| Sweet Paprika Stem Chips | 260 |

brussels sprouts
Brussels Sprout, Haloumi and Sauerkraut Sliders	120
Shaved Sprouts and Pecorino Salad	305
Stuffing 'n' All the Best Bits Salad	308

buckwheat
Bacon 'n' Egg Oatmeal	66
Crunchy Broccoli Buckwheat Tabbouli	187
Mushroom, Thyme and Hazelnut Oatmeal	64
My Allergy-Free Bread	113
Sprouted Cacao Pops	76

C

cabbage, red
Blaukraut	182
Greek San Choi Bau	146
Pickled Festive Red Slaw with Caramelized Ruby Grapefruit	309
Pink Sauerkraut (*use fresh cabbage only*)	337

cabbage
"But the Kitchen Sink" Kimchi	337
Okonomiyaki in a Tray	183
Shortcut Choucroute	258

| Simplicious Sauerkraut (*use fresh cabbage only*) | 337 |
| Thai Coconutty Cabbage | 182 |

carrot tops
Make a seaweed-style salad: Blanch once or twice, then toss in sesame oil and soy sauce.
Use small sprigs as a garnish.

carrots
Make orange "mayo": Cook, cool and blend carrots with macadamia oil, a little garlic and a hard-boiled egg.
Carrot "Bacon"	115
Easy Slaw	200
My Indian Kimchi	338
Nomato Sauce	51

cauliflower
Cauli Popcorn	100
Cauliflower Tartines with Green Goddess Dressing and Hazelnuts	184
Israeli Whole Baked Cauliflower	316
Moroccan Cauliflower, Chickpea and Quinoa Bake	238
SuperFoodie Lasagna Cake	140
Vegan "Ground Meat"	186
Vegan Watchagot Quiche	260

cauliflower stalks
| Leftovers Pesto | 55 |
| Sweet Paprika Stem Chips | 260 |

celeriac
Swedish Meatballs 145

celery
Add to stock bag and regrow the base. 33
| A Salad of Crushed Olives | 170 |
| Braised Celery with Leeks and Vanilla | 170 |

celery leaves
Add to your stock bag; use as a garnish for salads, Abundance Bowls etc.
| Celery Leaf Salt | 265 |
| Leftovers Pesto | 55 |

chard
Any Green Saag Paneer	177
A Super-Greens Couch Fondue	118
Super-Foodie Lasagna Cake	140
The Cheapest Stew Ever	212
Vata Balancing Bowl	133
Watercress "Colcannon"	178

chicken skin
Chicken Crackle Salt 204

chicken mince
Basic Meatballs 144

| Roast Chicken "Meffins" | 98 |

chickpeas
Moroccan Cauliflower, Chickpea and Quinoa Bake	238
Simplicious Sprouts in a Jar	352
Sweet Persian Tagine	224
The Whole Brassicus Hummus	187

coriander stems
Chop finely and use as you would the leaves.

cucumber
| Summer Probiotic Beet Soup | 244 |
| The Real Greek Yogurt | 74 |

E

eggplant
| Middle Eastern Eggplant | 148 |
| Baking-Sheet-Dinner-for-Two Eggplant Parmigiana | 228 |

eggs
| Not Quite Banana Bread | 69 |
| Okonomiyaki in a Tray | 183 |

eggs, boiled
Add to Leftover Mishmashes or Abundance Bowls.
Bacon 'n' Egg Oatmeal	66
Hipster Grandaddy Salad	176
Pink Devilish Googie Eggs	253
The Fish That Got Away Pie	261
Watercress Sauce and Some Eggs	176

eggs, poached
"But the Kitchen Sink" Breakfast Hash	82
Green Scraps Shakshouka	248
Poached Egg Floater	245

egg whites
Cacao Cayenne Pecans 312

egg yolks
Freeze straight up. 25

F

fennel
Add offcuts to your fish stock bag. 32
| The Green Counterbalance Salad | 309 |

G

green shallots
Use the green parts and put the rest in a jar of water to re-sprout; replenish the water regularly.

H

herbs, leaves
Freeze in ice-cube trays with oil,

stock or wine. 25

herbs, stems and stalks
Add to your stock bag; throw into a roasting pan with meat or root vegetables.
Leftovers Pesto 55
See also parsley, mint, coriander stems.

K

kale
A Super-Greens Couch Fondue 118
Kale Flakes 179
Massaged Kale 23
"Pizza" Bread-and-Butter Crumble 262
The Cheapest Stew Ever 212
Watercress "Colcannon" 178

kale stalks
Leftovers Pesto 55

L

lemon juice
Freeze in ice-cube trays and use for dressings.

lemon rind
Make gremolata: Add 1 whole rind to a blender and blend, adding a handful of leftover parsley and 1 clove garlic then freeze in ice-cube trays and use to splodge on meat and fish dishes.

lemons
Lemon and Turmeric Tonic-Ade 347
Sour Kiwi Immunity Boosters 350

lentils, red
Fermented Dosas 89

lentils, brown
Clean Bitters Bowl 129
Inside-Out Sprouted
  Kitcheri Loaf 114

lettuce
Sauté just-wilting lettuce in olive oil; season with garlic or shallot then serve with eggs.
Back to the 70s Lettuce Soup 172

M

milk
Use sour milk (not lumpy, rancid milk) to make pancakes or other baked goods that call for buttermilk.

mince meat
Basic Meatballs 144
"But the Kitchen Sink" Breakfast
  Hash 82
Cheeseburger Wontons 102
Greek San Choi Bau 146
Some Beefin' Good Jerky 209

mint
Steep the leaves in boiled water to make tea.
A Salad of Crushed Olives 170
Indian Sprout Raita 352
Minted Pea Pistou 240
The Green Counterbalance
  Salad 309

mushrooms
Beginner's Coq au Vin Pâté 196
Chinese Beef Cheeks 198
Mum's Steak and Kidney
  Stew with Herby Dumplings 194
Mushroom, Thyme
  and Hazelnut Oatmeal 64
Soothing Asian Poached Pot 216

mung beans
Inside-Out Sprouted Kitcheri Loaf 114

N

nuts
Bacon Granola 108
Beet Halwa 190
Beet Red Velvet
  Cheesecake 321
Nut Crumble 72
Raw Snickas Ice-Cream Bar 279
Vegan "Ground Meat" 186

O

onion tops and skins
Add to any stock bag.

olives
Use the brine or oil in dressings, sauces or Leftovers Pesto 55
A Salad of Crushed Olives 170

orange rind
Dry out and use as fire kindling – it releases a delightful aroma!

P

Parmesan rind
Add to soups (page 212), Homemade Stock (page 43) or cook it along with any sauce you'd serve with Parmesan.

parsley
Use the stems, chopped finely, as you would the leaves.
Basic Meatballs 144
Crunchy Broccoli Buckwheat
  Tabbouli 187
Green Scraps Shakshouka 248
The Fish That Got Away Pie 261

parsnips
Not Quite Banana Bread 69
Parsnip, Pear 'n' Thyme Soup 243
Pretty in Pastel Pink Parsnip
  Pasta 137

Roasted Roots 23
Puttanesca Festival 133

peaches
Cheesecake-Stuffed Peaches with
  Basil 294
Peach and Peanut Butter
  Frozen Yogurt 107 Summer Peach
  and Basil
  Colada 345
Vanilla Peach Kombucha Gums 351

potato
Watercress "Colcannon" 178

pumpkin
Pumpkin Spice-a-Chino 327
Pumpkin Spice Butter 79–80
Roast Chicken "Meffins" 98
Stuffing 'n' All the Best
  Bits Salad 308
Slow-Cooker Zucchini
  and Pumpkin Spice Breakfast
  Pudding 62

Q

quinoa
Bacon 'n' Egg Oatmeal 66
Crisp Skillet Bibimbap Pancake 250
Fermented Dosas 89
Moroccan Cauliflower,
  Chickpea and Quinoa Bake 238
Mushroom, Thyme
  and Hazelnut Oatmeal 64
One-Pan Moroccan Fish Pilaf 161

R

radishes
"But the Kitchen Sink" Kimchi 337

roast vegetables
Add to Abundance Bowls, Leftover Mishmashes, or make a quick soup: add to stock, bring to the boil then purée.
Baked Stuffing Loaf 305

S

seeds
'Bucha Mustard 336
Sesame-Crusted Haloumi and
  Strawberry Salad 179
Sunflower Strawberry Thumbles 298
The Fish That Got Away Pie 261

spinach
Any Green Saag Paneer 177
Green Apple Pie Smoothie Bowl
  (baby spinach only) 72
Green Smoothie Cake with Lemon
  Cheese Whip 330
"Pizza" Bread-and-Butter Crumble 262

spring onions, *see green shallots*

stock
Freeze in 1-cup portions or in ice-cube trays and use to make soups, stews, thin sauces, deglaze etc.

sugar
Use it to feed flowers, make cleaning products etc.
Ayurvedic Face Scrub 30–31

sweet potato
My Allergy-Free Bread 113
Sweet Potato, Miso
  and Sage Soup 244
Sweet Potato Nachos 230
Sweet Potato Skin Chips 23

T

turnip
Orange and Thyme
  Rainbow Chips 95
The Cheapest Stew Ever 212
Turnip Cheeseburgers 120

V

vegetable peels
What the hell are you peeling your veggies for?

W

watercress
Sesame-Crusted Haloumi and
  Strawberry Salad 179
The Green Counterbalance
  Salad 309
Watercress "Colcannon" 178
Watercress Sauce and
  Some Eggs 176

whey
Freeze in ice-cube trays to use in mayo, sauces, dressings etc.

wine, white
Beginner's Coq au Vin Pâté 196

wine, red
Blaukraut 182
Chocolate and Red Wine
  Creamsticks 326

Z

zucchini
"But the Kitchen Sink"
  Breakfast Hash 82
Chocolate Cherry Blitz 86
Green Spaghetti and Meatballs 145
My Gut-Healing Brew 87
Quick Zucchini Tzatziki 188
Slow-Cooker Zucchini and Pumpkin
  Spice Breakfast Pudding 62
Zucchini Bread Thickie 87
Zucchini Butter 189
Zucchini No-Carbonara 188

GENERAL INDEX
Page numbers in *italics* refer to photographs.

A
A really fat beet 190, *190*
A salad of crushed olives 170
A super-greens couch fondue 118, *119*
activated groaties 27, *27*, 358
  Buckwheat pops 242, *245*
  Cardamom and sea salt ganache tart 318, *319*
  Chocolate cake batter protein bowl 71, *72*
  Chocolate peanut butter crackles 280, *281*
  Crunchy broccoli buckwheat tabbouli 187, *187*
  Friday night chockito on a stick 286, *287*
  Golden happy times 296, *297*
  Pretty spring risotto *130*, 132
  Puttanesca festival 133, *135*
  Red velvet crunch bowl 71, *72*
agar 351
aioli 50
alcohol 363
almonds
  Bacon granola 108, *109*
  Beet red velvet cheesecake 320, 321–22
  Choc-ginger and pear muggin 288, *289*
  Chocolate cake batter protein bowl 71, *72*
  Clean bitters bowl 129, *129*
  Gingerbread muggin 288, *289*
  Golden happy times 296, *297*
  Green smoothie cake with lemon cheese whip 330, *331*
  Hot cross muffins 328, *329*
  Miso and walnut slow bros 282, *283*
  My totally messed-with Christmas cake *314*, 315
  Nut crumble 70, *72*
  organic 17
  One-pan Moroccan fish pilaf 161
  Party polenta cakes with popping topping 292, *293*
  Slow-cooker zucchini and pumpkin spice breakfast pudding 62, *63*
  Strawberry cheesecake muggin 288, *289*
anchovies
  Fridge-door tonnato 254, *255*
  Grilled caesar on the barbie 173, *173*
  Grilled sardines with chili, haloumi and lemony pesto 155, *157*
Any green saag paneer 177
apple cider vinegar 356, 358

apples
  Apple and blackberry cardamom fizz 347
  Apple and peanut butter with pumpkin spice butter 120, *121*
  Apple wedges with cream cheese 123
  Autumn apple pie kombucha 345
  Beet, beet leaf 'n' apple borscht 242, 244
  Blaukraut 182, *183*
  "But the kitchen sink" kimchi 337
  Caramelized leek, apple and rosemary socca *104*, 106
  Green apple pie smoothie bowl 70, *72*
  Shortcut choucroute 258, *259*
  Stuffing 'n' all the best bits salad 306, 308
  The green counterbalance salad 306, 309
artificial sweeteners 361
Asian cashew crisp 184, *184*
asparagus
  Asparagus stock 43
  Crunchy chicken satay in a pan 232, *233*
  My recalibrating pork meal 234, 235
  Nori roll in a bowl *131*, 132
  Pretty spring pot 216
  Pretty spring risotto *130*, 132
  Spring socca pizza 105, *106*
  The cheapest stew ever 212, *213*
Australiana mango flat white 327
avocados
  Clean bitters bowl 129, *129*
  Four-ingredient chicken shred-up 133, *134*
  Green minx dressing 54
  Green spaghetti and meatballs *143*, 145
  Margarita popsticks *325*, 326
  Misomite 54, 120, *121*
  Nori roll in a bowl *131*, 132
  Our office "emergency tuna" mishmash bowl 136, *136*
  Sweet potato nachos 230, *231*
  The BLAT 75, *75*
  The green goddess toastie 85, *85*
  Untinned sardines on avocado toast with chili flakes 154
Ayurveda 362

B
Back to the 70s lettuce soup 172, *172*
bacon
  Bacon bits 44
  Bacon granola 108, *109*
  Bacon 'n' egg oatmeal 66, *67*

Blaukraut 182, *183*
The BLAT 75, *75*
Hipster grandaddy salad 176, *176*
Homemade bacon 208
Lamb's fry and pear meatloaf 202, *203*
"Pizza" muggins 60, *61*
Watercress "colcannon" 178, *178*
Zucchini no-carbonara 188, *188*
Baked Mediterranean summer sardines *154–55*, 157
Baked stuffing loaf with mushroom sauce 304, 305
Baking-sheet-dinner-for-two eggplant parmigiana 228, *229*
bananas
  Chocolate cake batter protein bowl 71, *72*
  Kermit slushie *122*, 125
  Not quite banana bread 68, *69*
  Red velvet crunch bowl 71, *72*
  Warming berry 'n' beet smoothie 78, 80
  Zucchini bread thickie 87
Basic raw chocolate 56
basil
  Blueberry, basil and mozzarella toastie 85, *85*
  Cheesecake-stuffed peaches with basil 294, *295*
  Summer peach and basil colada 345
beans 26, *26–28*
  cooked beans and legumes 28
  see also green beans; lentils
beef
  Bloke beef 'n' beer with mash 206, *207*
  "But the kitchen sink" breakfast hash 82, *83*
  Cheeseburger wontons 102, *103*
  Chinese beef cheeks 198, *199*
  Coffee-and-cacao-cured pulled beef 223
  Homemade beef stock 42
  Kimchi instant noodles 116
  Lebanese roll pizza 186, *186*
  Mum's steak and kidney stew with herby dumplings 194, *195*
  organic 17
  Some beefin' good jerky 209
  Steak 'n' five veg 239
  sustainable steaks 239
  "Sweet" tacos with easy slaw 200, *201*
  The cheapest stew ever 212, *213*
  Vata balancing bowl 133, *134*
  see also ground meat
beet
  A really fat beet 190, *190*

Beet, beet leaf 'n' apple borscht 242, 244
Beet halwa 190, *190*
Beet that popstick salad 191, *191*
Beet red velvet cheesecake 320, 321–22
Cheeseburger wontons 102, *103*
Choc-beet allspice truffles 270, *271*
Chopped salad pickle 335, *335*
Cooked 'n' frozen beets 23
leaves 174, *174*, 177
Massaged kale or beet greens 23
My totally messed-with Christmas cake *314*, 315
Nomato sauce 51, *51*
Orange and thyme rainbow chips 94, *95*
Pickled festive red slaw with caramelized ruby grapefruit 307, 309
Pink beet and goat's cheese toastie 84, *84*
Pretty in pastel pink parsnip pasta 137, *137*
Pretty spring pot 216
Rainbow gado gado *130*, 132
Rainbow rolls *123*, 124
Red velvet crunch bowl 71, *72*
Warming berry 'n' beet smoothie 78, 80
Beginner's coq au vin pâté 196, *197*
bell peppers
  Baked Mediterranean summer sardines 157
  Chopped salad pickle 335, *335*
  Jerk pork shoulder roast 219, 222
  Lamb roast for two 240, *241*
  My brother Pete's app-and-entrée-in-one kokonda 158, *159*
  "Pizza" muggins 60, *61*
  "Sweet" tacos with easy slaw 200, *201*
berries
  Cardamom and sea salt ganache tart 318, *319*
  frozen 16
  organic 17
  Probiotic berries 'n' cream chews 351
  Warming berry 'n' beet smoothie 78, 80
"best before" dates 16
blackberries
  Apple and blackberry cardamom fizz 347
  Probiotic berries 'n' cream chews 351
  Warming berry 'n' beet smoothie 78, 80

BLAT 75, *75*
Blaukraut 182, *183*
blenders 13, *13*
Bloke beef 'n' beer with mash 206, *207*
blood oranges
　Blood orange tonic bombs 351
　Buttered blueberry and blood orange soup 284, 285
　Pickled festive red slaw with caramelized ruby grapefruit 307, 309
blueberries
　Blueberry banana bread 69
　Blueberry, basil and mozzarella toastie 85, *85*
　Buttered blueberry and blood orange soup 284, 285
　Probiotic berries 'n' cream chews 351
　Warming berry 'n' beet smoothie 78, 80
boiled eggs 44
bok choy
　"But the kitchen sink" kimchi 337
　growing your own 33
　Slow-cooker apple cider chicken 236, *237*
Bone marrow bombs 245, *245*
Bountiful slice 277, *279*
Braised celery and leeks with vanilla 170
breads
　choosing bread 82
　My allergy-free bread *112*, 113
　Not quite banana bread 68, 69
Broc bites 92, *93*
broccoli
　Asian cashew crisp 184, *184*
　Broc bites 92, *93*
　Broccoli and cheese melts toastie 85, *85*
　Broccoli rice 22
　Chopped salad pickle 335, *335*
　Crunchy broccoli buckwheat tabbouli 187, *187*
　Italian "pasta" noodles 116
　Lebanese roll pizza 186, *186*
　Parcooked 'n' frozen veggies 22
　"Pizza" muggins 60, *61*
　Pretty spring risotto *130*, 132
　Sweet paprika stem chips *186*, 260
　The whole brassicus hummus 187, *187*
　Two-minute desk lunch noodles 116, *117*
　Zesty caper crunch 185, *185*
broccolini
　Baking-sheet-dinner-for-two eggplant parmigiana 228, *229*
　Four-ingredient chicken shred-up 133, *134*
　Skillet fish 'n' superslaw 162

brown rice syrup 357, 359, 361
The bright side cocktail 310
Buttered blueberry and blood orange soup *284*, 285
Cacao cayenne pecans 312, *313*
Cardamom and sea salt ganache tart 318, *319*
Cheesecake-stuffed peaches with basil 294, *295*
Friday night chockito on a stick 286, *287*
The cultured mule cocktail 310
Da clean bee's knees cocktail *307*, 310
Green smoothie cake with lemon cheese whip 330, *331*
My totally messed-with Christmas cake *314*, 315
Party polenta cakes with popping topping 292, *293*
Raw snickas ice-cream bar *277*, 279
Thai lattes 323
brussels sprouts
　Brussels sprout, haloumi and sauerkraut sliders 120, *121*
　Shaved sprouts and pecorino salad *304*, 305
　Steak 'n' five veg 239
　Stuffing 'n' all the best bits salad *306*, 308
'Bucha mustard 336
buckinis *see* activated groaties
buckwheat 356
　Buckwheat pops *242*, 245
　Cooked buckwheat 27
　Crunchy broccoli buckwheat tabbouli 187, *187*
　My allergy-free bread *112*, 113
　Nori roll in a bowl *131*, 132
　"Pizza" bread-and-butter crumble 262, *263*
　raw groats 26
　sprouted 27, *27*
　Sprouted cacao pops 76
　Stuffing 'n' all the best bits salad *306*, 308
　versus quinoa 27
　Zesty caper crunch 185, *185*
see also activated groaties
Bulletproof coffee squares *349*, 351
"But the kitchen sink" breakfast hash 82, *83*
"But the kitchen sink" kimchi 337
Buttered blueberry and blood orange soup *284*, 285

C
cabbage
　Blaukraut 182, *183*
　"But the kitchen sink" breakfast hash 82, *83*
　"But the kitchen sink" kimchi 337

Clean bitters bowl 129, *129*
Crisp bibimbap skillet pancake 250, *251*
Greek san choi bau 146, *147*
Okonomiyaki in a tray 183, *183*
Pickled festive red slaw with caramelized ruby grapefruit *307*, 309
Shortcut choucroute 258, *259*
Simplicious sauerkraut 337
Soothing Asian poached pot 216
Steak 'n' five veg 239
Sweet potato nachos 230, *231*
"Sweet" tacos with easy slaw 200, *201*
Thai coconutty cabbage 182, *182*
types of 180–81, *180–81*
cacao powder 356
　Beet red velvet cheesecake *320*, 321–22
　Cacao cayenne pecans 312, *313*
　Choc-ginger and pear muggin 288, *289*
　Choc-nut spoon pops 120, *121*
　Chocolate and red wine creamsticks *325*, 326
　Chocolate cherry blitz 86, *86*
　Chocolate peanut butter crackles 280, *281*
　Coffee-and-cacao-cured pulled beef 234
　Miso and walnut slow bros 282, *283*
　My totally messed-with Christmas cake *314*, 315
　Raw snickas ice-cream bar *277*, 279
　Sprouted cacao pops 76
　Sugar-quitting butterscotch 'n' spice hot chocolate 79, 80
　Tam tims 274, *275*
Caesar salad boats 245, *245*
cakes 358
　Beet red velvet cheesecake *320*, 321–22
　Green smoothie cake with lemon cheese whip 330, *331*
　My spectacular popstick cake 324, *325*, 326
　My totally messed-with Christmas cake *314*, 315
　Party polenta cakes with popping topping 292, *293*
　Pull-apart caterpillar birthday cake 290, *291*
canned beans 356
capers 356
　Baked Mediterranean summer sardines 157
　Cheeseburger wontons 102, *103*
　Fridge-door tonnato 254, *255*
　Zesty caper crunch 185, *185*
Caramelized leek, apple and rosemary socca *104*, 106
cardamom

Apple and blackberry cardamom fizz 347
Cardamom and sea salt ganache tart 318, *319*
Salted cardamom caramel coffee 73
carrots
　Basic pot-au-feu 214, *215*
　Beet, beet leaf 'n' apple borscht *242*, 244
　"But the kitchen sink" breakfast hash 82, *83*
　"But the kitchen sink" kimchi 337
　Carrot "bacon" 115, *115*
　Chopped salad pickle 335, *335*
　Cucumber and carrot flowers 123, *123*
　My Indian kimchi 338, *339*
　Nomato sauce 51, *51*
　One-pan Moroccan fish pilaf 161
　Pickled festive red slaw with caramelized ruby grapefruit *307*, 309
　Rainbow gado gado *130*, 132
　Slow-cooked green peas and ham 217
　Sweet Persian tagine 224, *225*
　"Sweet" tacos with easy slaw 200, *201*
　The cheapest stew ever 212, *213*
　The fish that got away pie 261
　Vegan whatchagot quiche 260
　Watercress "colcannon" 178, *178*
cashews
　Asian cashew crisp 184, *184*
　Bacon granola 108, *109*
　Beet halwa 190, *190*
cauliflower
　Asian cashew crisp 184, *184*
　Cauli popcorn 100, *101*
　Cauliflower rice 22
　Cauliflower tartines with green goddess dressing and hazelnuts 184, *184*
　Chopped salad pickle 335, *335*
　Israeli whole-baked cauliflower 316, *317*
　Moroccan cauliflower, chickpea and quinoa bake 238
　Parcooked 'n' frozen veggies 22
　Superfoodie lasagna cake 140, *141*
　Sustainable sweet fish curry 164, *165*
　Sweet paprika stem chips *186*, 260
　The fish that got away pie 261
　The whole brassicus hummus 187, *187*
　Vegan "ground meat" 186
　Vegan whatchagot quiche 260
　Watercress "colcannon" 178, *178*

Zesty caper crunch 185, *185*
cavolo nero 174, *174*
celeriac 145
   Swedish meatballs *143*, 145
   Watercress "colcannon" 178, *178*
celery
   A salad of crushed olives 170, *170*
   Beet, beet leaf 'n' apple borscht 242, 244
   Braised celery and leeks with vanilla 170, *170*
   "But the kitchen sink" breakfast hash 82, *83*
   Celery and pink grapefruit granita 171, *171*
   Celery leaf salt 265
   Celery soda 171, *171*
   Clean bitters bowl 129, *129*
   growing your own 33
   Nomato sauce 51, *51*
   Puttanesca festival 133, *135*
   Slow-cooked green peas and ham 217
   Soothing Asian poached pot 216
   The cheapest stew ever 212, *213*
   The six-star waldorf 133, *135*
   Waldorf smash-up 75, *75*
chard 175, *175*
   A super-greens couch fondue 118, *119*
   Any green saag paneer 177, *177*
   pickled stems 335
   "Pizza" bread-and-butter crumble 262, *263*
   Steak 'n' five veg 239
   The cheapest stew ever 212, *213*
   Vata balancing bowl 133, *134*
Cheat's vitello tonnato 254
cheese 358
   A super-greens couch fondue 118, *119*
   Any green saag paneer 177, *177*
   Apple wedges with cream cheese *123*
   Baking-sheet-dinner-for-two eggplant parmigiana 228, *229*
   Blueberry, basil and mozzarella toasties 85, *85*
   Broc bites 92, *93*
   Broccoli and cheese melts toastie 85, *85*
   Brussels sprout, haloumi and sauerkraut sliders 120, *121*
   Cheeseburger wontons 102, *103*
   Cheeseburgers *122*
   Cheesy cauli popcorn 100
   Chicken caesar on a stick *123*, 125
   Cream cheese frosting 56
   Golden oatmeal wedges 253, *253*
   Greek lamb salad *218*, 221

Green scraps shakshouka 248, *249*
Grilled sardines with chili, haloumi and lemony pesto 155, 157
Haloumi crisps 242, 245
Homemade cream cheese and whey 46, *47*
Homemade paneer 48, *49*
Lamb roast for two 240, *241*
Lebanese roll pizza 186, *186*
Marinated goat's cheese 46
Monster-mash roll-ups 122, 124
Mushroom, thyme and hazelnut oatmeal 64, *65*
Pink beet and goat's cheese toastie 84, *84*
"Pizza" bread-and-butter crumble 262, *263*
Prosciutto-Parmesan stock 43
Sesame-crusted haloumi and strawberry salad 179, *179*
Shaved sprouts and pecorino salad *304*, 305
Spiced paneer 'n' peas 110, *111*
Superfoodie lasagna cake 140, *141*
Sweet potato nachos 230, *231*
The green goddess toastie 85, *85*
The six-star waldorf 133, *135*
Totally gaudy Christmas tree cheese ball 302, *303*
Turnip cheeseburger 120, *121*
Waldorf smash-up 75, *75*
Zesty caper crunch 185, *185*
cheesecake
   Beet red velvet cheesecake *320*, 321–22
   Cheesecake-stuffed peaches with basil 294, *295*
   Strawberry cheesecake muggin 288, *289*
chia seeds 356, 358
   Bacon granola 108, *109*
   Lebanese roll pizza 186, *186*
   Monster-mash roll-ups 122, 124
   My allergy-free bread *112*, 113
   Not quite banana bread 68, 69
   Rainbow rolls *123*, 124
   Strawberry chia jam 57, *57*, *143*
   Vegan whatchagot quiche 260
   Vietnamese turkey pancakes 150, *151*
chicken
   Basic pot-au-feu 214, *215*
   Beginner's coq au vin pâté 196, *197*
   Chicken caesar on a stick *123*, 125
   Chicken crackle salt 204, *205*
   Crunchy chicken satay in a pan 232, *233*
   Four-ingredient chicken shred-up 133, *134*
   Grilled caesar on the barbie 173, *173*

Homemade chicken stock 42
Italian "pasta" noodles 116
Kimchi chicken choucroute 258
Leftovers kimchi soup 264
Moroccan chicken and cauliflower bake 238
organic 17
precooked chickens 16
Pretty spring pot 216
Rainbow rolls *123*, 124
Roast chicken "meffins" 98, *99*, *123*
Slow-cooker apple cider chicken 236, *237*
Soothing Asian poached pot 216
Sweet potato nachos 230, *231*
chickpeas
   Fermented socca *104–05*, 106
   how to sprout 352, *353*
   Moroccan cauliflower, chickpea and quinoa bake 238
   Sweet Persian tagine 224, *225*
chilies
   "But the kitchen sink" kimchi 337
   Cacao cayenne pecans 312, *313*
   Grilled sardines with chili, haloumi and lemony pesto 155, 157
   My Indian kimchi 338, *339*
   Thai lattes 323
Chinese cabbage 181, *181*
chips
   Orange and thyme rainbow chips 94, 95
   Sweet paprika stem chips 260
Choc-beet allspice truffles 270, *271*
Choc-ginger and pear muggin 288, *289*
Choc-nut spoon pops 120, *121*
chocolate 363
   Basic raw chocolate 56
   Beet red velvet cheesecake *320*, 321–22
   Bountiful slice *277*, 279
   Cardamom and sea salt ganache tart 318, *319*
   Choc-beet allspice truffles 270, *271*
   Chocolate and red wine creamsticks *325*, 326
   Chocolate cake batter protein bowl *71*, 72
   Chocolate cherry blitz 86, *86*
   Chocolate peanut butter crackles 280, *281*
   Friday night chockito on a stick 286, *287*
   Golden happy times 296, *297*
   Hot cross muffins 328, *329*
   Lamington ice creams 268, *269*
   Miso and walnut slow bros 282, *283*
   My totally messed-with Christmas cake 314, 315
   Off the wagon wheel *276*, 278
   Raspberry ripe bites *271*, 273

Raw snickas ice-cream bar *277*, 279
Sugar-quitting butterscotch 'n' spice hot chocolate 79, 80
Tam tims 274, *275*
Chopped salad pickle 335, *335*
Christmas cake 314, 315
Christmas day *306–07*, 308–09
Christmas tree cheese ball 302, *303*
Clean bitters bowl 129
cocktails 310
coconut 356
   Beet red velvet cheesecake *320*, 321–22
   Bountiful slice *277*, 279
   Cardamom and sea salt ganache tart 318, *319*
   Choc-ginger and pear muggin 288, *289*
   Chocolate and red wine creamsticks *325*, 326
   Chocolate peanut butter crackles 280, *281*
coconut cream 356
coconut flakes 358
coconut milk 359
Coconut "marshmallows" 351
coconut oil 31, 356
Gingerbread muggin 288, *289*
Golden happy times 296, *297*
Green apple pie smoothie bowl *70*, 72
Kermit slushie 122, 125
Lamington ice creams 268, *269*
Lemon syrup and poppy seed muggin 288, *289*
Mango and coconut squares *349*, 351
Margarita popsticks *325*, 326
My brother Pete's app-and-entrée-in-one kokonda 158, *159*
My totally messed-with Christmas cake 314, 315
Off the wagon wheel *276*, 278
Pomegranate and coconut vodka popsticks 324, *325*
Raspberry ripe bites *271*, 273
Raw snickas ice-cream bar *277*, 279
Strawberry cheesecake muggin 288, *289*
Strawberry frozen yogurt 125
Sugar-quitting butterscotch 'n' spice hot chocolate 79, 80
Supercharged coconut frosting 56
Sustainable sweet fish curry 164, *165*
Thai coconutty cabbage 182, *182*
Thai lattes 323
Two-minute desk lunch noodles 116, *117*
Whipped coconut frosting 56

coffee
 Bulletproof coffee squares *349*, 351
 Coffee-and-cacao-cured pulled beef 223
 Salted caramel cardamom coffee 73
coleslaw
 Pickled festive red slaw with caramelized ruby grapefruit *307*, 309
 Shortcut choucroute 258, *259*
 Skillet fish 'n' superslaw 162
 Sweet potato nachos 230, *231*
 "Sweet" tacos with easy slaw 200, *201*
condiment leftovers, how to use 32
constipation 23
Cooked 'n' frozen beets 23
cookies 276–67, 278–79
coriander
 Green minx dressing 54
 Vietnamese turkey pancakes 150, *151*
corn
 Corn cob stock 43
 Sweet potato nachos 230, *231*
cream cheese
 Apple wedges with cream cheese *123*
 Beet red velvet cheesecake *320*, 321–22
 Cream cheese frosting 56
 Green smoothie cake with lemon cheese whip 330, *331*
 Homemade cream cheese and whey 46, *47*
 Totally gaudy Christmas tree cheese ball 302, *303*
Crisp bibimbap skillet pancake 250, *251*
Crunchy broccoli buckwheat tabbouli 187, *187*
Crunchy chicken satay in a pan 232, *233*
cucumbers
 Chicken caesar on a stick *123*, 125
 Cucumber and carrot flowers *123, 123*
 Greek san choi bau 146, *147*
 My brother Pete's app-and-entrée-in-one kokonda 158, *159*
 The real Greek yogurt 74, *74*
curry pastes 16, 356

D

Da clean bee's knees cocktail *307*, 310
daikon, in Indian kimchi 338, *339*
daily requirements 36
dairy products 356
 organic 17
dandelion greens 175, *175*
 Any green saag paneer 177, *177*

Dosas *88, 89*
doshas 362
double steamers 10, *10*
dressings
 Caesar dressing 173
 Green goddess dressing 184
 Green minx dressing 54
 Powerhouse dressing 53
 TMT dressing 53
 Whey-good mayo 50
drinks *see* cocktails; kombucha; smoothies
dukkah *see* Seaweed dukkah

E

Easiest-ever Korean breakfast custard 264
Easy slaw 200
eggplants
 Baked Mediterranean summer sardines 157
 Baking-sheet-dinner-for-two eggplant parmigiana 228, *229*
 Greek san choi bau 146, *147*
 Middle Eastern eggplant 148, *149*
eggs 358
 Baked stuffing loaf with mushroom sauce *304*, 305
 boiled 44, 125
 Broc bites 92, *93*
 Chicken caesar on a stick *123*, 125
 Easiest-ever Korean breakfast custard 264
 Egg-drop soup 264
 Egg 'n' bacon oatmeal 66, *67*
 Green scraps shakshouka 248, *249*
 Green smoothie cake with lemon cheese whip 330, *331*
 hard-boiled *123*
 Hipster grandaddy salad 176, *176*
 Hot cross muffins 328, *329*
 Last night's dinner with an egg stuck in it 256, *257*
 Monster-mash roll-ups *122*, 124
 Not quite banana bread 68, *69*
 Okonomiyaki in a tray 183, *183*
 organic 17
 Party polenta cakes with popping topping 292, *293*
 Pink devilish googie eggs 253, *253*
 "Pizza" muggins 60, *61*
 poached 44
 Poached egg floater 242, *245*
 Rainbow gado gado 130, *132*
 Sprouted kitcheri loaf 114
 The fish that got away pie 261
 Watercress sauce and some eggs 176, *177*
 Zucchini no-carbonara 188, *188*
endive 120, *121*
 in Clean bitters bowl 129, *129*

Caesar salad boats 245, *245*
equipment 10–13

F

fennel
 Basic pot-au-feu 214, *215*
 Clean bitters bowl 129, *129*
 Green scraps shakshouka 248, *249*
 My recalibrating pork meal 234, *235*
 My sausage and fennel lunch bowl 136, *136*
 Pretty spring pot 216
 Pretty spring risotto 130, *132*
 The cheapest stew ever 212, *213*
 The green counterbalance salad *306*, 309
 Untinned sardines 156
fenugreek, in Fermented dosas *88, 89*
ferment brine 358
Fermented dosas *88, 89*
Fermented socca *104–05*, 106
Fermented turmeric paste 340
fermented vegetables 334–41
feta
 Greek lamb salad *218*, 221
 Lamb roast for two 240, *241*
 Monster-mash roll-ups *122*, 124
 Mushroom, thyme and hazelnut oatmeal 64, *65*
 The six-star waldorf 133, *135*
 Totally gaudy Christmas tree cheese ball 302, *303*
fish 153–65
 Gift-wrapped miso cod 166, *167*
 Homemade fish stock 42
 My brother Pete's app-and-entrée-in-one kokonda 158, *159*
 One-pan Moroccan fish pilaf 161
 Simplicious smoked salmon 160
 Skillet fish 'n' coleslaw 162, *163*
 Sustainable sweet fish curry 164, *165*
 The fish that got away pie 261
 see also sardines; tuna
flours 358
Flu tonic 346
Four-ingredient chicken shred-up 133, *134*
freezing, of food 20–21, *20–21*, 24–25, *24–25*, 29
Friday night chockito on a stick 286, *287*
Fridge-door tonnato 254, *255*
frostings
 Cream cheese frosting 56
 Supercharged coconut frosting 56
 Whipped coconut frosting 56
fructose 360
fruit 363
 freezing of 21, *21*
 organic 17

G

garlic 358
 "But the kitchen sink" kimchi 337
 Good for your guts garlic 340, *341*
gelatin 348, *349–50*, 351, 356
 Pumpkin spice-a-chino 327
 Thai lattes 323
Gift-wrapped miso cod 166, *167*
ginger
 "But the kitchen sink" kimchi 337
 Choc-ginger and pear muggin 288, *289*
 Gingerbread muggin 288, *289*
 growing your own 33
goat
 Bloke beef 'n' beer with mash 206
 Sweet Persian tagine 224
 "Sweet" tacos with easy slaw 200
goat's cheese
 Pink beet and goat's cheese toastie 84, *84*
 Marinated 46
"Gochujang" sauce 250, *251*
Golden happy times 296, *297*
Golden oatmeal wedges 253, *253*
Good for your guts garlic 340, *341*
grains 26–8
grapefruit
 Celery and pink grapefruit granita 171, *171*
 Pickled festive red slaw with caramelized ruby grapefruit *307*, 309
 Ruby grapefruit tonic bombs *349*, 351
 The bright side cocktail 310
Greek lamb salad *218*, 221
Greek san choi bau 146, *147*
Green apple pie smoothie bowl 70, *72*
green beans
 Bloke beef 'n' beer with mash 206, *207*
 "But the kitchen sink" breakfast hash 82, *83*
 Chopped salad pickle 335, *335*
 Gift-wrapped miso cod 166
 Jerk pork shoulder roast *219*, 222
 Middle Eastern eggplant 148, *149*
 Parcooked 'n' frozen veggies 22
 Persian lamb salad *218*, 221
 Sustainable sweet fish curry 164, *165*
 Sweet Persian tagine 224, *225*
Green goddess dressing 184
Green gumbo 265
Green juice detox jellies 351
Green minx dressing 54
Green scraps shakshouka 248, *249*
Green smoothie cake with lemon cheese whip 330, *331*

green smoothies 86–87, *86–87*, 351
Green spaghetti and meatballs *143*, 145
greens
  A super-greens couch fondue 118, *119*
  Any green saag paneer 177, *177*
  Green gumbo 265
  Green scraps shakshouka 248, *249*
  Kermit slushie *122*, 125
  Massaged kale or beet greens 23
  Mum's steak and kidney stew with herby dumplings 194, *195*
  Our office "emergency tuna" mishmash bowl 136, *136*
  Parcooked 'n' frozen veggies 22
  Rainbow rolls *123*, 124
  Slow-cooker apple cider chicken 236, *237*
  Swedish meatballs *143*, 145
  see also specific greens, e.g. spinach
Gribiche sauce plate *252*, 252
Grilled caesar on the barbie 173, *173*
Grilled sardines with chili, haloumi and lemony pesto *155*, 157
groaties *see Activated groaties*
Grounding crimson tonic 347
ground meat 140–51, 359
  "But the kitchen sink" breakfast hash 82, *83*
  Greek san choi bau 146, *147*
  Lebanese roll pizza 186, *186*
  Meatballs *142–43*, 144–45
  Middle Eastern eggplant 148, *149*
  Some beefin' good jerky 209
  Superfoodie lasagna cake 140, *141*
  Vietnamese turkey pancakes 150, *151*
gummies 348, *349–50*, 351
Gut-healing brew, My 87, *87*

H
haloumi
  Brussels sprout, haloumi and sauerkraut sliders 120, *121*
  Grilled sardines with chili, haloumi and lemony pesto *155*, 157
  Haloumi crisps *242*, 245
  Sesame-crusted haloumi and strawberry salad 179, *179*
ham
  Green gumbo 265
  Slow-cooked green peas and ham 217
  Sugar-free glazed Christmas ham *306*, 308
Hardcore flu tonic 346
Harissa cream cheese bombs 245

Have some lettuce with your dressing 173
hazelnuts
  Cauliflower tartines with green goddess dressing and hazelnuts 184, *184*
  Mushroom, thyme and hazelnut oatmeal 64, *65*
herbs 358
  storing 19
Hipster grandaddy salad 176, *176*
Homemade bacon 208
Hot cross muffins 328, *329*

I
ice cream
  Golden happy times 296, *297*
  Lamington ice creams 268, *269*
  Raw snickas ice-cream bar 277, *279*
ice-cube trays 13, *13*, 24–25, *24–25*
ingredients, guidelines for buying 15–17
Inside-out sprouted kitcheri loaf 114
Israeli whole-baked cauliflower 316, *317*
Italian "pasta" noodles 116

J
jam, strawberry chia 57, *57*
Jerk pork shoulder roast 219, *222*
jerky
  Some beefin' good jerky 209
  Some beefin' good jerky wrapped in a mustard leaf 120, *121*
juices, versus smoothies 86

K
kale 175, *175*
  Any green saag paneer 177, *177*
  Greek lamb salad *218*, 221
  Hipster grandaddy salad 176, *176*
  Kale flakes 179, *179*
  Massaged kale or beet greens 23
  "Pizza" bread-and-butter crumble 262, *263*
  Steak 'n' five veg 239
  The cheapest stew ever 212, *213*
  The six-star waldorf 133, *135*
  Kapha types 362
Kermit slushie *122*, 125
kimchi 356
  "But the kitchen sink" kimchi 337
  Crisp bibimbap skillet pancake 250, *251*
  Kimcheese toastie 84, *84*
  Kimchi chicken choucroute 258
  Kimchi instant noodles 116
  My Indian kimchi 338, *339*
Kitcheri loaf 114

kiwi
  Kiwi and raspberry kebabs *123*
  Sour kiwi immunity boosters *349*, 350
knives 10, *10*
kokonda, My brother Pete's app-and-entrée-in-one 158, *159*
kombucha 356
  Autumn apple pie kombucha 345
  'Bucha mustard 336
  Plain kombucha *342*, 344
  Spring strawberry and vanilla kombucha 345
  Summer peach and basil colada 345
  The cultured mule cocktail 310
  Vanilla peach kombucha gums 351
  Winter chai kombucha *342*, 345

L
lamb
  Greek lamb salad *218*, 221
  Lamb's fry and pear meatloaf 202, *203*
  Lamb roast for two 240, *241*
  Persian lamb salad *218*, 221
  Roast lamb shoulder 220
  Shredded 224
  Sweet Persian tagine 224, *225*
  Vata balancing bowl 133, *134*
  see also ground meat
Lamington ice creams 268, *269*
Last night's dinner with an egg stuck in it 256, *257*
lattes, Thai 323
Lebanese roll pizza 186, *186*
leeks
  Braised celery and leeks with vanilla 170, *170*
  Caramelized leek, apple and rosemary socca *104*, 106
  Pretty spring pot 216
  The fish that got away pie 261
  Watercress "colcannon" 178, *178*
Leftovers kimchi soup 264
Leftovers pesto 55
legumes, how to sprout 352, *353*
lemongrass
  growing your own 33
  Thai lattes 323
lemons
  Da clean bee's knees cocktail 307, *310*
  Green smoothie cake with lemon cheese whip 330, *331*
  Grilled sardines with chili, haloumi and lemony pesto *155*, 157
  Lemon and turmeric tonic-ade 347
  Lemon syrup and poppy seed muggin 288, *289*
  My brother Pete's app-and-entrée-in-one kokonda 158, *159*

lentils
  Clean bitters bowl 129, *129*
  Fermented dosas 88, 89
  Golden oatmeal wedges 253, *253*
  how to sprout 352, *353*
  Inside-out sprouted kitcheri loaf 114
  Slow-cooked green peas and ham 217
lettuce
  Back to the 70s lettuce soup 172, *172*
  Chicken caesar on a stick *123*, 125
  Green minx dressing 54
  Grilled caesar on the barbie 173, *173*
  growing your own 33
  Have some lettuce with your dressing 173
  Kermit slushie *122*, 125
limes
  Crunchy chicken satay in a pan 232, *233*
  Margarita popsticks *325*, 326
  Sweet potato nachos 230, *231*
  The cultured mule cocktail 310
liver
  Beginner's coq au vin pâté 196, *197*
  Lamb's fry and pear meatloaf 202, *203*
lunchbox fillers *122–23*, 124–25, 369

M
macadamias
  Seaweed dukkah 45
  Skillet fish 'n' superslaw 162
mandoline 13, *13*
mangoes
  Australiana mango flat white 327
  Mango and coconut squares *349*, 351
"Maple syrup" pork belly with pecans 311
Margarita popsticks *325*, 326
mayonnaise, whey-good 50
meals, planning proportions for 35
meat
  freezing of 21, *21*
  "Pizza" bread-and-butter crumble 262, *263*
  "Pizza" muggins 60, *61*
  storing 19
  what to do with scraps 32
  see also ground meat
meatballs *142–43*, 144–45, 258, 359
meatloaf 202
"meffins" 98, *99*, *123*
microwaves 12
Middle Eastern eggplant 148, *149*
Middle Eastern groaties 27

milk
  Beet halwa 190, *190*
  Chocolate cherry blitz 86, *86*
  coconut milk 359
  Swedish meatballs *143*; 145
  Warming berry 'n' beet smoothie 78, *80*
  Warming golden milk 81
  Zucchini bread thickie 87
  see also smoothies
mint
  A salad of crushed olives 170, *170*
  Crunchy broccoli buckwheat tabbouli 187, *187*
  Kermit slushie *122*, 125
  Middle Eastern eggplant 148, *149*
  Minted pea pistou 240, *241*
  One-pan Moroccan fish pilaf 161
  The green counterbalance salad *306*, 309
  Vietnamese turkey pancakes 150, *151*
miso 356, 359
  Gift-wrapped miso cod 166, *167*
  Miso and walnut slow bros 282, *283*
  Misomite 54, 120, *121*
  MT dressing 53
  Slice 'n' bake miso butter biscuits 96, *96–97*
  Sweet potato, miso and sage soup 242, *244*
Monster-mash roll-ups *122*, 124
Moroccan cauliflower, chickpea and quinoa bake 238
mozzarella
  Baking-sheet-dinner-for-two eggplant parmigiana 228, *229*
  Blueberry, basil and mozzarella toastie 85, *85*
muffins 328, *329*, 358
mug cakes 288, *289*
Mum's steak and kidney stew with herby dumplings 194, *195*
mung beans
  how to sprout 352, *353*
  Sprouted kitcheri loaf 114
mushrooms
  Baked stuffing loaf with mushroom sauce *304*, 305
  Beginner's coq au vin pâté 196, *197*
  Chinese beef cheeks 198, *199*
  Lamb's fry and pear meatloaf 202, *203*
  Mushroom, thyme and hazelnut oatmeal 64, *65*
  Soothing Asian poached pot 216
mustard greens, in Any green saag paneer 177, *177*
mustard, 'Bucha 33
My allergy-free bread *112*, 113
My brother Pete's app-and-entrée-in-one kokonda 158, *159*
My gut-healing brew 87, *87*

My Indian kimchi *135*, 338, *339*
My recalibrating pork meal 234, *235*
My sausage and fennel lunch bowl 136, *136*
My spectacular popstick cake 324, *325*, 326
My totally messed-with Christmas cake 314, *315*

N

nachos, Sweet potato 230, *231*
napa cabbage 181, *181*
Nomato sauce 51, *51*
  Italian "pasta" noodles 116
  One-pot spaghetti and meatballs 142, *144*
  Socettes *104*, 106
  Superfoodie lasagna cake 140, *141*
noodles 116
nori
  Nori roll in a bowl *131*, 132
  Superfoodie lasagna cake 140, *141*
Not quite banana bread 68, *69*
nut butters 356
nutrition guidelines 7, 35
nuts 28
  Bacon granola 108, *109*
  Beet red velvet cheesecake *320*, 321–22
  Leftovers pesto 55
  Nut crumble 70, *72*
  Raw snickas ice-cream bar *277*, 279
  Seaweed dukkah 45
  see also specific nuts, e.g. walnuts

O

oatmeal
  Bacon 'n' egg oatmeal 66, *67*
  Golden oatmeal wedges 253, *253*
  Mushroom, thyme and hazelnut oatmeal 64, *65*
oats 358
  Bacon 'n' egg oatmeal 66, *67*
  Mushroom, thyme and hazelnut oatmeal 64, *65*
Off the wagon wheel *276*, 278
Okonomiyaki in a tray *183*, 183
olive oil 356
olives 356
  A salad of crushed olives 170, *170*
  Greek lamb salad *218*, 221
  Nomato sauce 51, *51*
  Puttanesca festival 133, *135*
  Spring socca pizza *105*, 106
  Sweet Persian tagine 224, *225*
  The real Greek yogurt 74, *74*
  Vegan whatchagot quiche 260

omega-3 fats 157
One-pan Moroccan fish pilaf 161
One-pot spaghetti and meatballs 142, *144*
onions
  A super-greens couch fondue 118, *119*
  Baked Mediterranean summer sardines 157
  Baked stuffing loaf with mushroom sauce *304*, 305
  Bloke beef 'n' beer with mash 206, *207*
  "But the kitchen sink" kimchi 337
  Chopped salad pickle 335, *335*
  Green scraps shakshouka 248, *249*
  Jerk pork shoulder roast *219*, 222
  Lamb roast for two 240, *241*
  Lamb's fry and pear meatloaf 202, *203*
  Middle Eastern eggplant 148, *149*
  Moroccan cauliflower, chickpea and quinoa bake 238
  My allergy-free bread *112*, 113
  Nomato sauce 51, *51*
  Onion curry dosa 89
  Pickled festive red slaw with caramelized ruby grapefruit *307*, 309
  Puttanesca festival 133, *135*
  Shortcut choucroute 258, *259*
  Slow-cooked green peas and ham 217
  Soothing Asian poached pot 216
  Steak 'n' five veg 239
  Superfoodie lasagna cake 140, *141*
  Sustainable sweet fish curry 164, *165*
  Sweet Persian tagine 224, *225*
  Sweet potato, miso and sage soup 242, *244*
  Sweet potato nachos 230, *231*
  "Sweet" tacos with easy slaw 200, *201*
  The cheapest stew ever 212, *213*
  The fish that got away pie 261
  The green counterbalance salad *306*, 309
  The real Greek yogurt 74, *74*
  Vegan whatchagot quiche 260
  Zesty caper crunch 185, *185*
Orange and thyme rainbow chips 94, 95, *122*
organic foods 17
Our office "emergency tuna" mishmash bowl 136, *136*

P

pancakes
  Crisp bibimbap skillet pancake 250, *251*
  Fermented dosas 88, 89
  Vietnamese turkey pancakes 150, *151*
pancetta, in Stuffing 'n' all the best bits salad *306*, 308
paneer
  Any green saag paneer 177, *177*
  Homemade paneer 48, *49*
  Spiced paneer 'n' peas 110, *111*
parchment paper 13
Parcooked 'n' frozen veggies 22
Parmesan
  Baking-sheet-dinner-for-two eggplant parmigiana 228, *229*
  Broc bites 92, *93*
  Cheesy cauli popcorn 100
  Golden oatmeal wedges 253, *253*
  Prosciutto-Parmesan stock 43
  Superfoodie lasagna cake 140, *141*
  Zesty caper crunch 185, *185*
parsnips
  Basic pot-au-feu 214, *215*
  Bloke beef 'n' beer with mash 206, *207*
  Not quite banana bread 68, *69*
  Orange and thyme rainbow chips 94, 95
  Parsnip, pear 'n' thyme soup 242, *243*
  Pretty in pastel pink parsnip pasta 137, *137*
  Roasted roots 23
  Steak 'n' five veg 239
  Stuffing 'n' all the best bits salad *306*, 308
  The cheapest stew ever 212, *213*
  Vegan whatchagot quiche 260
  Watercress "colcannon" 178, *178*
Party polenta cakes with popping topping 292, *293*
pâté, Beginner's coq au vin 196, *197*
patta gobi 181
peaches
  Cheesecake-stuffed peaches with basil 294, *295*
  Peach and peanut butter frozen yogurt 107
  Skillet fish 'n' superslaw 162
  Summer peach and basil colada 345
  The six-star waldorf 133, *135*
  Vanilla peach kombucha gums 351
peanut butter 357
  Apple and peanut butter with pumpkin spice butter 120, *121*

Chocolate peanut butter crackles 280, *281*
organic 17
Peach and peanut butter frozen yogurt 107
Raw snickas ice-cream bar *277*, 279
versus tahini 53
peanuts
Crunchy chicken satay in a pan 232, *233*
versus seeds 125
Thai lattes 323
pears
Choc-ginger and pear muggin 288, *289*
Lamb's fry and pear meatloaf 202, *203*
Parsnip, pear 'n' thyme soup 242, *243*
Waldorf smash-up 75, *75*
peas
"But the kitchen sink" breakfast hash 82, *83*
frozen 16
Green gumbo 265
Italian "pasta" noodles 116
Minted pea pistou 240, *241*
My gut-healing brew 87, *87*
My sausage and fennel lunch bowl 136, *136*
One-pan Moroccan fish pilaf 161
"Pizza" muggins 60, *61*
Pretty spring pot 216
Roast chicken "meffins" 98, *99*
Slow-cooked green peas and ham 217
Spiced paneer 'n' peas 110, *111*
Spring socca pizza 105, *106*
Sustainable sweet fish curry 164, *165*
The fish that got away pie 261
Two-minute desk lunch noodles 116, *117*
Vata balancing bowl 133, *134*
pecans
Bacon granola 108, *109*
Cacao cayenne pecans 312, *313*
Gingerbread muggin 288, *289*
Hot cross muffins 328, *329*
"Maple syrup" pork belly with pecans 311
Stuffing 'n' all the best bits salad 306, *308*
The six-star waldorf 133, *135*
pepitas
Bacon granola 108, *109*
Crunchy broccoli buckwheat tabbouli 187, *187*
Persian lamb salad *218*, 221
pesto
Grilled sardines with chili, haloumi and lemony pesto 155, *157*

Leftovers pesto 55
The green goddess toastie 85, *85*
Pickled festive red slaw with caramelized ruby grapefruit *307*, 309
Pickled roast veggies 252
pickles, in Cheeseburger wontons 102, *103*
pine nuts
Middle Eastern eggplant 148, *149*
The real Greek yogurt 74, *74*
pineapple, growing your own 33
Pink devilish googie eggs 253, *253*
pistachios
Baked stuffing loaf with mushroom sauce *304*, 305
Beet halwa 190, *190*
One-pan Moroccan fish pilaf 161
Strawberry cheesecake muggin 288, *289*
Pitta types 362
pizza
Lebanese roll pizza 186, *186*
"Pizza" bread-and-butter crumble 262, *263*
"Pizza" muggins 60, *61*
Spring socca pizza 105, *106*
Plain kombucha 344
plants, growing your own 33, *33*
Poached egg floater 242, *245*
poached eggs 44
pomegranate seeds 128
pomegranates
Pomegranate and coconut vodka popsticks 324, *325*
Turkish delightfuls *271*, 272
popcorn
Cauli popcorn 100, *101*
Party polenta cakes with popping topping 292, *293*
pork
Homemade bacon 208
Jerk pork shoulder roast *219*, 222
Lamb's fry and pear meatloaf 202, *203*
"Maple syrup" pork belly with pecans 311
My recalibrating pork meal 234, *235*
Pulled pork 222, 224
Shortcut choucroute 258, *259*
Sweet Persian tagine 224, *225*
Sweet potato nachos 230, *231*
Vata balancing bowl 133, *134*
see also mince
Pot-au-feu 214
potatoes
Bloke beef 'n' beer with mash 206, *207*
Skillet fish 'n' superslaw 162
The cheapest stew ever 212, *213*

Watercress "colcannon" 178, *178*
Powerhouse dressing 53
Pretty in pastel pink parsnip pasta 137, *137*
Pretty spring pot 216
Pretty spring risotto 130, *132*
Probiotic berries 'n' cream chews 351
proportions, for meals 35
Prosciutto-Parmesan stock 43
protein powder 357
Pull-apart caterpillar birthday cake 290, *291*
pumpkin
Jerk pork shoulder roast *219*, 222
"Pizza" muggins 60, *61*
Pumpkin spice-a-chino 327
purée 23
Rainbow gado gado 130, *132*
Roasted roots 23
Slow-cooker zucchini and pumpkin spice breakfast pudding 62, *63*
Stuffing 'n' all the best bits salad 306, *308*
Superfoodie lasagna cake 140, *141*
Sustainable sweet fish curry 164, *165*
Pumpkin spice mix 45, 359
Apple and peanut butter with pumpkin spice butter 120, *121*
Bacon granola 108, *109*
Gingerbread muggin 288, *289*
Not quite banana bread 68, 69
Pumpkin spice butter 79, 80
Pumpkin spice butter, walnut and sauerkraut toastie 84, *84*
Slow-cooker zucchini and pumpkin spice breakfast pudding 62, *63*
Socettes 104, *106*
Sugar-quitting butterscotch 'n' spice hot chocolate 79, 80
Warming berry 'n' beet smoothie 78, 80
Puttanesca festival 133, *135*
Pyrex dishes 13, *13*

Q
quinoa 27, 357
Chocolate peanut butter crackles 280, *281*
cooked 26, *26*
Crisp bibimbap skillet pancake 250, *251*
Fermented dosas 88, 89
Four-ingredient chicken shred-up 133, *134*
Golden oatmeal wedges 253, *253*
Italian "pasta" noodles 116
Jerk pork shoulder roast *219*, 222

Moroccan cauliflower, chickpea and quinoa bake 238
One-pan Moroccan fish pilaf 161
"Pizza" bread-and-butter crumble 262, *263*
Slow-cooker apple cider chicken 236, *237*
Zesty caper crunch 185, *185*
Zucchini bread thickie 87

R
radishes
"But the kitchen sink" kimchi 337
Chopped salad pickle 335, *335*
Nori roll in a bowl 131, *132*
The green counterbalance salad 306, *309*
Rainbow gado gado 130, *132*
Rainbow rolls 123, *124*
Ras el hanout mix 45, 359
raspberries
Kiwi and raspberry kebabs 123
Off the wagon wheel 276, *278*
Probiotic berries 'n' cream chews 351
Raspberry chia jam 57
Raspberry ripe bites *271*, 273
Red velvet crunch bowl 71, *72*
Turkish delightfuls *271*, 272
Warming berry 'n' beet smoothie 78, 80
Raw snickas ice-cream bar *277*, 279
red cabbage 180, *180*
Red velvet crunch bowl 71, *72*
rice
Broccoli and cauliflower rice 22
Golden oatmeal wedges 253, *253*
Inside-out sprouted kitcheri loaf 114
rice paper
Rainbow rolls 123, *124*
Superfoodie lasagna cake 140, *141*
Roast chicken "meffins" 98, *99*, 123
roast dinners 218–19, 220–22
Ruby grapefruit tonic bombs 349, 351

S
salads
A salad of crushed olives 170, *170*
Beet that popstick salad 191, *191*
Chopped salad pickle 335, *335*
Greek lamb salad *218*, 221
Hipster grandaddy salad 176, *176*
Persian lamb salad *218*, 221
Stuffing 'n' all the best bits salad 306, *308*
The green counterbalance salad 306, *309*

salt 337, 357
Salted caramel cardamom coffee 73
Salted caramel groaties 27
salmon 160
  Simplicious smoked salmon 160
sardines
  Baked Mediterranean summer sardines 154–55, 157
  Grilled sardines with chili, haloumi and lemony pesto 155, 157
  Puttanesca festival 133, 135
  Untinned sardines 120, 121, 154, 156
  ways to eat 156
sauces
  Leftovers pesto 55
  Nomato sauce 51, 51
sauerkraut 357
  Brussels sprout, haloumi and sauerkraut sliders 120, 121
  Pink sauerkraut 134
  Pumpkin spice butter, walnut and sauerkraut toastie 84, 84
  Shortcut choucroute 258, 259
  Simplicious sauerkraut 337
Sausage and fennel lunch bowl 136, 136
savory yogurts 74–75, 74–75
savoy cabbage 181
SCOBY 342, 344
Seaweed dukkah 45
  Four-ingredient chicken shred-up 133, 134
  Rainbow gado gado 130, 132
seeds 28, 125, 359
servings 36
sesame oil 357
sesame seeds
  Crunchy chicken satay in a pan 232, 233
  Sesame-crusted haloumi and strawberry salad 179, 179
shallots
  Chinese beef cheeks 198, 199
  Crisp bibimbap skillet pancake 250, 251
  Crunchy chicken satay in a pan 232, 233
  growing your own 33
  Soothing Asian poached pot 216
  Totally gaudy Christmas tree cheese ball 302, 303
  Two-minute desk lunch noodles 116, 117
Shaved sprouts and pecorino salad 304, 305
Shortcut choucroute 258, 259
Simple "Gochujang" sauce 250, 251
Skillet fish 'n' superslaw 162, 163
skillets 11, 11
Slice 'n' bake miso butter biscuits 96, 96–97
slow cookers 10, 10

Slow-cooker apple cider chicken 236, 237
Slow-cooker zucchini and pumpkin spice breakfast pudding 62, 63
Simplicious smoked salmon 160
Simplicious sprouts in a jar 352
smoothies
  green smoothies 86–87, 86–87
  smoothie bowls 70–71, 72
  versus juices 86
  Warming berry 'n' beet smoothie 78, 80
snacks 120, 121
snow peas
  Rainbow rolls 123, 124
  The six-star waldorf 133, 135
Socca, fermented 104–05, 106
Socettes 104, 106
Some beefin' good jerky 209
Soothing Asian poached pot 216
soups
  Back to the 70s lettuce soup 172, 172
  Beet, beet leaf 'n' apple borscht 242, 244
  Buttered blueberry and blood orange soup 284, 285
  Egg-drop soup 264
  Leftovers kimchi soup 264
  Parsnip, pear 'n' thyme soup 242, 244
  Slow-cooked green peas and ham 217
  soup toppers 242, 244
  Sweet potato, miso and sage soup 242, 244
Sour kiwi immunity boosters 349, 350
spaghetti
  Green spaghetti and meatballs 143, 145
  One-pot spaghetti and meatballs 142, 144
spice mixes 45, 359
Spiced paneer 'n' peas 110, 111
spices 357
spinach 174, 174
  A super-greens couch fondue 118, 119
  Any green saag paneer 177, 177
  Chocolate cherry blitz 86, 86
  Green apple pie smoothie bowl 70, 72
  Green smoothie cake with lemon cheese whip 330, 331
  Kermit slushie 122, 125
  Middle Eastern eggplant 148, 149
  Monster-mash roll-ups 122, 124
  Parcooked 'n' frozen veggies 22
  Superfoodie lasagna cake 140, 141
  Swedish meatballs 143, 145
  The green goddess toastie 85, 85
Spring socca pizza 105, 106

Sprouted cacao pops 76
Sprouted kitcheri loaf 114
sprouts, how to grow 352, 353
steak see beef
stevia 357, 359, 361
  Chocolate and red wine creamsticks 325, 326
  Margarita popsticks 325, 326
stew
  Mum's steak and kidney stew with herby dumplings 194, 195
  Slow-cooked green peas and ham 217
  The cheapest stew ever 212, 213
stock 359
  Asparagus 43
  Beef 42
  Chicken 42
  Corn cob 43
  Fish 42
  healing qualities of 43
  healing recipes 264
  My gut-healing brew 87, 87
  Prosciutto-Parmesan 43
  veggie variations 43
storing, of food 18–19, 18–21, 21, 24–25, 24–25
strawberries
  Pretty spring risotto 130, 132
  Sesame-crusted haloumi and strawberry salad 179, 179
  Spring strawberry and vanilla kombucha 345
  Strawberry cheesecake muggin 288, 289
  Strawberry chia jam 57, 57, 143
  Strawberry delight 351
  Strawberry frozen yogurt 122, 123, 125
  Sunflower strawberry thumbles 298, 299
Stuffing loaf with mushroom sauce 304, 305
Stuffing 'n' all the best bits salad 306, 308
substitutions 358–59
sugar 360–61, 363
  Ayurvedic face scrub 31
  how to use leftover sugar 30–32
  safe levels of consumption 34
Sugar-free glazed Christmas ham 306, 308
Sugar-quitting butterscotch 'n' spice hot chocolate 79, 80
sugar snap peas, in Crunchy chicken satay in a pan 232, 233
sunflower seeds
  how to sprout 352, 353
  Sunflower strawberry thumbles 298, 299
Supercharged coconut frosting 56
Superfoodie lasagna cake 140, 141

Sustainable sweet fish curry 164, 165
Swedish meatballs 143, 145
Sweet paprika stem chips 186, 260
sweet potatoes
  "But the kitchen sink" breakfast hash 82, 83
  Gingerbread muggin 288, 289
  My allergy-free bread 112, 113
  My recalibrating pork meal 234, 235
  Okonomiyaki in a tray 183, 183
  Orange and thyme rainbow chips 94, 95
  Roast chicken "meffins" 98, 99
  Roasted roots 23
  Sprouted kitcheri loaf 114
  Steak 'n' five veg 239
  Sustainable sweet fish curry 164, 165
  Sweet Persian tagine 224, 225
  Sweet potato chips 133
  Sweet potato croutons 245
  Sweet potato, miso and sage soup 242, 244
  Sweet potato nachos 230, 231
  Sweet potato purée 23
  Sweet potato skins 23
  The cheapest stew ever 212, 213
  The fish that got away pie 261
  Vata balancing bowl 133, 134
  Vegan whatchagot quiche 260
  Watercress "colcannon" 178, 178
Sweet Persian tagine 224, 225
Sweet spice groaties 27
sweetbreads 200
sweeteners 359, 360–61
sweets
  Bountiful slice 277, 279
  Buttered blueberry and blood orange soup 284, 285
  Cheesecake-stuffed peaches with basil 294, 295
  Choc-beet allspice truffles 270, 271
  Chocolate peanut butter crackles 280, 281
  cookies 276–77, 278–79
  Friday night chockito on a stick 286, 287
  Golden happy times 296, 297
  Lamington ice creams 268, 269
  Miso and walnut slow bros 282, 283
  mug cakes 288, 289
  Party polenta cakes with popping topping 292, 293
  Pull-apart caterpillar birthday cake 290, 291
  Raspberry ripe bites 271, 273
  Sunflower strawberry thumbles 298, 299

Tam tims 274, *275*
Turkish delightfuls *271, 272*
"Sweet" tacos with easy slaw 200, *201*

T

tabbouli 187, *187*
tacos
  "Sweet" tacos with easy slaw 200, *201*
tahini 357
  Friday night chockito on a stick 286, *287*
  TMT dressing 53
  versus peanut butter 53
Tam tims 274, *275*
tamari 357
tempeh, in Nori roll in a bowl *131*, 132
tequila, in Margarita popsticks *325*, 326
Thai coconutty cabbage 182, *182*
Thai lattes 323
The BLAT 75
The bright side cocktail 310
The cheapest stew ever 212, *213*
The cultured mule cocktail 310
The fish that got away pie 261
The green counterbalance salad *306*, 309
The green goddess toastie 85, *85*
The real Greek yogurt 74, *74*
The six-star waldorf 133, *135*
The whole brassicus hummus 187, *187*
thickeners 359
thyme
  Mushroom, thyme and hazelnut oatmeal 64, *65*
  Parsnip, pear 'n' thyme soup *242*, 243
  TMT dressing 53
toasties 84–85, *84–85*
tomatoes
  Baked Mediterranean summer sardines 157
  The BLAT 75, *75*
  Chicken caesar on a stick *123*, 125
  Greek san choi bau 146, *147*
  Greek lamb salad 218, *221*
  Lamb roast for two 240, *241*
  My brother Pete's app-and-entrée-in-one kokonda 158, *159*
  "Pizza" muggins 60, *61*
  Puttanesca festival 133, *135*
  Sweet potato nachos 230, *231*
  The real Greek yogurt 74, *74*
tonics 346–47
Totally gaudy Christmas tree cheese ball 302, *303*
tuna
  Fridge-door tonnato 254, *255*
  Nori roll in a bowl *131*, 132

Our office "emergency tuna" mishmash bowl 136, *136*
  tinned tuna 357
turkey pancakes, Vietnamese 150, *151*
Turkish delightfuls *271, 272*
turmeric 359
  Fermented turmeric paste 124, 340
  growing your own 33
  Lemon and turmeric tonic-ade 347
  My Indian kimchi 338, *339*
  Sustainable sweet fish curry 164, *165*
  TMT dressing 53
  turmeric paste 357
  Warming golden milk 81
turnips
  Basic pot-au-feu 214, *215*
  Chopped salad pickle 335, *335*
  Orange and thyme rainbow chips *94*, 95
  The cheapest stew ever 212, *213*
Turnip cheeseburger 120, *121*
Watercress "colcannon" 178, *178*
Two-minute desk lunch noodles 116, *117*

U

Untinned sardines 120, *121*, *154*, 156
"use by" dates 16

V

vanilla 359
  Braised celery and leeks with vanilla 170, *170*
  Chocolate cherry blitz 86, *86*
  Never-ending vanilla extract 45
  Spring strawberry and vanilla kombucha 345
  Vanilla peach kombucha gums 351
Vata balancing bowl 133, *134*
Vata types 362
Vegan "ground meat" 186
Vegan whatchagot quiche 260
vegetables 170–91
  Baked stuffing loaf with mushroom sauce *304*, 305
  "But the kitchen sink" breakfast hash 82, *83*
  Chopped salad pickle 335, *335*
  Crisp bibimbap skillet pancake 250, *251*
  fermented vegetables 334–41
  Green scraps shakshouka 248, *249*
  Homemade stock 42
  organic 17
  Parcooked 'n' frozen veggies 22
  Pickled roast veggies 252, *252*

Pretty spring risotto *130*, 132
Roasted roots 23
Steak 'n' five veg 239
storing 18–19
Sustainable sweet fish curry 164, *165*
The cheapest stew ever 212, *213*
what to do with scraps 32
Vietnamese turkey pancakes 150, *151*
vodka
  Da clean bee's knees cocktail 307, 310
  Pomegranate and coconut vodka popsticks 324, *325*
  The bright side cocktail 310
  The cultured mule cocktail 310

W

Waldorf smash-up 75, *75*
walnuts
  Bacon granola 108, *109*
  Beet that popstick salad 191, *191*
  Miso and walnut slow bros 282, *283*
  My totally messed-with Christmas cake 314, *315*
  Pretty in pastel pink parsnip pasta 137, *137*
  Pumpkin spice butter, walnut and sauerkraut toastie 84, *84*
  Vegan "ground meat" 186
  Waldorf smash-up 75, *75*
Warming berry 'n' beet smoothie *78*, 80
Warming golden milk 81
watercress 174, *174*
  Any green saag paneer 177, *177*
  The BLAT 75, *75*
  how to dry 19
  Persian lamb salad 218, *221*
  Puttanesca festival 133, *135*
  Spring socca pizza *105*, 106
  The green counterbalance salad *306*, 309
  The green goddess toastie 85, *85*
  Watercress "colcannon" 178, *178*
  Watercress sauce and some eggs 176, *177*
whey
  Homemade whey and cream cheese 46, *47*
  versus salt 337
  Whey-good mayo 50
white cabbage 181, *181*
Winter chai kombucha *342*, 345

Y

yogurt 357
  Greek san choi bau 146, *147*
  Israeli whole-baked cauliflower 316, *317*

Middle Eastern eggplant 148, *149*
Peach and peanut butter frozen yogurt 107
Persian lamb salad 218, *221*
Pretty in pastel pink parsnip pasta 137, *137*
savory yogurts 74–75, *74–75*
Strawberry frozen yogurt *122*, *123*, 125
Zucchini tzatziki 188, *188*

Z

Zesty caper crunch 185, *185*
zip-lock bags 10
zucchini
  Baked Mediterranean summer sardines 157
  "But the kitchen sink" breakfast hash 82, *83*
  Chocolate cherry blitz 86, *86*
  Chopped salad pickle 335, *335*
  Greek san choi bau 146, *147*
  Green minx dressing 54
  Green scraps shakshouka 248, *249*
  Green smoothie cake with lemon cheese whip 330, *331*
  Green spaghetti and meatballs *143*, 145
  in salads 133
  Italian "pasta" noodles 116
  Kermit slushie *122*, 125
  Lamb roast for two 240, *241*
  Lamb's fry and pear meatloaf 202, *203*
  My gut-healing brew 87, *87*
  Pretty spring risotto *130*, 132
  Puttanesca festival 133, *135*
  Sustainable sweet fish curry 164, *165*
  "Sweet" tacos with easy slaw 200, *201*
  The cheapest stew ever 212, *213*
  The fish that got away pie 261
  Vata balancing bowl 133, *134*
  Vegan whatchagot quiche 260
  Zucchini bread thickie 87
  Zucchini butter 188, *188*
  Zucchini no-carbonara 188, *188*
  Zucchini tzatziki 188, *188*

To everyone mentioned on this page, thanks for enduring my scraps + OBSESSED drive to make a book dedicated to getting us responsible.

THANK YOU ...

To the I Quit Sugar team: my kitchen crew, Kate Kneipp (@cake_kat), Stephanie Hinton (@highlystef), Renee Lynch (@iloveapplepie) and Megan Yonson (@megandveg); Jo Foster for her timeline and support prowess; Zoe Eaton (Rouchie), my mate and business partner. — *Let's FLOW!*

To the lovely I Quit Sugar community around the world who tested some of the recipes to make sure they tasted good: Nicky Burrell (@nickyburrell), Lana Jankovic (@lanajankovic), Alexx Stuart (@alexx_stuart), Charlotte Dupont (@aipxwhole30) and Marisa Alvarsson (@missmarzipancom). — *Readers who quit sugar via my 8 week Program + asked to help ♡*

Special props to the Little People who helped out: Mia, Isaac, Sarah, Robbie, Charlotte and Emil.

A special nod to my bro Pete (Emil's dad), who gave me his Kokonda recipe and Matt Preston, who gave me the recipe for Bone Marrow Bombs (in exchange for me introducing him to kale chips), and to Kate Gibbs, Byron Woolfrey (@trolleyed) and Jordanna Levin (@theinspiredtable).

Thanks to Dr. John Richmond Ford, Marine Research Fellow at the University of Melbourne, and Oliver Edwards from GoodFishBadFish for checking the sustainable fish guff; Feather and Bone Providore (@featherandboneprovidore) for their mindful meat advice; Marieke Rodenstein for her dietary diligence (checking the nutrition profile of my meals); and Nadia Marshall for her Ayurvedic feedback.

Big love to the Shoot Crew: Rob Palmer, David Morgan, Olivia Andrews, Claire Dickson-Smith, Maxwell Adey and Paulie Bedggood. And to Aaron Teece from Studio Neon, who helped me build my scraps dress and bouquet.

Finally, a big thanks to the ever-loyal and caring Pan Macmillan team: Ariane Durkin, Charlotte Bachali, Charlotte Ree, Sally Devenish, Emma Rafferty, Megan Ellis, Cate Paterson, Trisha Garner and Miriam Cannell (darling Mizza, I love that your cockatiel ate your activated groaties and that you cooked almost every recipe in the book as you edited them). Thanks to the Clarkson Potter team and my gorgeous martini-drinking teammate and agent Laurie Liss. And, finally, thank you Ingrid Ohlsson for being my mate and "getting me." Couldn't have done it without you. Literally.

AN INSIDE FLAP dedicated to the people who SO GENEROUSLY stuck their hand up to be part of this project.